Recent Results in Cancer Research

Volume 205

More information about this series at http://www.springer.com/series/392

Gabriella Pichert · Chris Jacobs
Editors

Rare Hereditary Cancers

Diagnosis and Management

Springer

Editors
Gabriella Pichert
London Bridge Hospital
London
UK

Chris Jacobs
Guy's and St. Thomas' NHS Foundation Trust
University College London
London
UK

ISSN 0080-0015 ISSN 2197-6767 (electronic)
Recent Results in Cancer Research
ISBN 978-3-319-29996-9 ISBN 978-3-319-29998-3 (eBook)
DOI 10.1007/978-3-319-29998-3

Library of Congress Control Number: 2016931320

Printed on acid-free paper

This Springer imprint is published by SpringerNature
The registered company is Springer International Publishing AG Switzerland

Preface

Alongside rapid advances in scientific understanding about cancer genomics, there have been huge steps forward in genetic testing for pathogenic mutations in cancer predisposing genes, as well as the management of cancer risks associated with these mutations.

Until recently, families with a history of cancer suggesting high risk cancer predisposition genes as their cause have been counselled and managed within specialised genetic services. As the number of individuals eligible for cancer predisposition testing is rapidly increasing and more management options and treatments tailored to pathways disrupted by mutated cancer predisposition genes are developed, oncologists, surgeons and other healthcare specialists treating these patients have to become more involved in genetic testing and managing cancer risks in their patients.

Much has been written about the diagnosis and management of patients with common hereditary cancer such as breast/ovarian and colorectal cancer syndromes. However, there is limited information available to health professionals who diagnose and manage rare hereditary cancer syndromes, some of which present in childhood.

This book approaches the issue of the differential diagnosis and management of rare hereditary cancer syndromes from a practical angle, addressing the issues for each tumour type as seen by health professionals in their day-to-day practice.

The first chapter aims to update cancer specialists on the newest developments in genetic testing technology. It describes the strengths, limitations and caveats of these technologies to enable cancer specialists to use these tests safely and effectively for the benefit of their patients.

The subsequent chapters describe how patients with specific rare hereditary cancer syndromes may be identified through their personal and family history of cancer, which genes should be tested based on these criteria, the clinical picture of the respective cancer syndromes caused by mutations in these genes, as well as the appropriate management options.

The final chapter deals with the wider issues involved in genetic counselling and testing for cancer susceptibility for patients, families and health professionals.

In summary, this book has been written by leading specialists in the field to enable health professionals to correctly identify patients with these rare syndromes who will benefit from genetic counselling and testing and to provide them with the knowledge to manage patients and advise family members who may be at risk of an inherited cancer predisposition.

Contents

Contributors

Anna Angelousi Section on Endocrinology and Genetics, Program on Developmental Endocrinology and Genetics, Eunice Kennedy Shriver National Institute of Child Health and Human Development, National Institutes of Health, Bethesda, MD, USA

Mandy L. Ballinger The Kinghorn Cancer Centre, Garvan Institute of Medical Research, Darlinghurst, NSW, Australia

Gul Bano Thomas Addison Unit, Department of Endocrinology and Diabetes, St George's Healthcare NHS Trust, Tooting, London, UK

Sarah Benafif The Institute of Cancer Research, Sutton, Surrey, UK; Royal Marsden NHS Foundation Trust, Sutton, Surrey, UK

Annabel Berthon Section on Endocrinology and Genetics, Program on Developmental Endocrinology and Genetics, Eunice Kennedy Shriver National Institute of Child Health and Human Development, National Institutes of Health, Bethesda, MD, USA

Andrew V. Biankin The Kinghorn Cancer Centre, Cancer Research Program, Darlinghurst, NSW, Australia

Rosalind Eeles The Institute of Cancer Research, Sutton, Surrey, UK

Stéphanie Espiard Section on Endocrinology and Genetics, Program on Developmental Endocrinology and Genetics, Eunice Kennedy Shriver National Institute of Child Health and Human Development, National Institutes of Health, Bethesda, MD, USA

Shirley Hodgson St. George's, University of London, London, UK

Laura Hopkins Family History of Bowel Cancer Clinic, Gastroenterology Department, West Middlesex University Hospital, Chelsea and Westminster Hospitals NHS Trust, London, UK

Jeremy L. Humphris The Kinghorn Cancer Centre, Cancer Research Program, Darlinghurst, NSW, Australia

Chris Jacobs Department of Clinical Genetics, Guy's and St Thomas' NHS Foundation Trust, London, UK

Fiona Lalloo Manchester Centre for Genomic Medicine, St Mary's Hospital, Central Manchester University Hospitals NHS Foundation Trust, Manchester Academic Health Science Centre, Manchester, UK

Eamonn R. Maher Department of Medical Genetics, University of Cambridge, Cambridge, UK

Christopher McCormack Dermatology Unit, Department of Surgical Oncology, Peter MacCallum Cancer Centre, Melbourne, Australia

Fred H. Menko Antoni van Leeuwenhoek, Netherlands Cancer Institute, Amsterdam, The Netherlands

Shehla Mohammed Department of Clinical Genetics, Guy's and St Thomas' NHS Foundation Trust, London, UK

Kevin John Monahan Gastroenterology Department, Family History of Bowel Cancer Clinic, West Middlesex University Hospital, Chelsea and Westminster Hospitals NHS Trust, London, UK

Gabriella Pichert London Bridge Hospital, London, UK

Susan Shanley Familial Cancer Clinic, Peter MacCallum Cancer Centre, Melbourne, Australia

Adam Shaw Department of Clinical Genetics, Guy's and St Thomas' NHS Foundation Trust, London, UK

Constantine A. Stratakis Section on Endocrinology and Genetics, Program on Developmental Endocrinology and Genetics, Eunice Kennedy Shriver National Institute of Child Health and Human Development, National Institutes of Health, Bethesda, MD, USA

David M. Thomas The Kinghorn Cancer Centre, Garvan Institute of Medical Research, Darlinghurst, NSW, Australia

Ellen Thomas Department of Clinical Genetics, Guy's and St Thomas' NHS Foundation Trust, London, UK

Mihail Zilbermint Section on Endocrinology and Genetics, Program on Developmental Endocrinology and Genetics, Eunice Kennedy Shriver National Institute of Child Health and Human Development, National Institutes of Health, Bethesda, MD, USA

Abbreviations

^{123}I-MIBG	Metaiodobenzyleguanindine
ACCs	Adrenocortical carcinomas
ACT	Adrenocortical tumours
AD	Autosomal dominant
AF	Aggressive fibromatosis
APC	Adenomatous polyposis coli
Array-CGH	Comparative genome hybridisation
ATM	Ataxia telangiectasia
BAP1	BRCA1 associated protein 1
BCC	Basal cell carcinoma
BHD	Birt–Hogg–Dubé syndrome
BRRS	Bannayan–Riley–Ruvalcaba syndrome
BWS	Beckwith–Wiedemann syndrome
(CAPS) consortium	Cancer of the pancreas screening
CCH	C-cell hyperplasia
ccRCC	Clear cell renal cell cancer
ccRCC	Renal cell carcinomas
CDKN1C	Cyclin-dependent kinase inhibitor 1C
CDKNIK1	Cyclin-dependent kinase inhibitor 1C
CEA	Carcinoembryonic antigen
CHRPE	Congenital hypertrophy of the retinal pigment epithelium
CLA	Cutaneous lichen amyloidosis
CNC	Carney complex
CRC	Colorectal cancer
CT	Calcitonin
CT	Computerised tomography
CTNNB1	Catenin-beta 1
DBC	Invasive ductal cancer
DGC	Diffuse gastric cancer
dHPLC	High performance liquid chromatography
DTC	Differentiated thyroid carcinoma
EB	Epidermolysis bullosa
EC	Endomentrial cancer
EGF	Epidermal growth factor
ENCODE	The Encyclopedia of DNA Elements

EUS	Endoscopic ultrasound
FAMMM	Familial atypical multiple mole melanoma
FAP	Familial adenomatous polyposis
FDA	United States Food and Drug Administration
FDG-PET/CT	^{18}Fluorodeoxyglucose-positron emission tomography/computed tomography
FDR	First degree relative
FFPE	Formalin fixed paraffin embedded
FH	Fumarate hydratase
FIHP	Familial isolated hyperparathyroidism
FISH	Fluorescence in situ hybridisation
FLCN	Folliculin
FMTC	Familial medullary thyroid carcinoma
FNA	Fine needle aspiration
FNMTC	Familial non-medullary thyroid cancer
FPC	Familial pancreatic cancer
FPTC	Familial papillary thyroid cancer
FRCC	Familial non-syndromic renal cell cancer
FTC	Follicular thyroid cancer
GC	Gastric cancer
GEP	Gastroenteropancreatic
GIST	Gastrointestinal stromal tumours
GWAS	Genome-wide association studies
H&E	Haematoxylin and eosin
HBOC	Hereditary breast ovarian cancer
hCG	Beta-human chorionic gonadotropin
HDGC	Hereditary diffuse gastric cancer
HIF	Hypoxia inducible factor
HNPCC	Hereditary non-polyposis colorectal cancer
HP	Helicobacter pylori
HPT-JT	Hyperparathyroidism-jaw tumour syndrome
IC1	Imprinting centre 1
IC2	Imprinting centre 2
ICGC	International Cancer Genome Consortium
IGF2	Insulin growth factor-2
IM	Intestinal metaplasia
IPMK	Inositol polyphosphate multikinase
IPMN	Intraductal papillary mucinous neoplasm
JPS	Juvenile-polyposis syndrome
KCOT	Keratocystic odontogenic tumours
LAM	Lyphangioleiomyomatosis
LBC	Lobular breast cancer
LCCSCT	Large cell calcifying Sertoli cell tumours
LFLS	Li-Fraumeni-like-syndrome
LFS	Li Fraumeni syndrome

LOH	Loss of heterozygosity
LT4	Levothyroxine
MAP	MUTYH-associated polyposis
MCR1	Melanocortin receptor1
MDT	Multidisciplinary team
MEN1	Multiple endocrine neoplasia 1
MEN2/MENII	Multiple endocrine neoplasia 2
MEN2a/IIA	Multiple endocrine neoplasia type 2a
MEN2B/IIB	Multiple endocrine neoplasia type 2b
MEN4	Multiple endocrine neoplasia type 4
MET	Mesenchymal epithelial transition factor
MMR	Mismatch repair
MPLA	Multiplex ligation-dependent probe amplification
MPNST	Malignant transformation of peripheral nerve sheath tumours
MRCP	Magnetic resonance cholangiopancreatography
MRI	Magnetic resonance Imaging
MS	Methylation-specific
MTC	Medullary thyroid carcinoma
mTOR	mammalian target of rapamycin
MTTs	Molecular targeted therapeutics
NANETS	North American Neuroendocrine Tumor Society
NBI	Narrow band imaging
NBS1	Nijmegen breakage syndrome
NCCN	National Comprehensive Cancer Network
NCR	Netherlands Cancer Registry
NET	Neuroendocrine tumour
NF1	Neurofibromatosis type 1
NF2	Neurofibromatosis type II
NFPTR	National Familial Pancreatic Tumor Registry
NGF	Nerve growth factor
NGS	Next generation sequencing
NIH	National Institutes of Health
NMTC	Non-medullary thyroid cancer
OCA	Oculocutaneous albinism
OGD	Oesophago-gastroduodenoscopy
OPG	Orthopantomogram
OR	Odds ratio
PALLD	Palladin
PanIN	Pancreatic intraepithelial neoplasia
PARP	Poly ADP ribose polymerase
PAS	Periodic acid-Schiff
PCR	Polymerase chain reaction
PDGF	Platelet derived growth factor
PDT	Photodynamic therapy
PEComas	Perivascular epithelioid cell sarcomas

PG	Paraganglioma
PHTS	PTEN hamartoma tumour syndrome
PJS	Peutz–Jeghers syndrome
PKA	Protein kinase A
PPNAD	Primary pigmented nodular adrenocortical hyperplasia
PRKAR1A	Protein kinase regulatory subunit type 1 alpha gene
PTC	Papillary thyroid cancer
RB1	Retinoblastoma gene
RCC	Renal cell cancer
SCC	Squamous cell carcinomas
SDH	Succinate dehydrogenase
SDHAF2	Succinate dehydrogenase assembly factor 2
SDHB	SDH subunit B
SEER	Surveillance, Epidemiology and End Results Program
SI NET	Small intestinal NET
SMO	Smoothened
SNP	SNP single nucleotide polymorphism
SUFU	Suppressor of fused
TCA	Tricarboxylic acid
TCF	T-cell factor
TCO	Thyroid cancer with oxyphilia
Tg	Thyroglobulin
TGCA	The Cancer Genome Atlas Research
TSH	Thyroid stimulating hormone
TSC	Tuberous sclerosis complex
TYR	Tyrosinase gene
UDP	Uniparental disomy
USS	Ultrasound scan
UV	Ultraviolet
VEGF	Vascular endothelial growth factor
VHL	Von Hippel–Lindau
VHL	Von Hippel–Lindau disease
VHL	Von Hippel–Lindau syndrome
VS	Vestibular schwannoma
VUS	Variant of uncertain significance
VUS/VUCS	Variant of unknown clinical significance
WBS	Whole body scan
WDTC	Well-differentiated thyroid cancer
WES	Whole Exome Sequencing
WGS	Whole Genome Sequencing
XP	Xerodermapigmentosum

Advances in Genetic Testing for Hereditary Cancer Syndromes

Ellen Thomas and Shehla Mohammed

Abstract

The ability to identify genetic mutations causing an increased risk of cancer represents the first widespread example of personalised medicine, in which genetic information is used to inform patients of their cancer risks and direct an appropriate strategy to minimise those risks. Increasingly, an understanding of the genetic basis of many cancers also facilitates selection of the most effective therapeutic options. The technology underlying genetic testing has been revolutionised in the years since the completion of the Human Genome Project in 2001. This has advanced knowledge of the genetic factors underlying familial cancer risk, and has also improved genetic testing capacity allowing a larger number of patients to be tested for a constitutional cancer predisposition. To use these tests safely and effectively, they must be assessed for their ability to provide accurate and useful results, and be requested and interpreted by health professionals with an understanding of their strengths and limitations. Genetic testing is increasing in its scope and ambition with each year that passes, requiring a greater proportion of the healthcare workforce to acquire a working knowledge of genetics and genetic testing to manage their patients safely and sensitively.

Keywords

Genetic testing · Molecular diagnosis of inherited cancer · Diagnostic use of next-generation sequencing

E. Thomas (✉) · S. Mohammed
Department of Clinical Genetics, Guy's and St Thomas' NHS Foundation Trust, London, UK
e-mail: ellen.thomas@kcl.ac.uk

E. Thomas
King's College London, London, UK

G. Pichert and C. Jacobs (eds.), *Rare Hereditary Cancers*,
Recent Results in Cancer Research 205, DOI 10.1007/978-3-319-29998-3_1

Contents

1 Introduction

The genetics of cancer has been the focus of a huge research effort for several decades. This can be divided into two main areas: firstly, the study of how genetic changes within a particular organ arise and accumulate, causing the development of an individual tumour; and secondly, the search for inherited genetic changes which increase a person's chance of developing cancer. The first category, known as 'somatic' genetic changes, occurs only in tumour cells and the tissue they developed from, while the second category, known as 'germline' or 'constitutional' genetic variants, is present in every cell in the body, including the germ cells (eggs and sperm) which pass on DNA to the next generation.

Cancers are initiated and driven by changes in a cell's DNA which cause it to divide uncontrollably, and to this extent, all cancers are genetic diseases. However, the majority of cancers are caused by a combination of lifestyle, environmental and stochastic (chance) influences with only a minor contribution from constitutional inherited genetic variation.

A significant minority of cancers (a variable proportion depending on the cancer type) are caused more directly by a rare single mutation, which is usually inherited in an autosomal dominant way. Diagnostic genetic testing can identify such mutations in individuals with a personal and family history of cancer. These tests must examine the entire sequence of the relevant gene(s) looking for the single mutation which could be causing the family's cancers. In some cases, even when there is a high suspicion of an inherited predisposition to cancer, no genetic cause is found, and the reasons for this will be discussed later in this chapter. Diagnostic tests can be carried out in individuals with a family history but no personal history of cancer. However, a negative test result in this situation is **uninformative and of limited value**, as it is not possible to tell whether there is a mutation in a known cancer gene in the family which has not been inherited by the individual tested, or whether there is no mutation in a known gene and the tested individual could still be at risk from an unidentified gene mutation.

Once a cancer-predisposing mutation has been identified in a patient with cancer, their relatives can be offered predictive testing to find out whether they have inherited the mutation and may be at increased risk of developing cancer in the future. This is a highly accurate test, because only the single genetic variant identified in the family needs to be tested. In general, predictive tests are cheaper and quicker than diagnostic tests, although their health implications are significant and appropriate counselling is always required. Individuals in these families who have inherited the mutation may have a very high risk of developing cancer—up to 100 % in some cases such as classical familial adenomatous polyposis. In addition, the cancers are likely to occur at a younger age than sporadic non-familial cancers, and may be of particular histological subtypes. A test showing that an individual has not inherited the familial mutation removes any increased risk for that individual related to their family history, unless they have a family history of cancers which cannot be accounted for by the familial mutation, for example if relatives of their unaffected parent have also had significant cancers. These individuals can be reassured, and additional surveillance for that cancer is not required following this test result.

Individuals who have a positive predictive testing result will be offered a range of strategies to try to reduce their future cancer risks. Demand for genetic testing is therefore increasing, from patients and healthcare professionals, and advances in genetic testing technology described in this chapter have been introduced into clinical practice with the aim of making access to genetic testing broader and more equitable.

In between sporadic and inherited cancers are another loosely defined group where the patient has a family history which is likely to be relevant to their own cancer, but no mutation is detectable in a known gene. These families are likely to have one or several variants which are contributing to an increased cancer risk, but the level of risk is lower than with the inherited cancer gene faults. These families may be offered some additional surveillance, but genetic testing is usually not contributory or informative in this situation. However, this may change as our understanding of the whole spectrum of constitutional genetic predisposition to cancer improves with further large-scale genetic research projects.

2 Advances in Genetic Testing Technology

Traditionally, genetic testing for cancer predisposition genes has used capillary sequencing (also known as Sanger sequencing), which is a highly accurate but labour-intensive and expensive way of working through each individual exon of the gene of interest, requiring a large DNA specimen. Genetic testing has therefore been limited by cost and throughput to individuals with a clinical picture indicating a high likelihood of a cancer-predisposing gene mutation (Table 1).

Table 1 Comparison of tests used to make genetic diagnoses

Test	Use	Strengths	Limitations
Capillary (Sanger) sequencing	Sequencing of small genomic regions, e.g. individual exons	Highly accurate	Low throughput, labour intensive, expensive
Panel testing using next-generation sequencing	Simultaneous sequencing of genes causing a particular phenotype (up to several hundred genes)	Allows multipanel gene testing Useful in heterogeneous conditions	Needs adjusting when new genes are discovered, and coverage of each gene may not be as good as capillary sequencing
Array CGH	Detection of large structural chromosome rearrangements	Highly accurate, high throughput	
Exome sequencing	Simultaneous sequencing of all coding regions of the genome	Streamlines lab workflow and useful extension of the panel test	Coverage of some genes is inadequate, no information on structural rearrangements
Genome sequencing	Sequencing of the whole genome	More even coverage of all genes	Expensive, data storage and analysis costs are high, and non-coding regions hard to interpret

In the last 15 years, rapid advances have been made in genetic and genomic research and technology development, initially driven by the Human Genome Project which was completed in the year 2000 (Lander et al. 2001). The HapMap project then identified sites of common variation in different human populations (The International HapMap Consortium 2005), which led to the development of high-throughput accurate genotyping platforms.

This work laid the foundations for genome-wide association studies (GWAS), a large-scale population-based case-control study design exploiting linkage disequilibrium between ancient common variants to compare allele and haplotype frequencies in large cohorts of patient and control subjects. The GWAS design is based on the 'common disease–common variant' hypothesis that multiple small genetic effects combine to predispose individuals to complex diseases. Several thousand loci have now been reliably identified as contributing to a large range of common diseases and other phenotypes by this method, and this has provided insights into novel disease pathways and mechanisms (Hirschhorn and Gajdos 2011). However, in only a minority of cases has the precise gene or variant giving rise to the association signal been identified and its mechanism of action has been established, and the odds ratios for disease development associated with each individual variant identified on GWAS tend to be in the region of 1.1–1.5, indicating that their effect on disease risk in any individual person is small. Even when an individual's genotype at multiple risk single nucleotide polymorphisms (SNPs) is taken into account, these results only account for a small amount of the variation in cancer risk between individuals. The GWAS effort has contributed to our understanding of the molecular processes and pathways underlying many diseases, and it is hoped that this will be translated into therapeutic advances. However, common SNP genotype tests have not been adopted as clinical tools due to their limited clinical utility, and therefore, the original hope that GWAS would lead to the use of SNP genotyping to stratify risk and deliver personalised medicine has not been realised.

In parallel with the technology used for large-scale SNP genotyping, similar protocols were developed to study larger changes in the genome known as structural variation (deletions—missing regions of the genome; duplications—extra copies of regions of the genome; and inversions—sections of the genome which have become rotated). It used to be thought that the overall structure of the healthy human genome was relatively invariant, because large genome rearrangements visible down the microscope were nearly all associated with significant medical and developmental difficulties (in a constitutional form) or were found as somatic changes in tumour cell genomes. However, once microarray techniques such as comparative genome hybridisation (known as array CGH) were developed to study copy number variation in more detail, it was discovered that smaller scale structural changes are often well tolerated and may not lead to any detectable phenotype. Array-CGH results have also led to the understanding that a significant minority of monogenic disease is caused by a structural variant affecting an important gene, and some families whose condition remained unexplained by DNA sequencing have a whole gene deletion; for example, deletions of the *APC* gene cause classic familial adenomatous polyposis.

The most recent major advance in genetic technology has been the exponential increase in sequencing capacity brought about in the last decade by the high-throughput platforms developed by Illumina (Bentley et al. 2008), Roche 454 (Margulies et al. 2005), ABI SOLiD (McKernan et al. 2009), and Complete Genomics (Peters et al. 2012). This has been made possible by the use of massively parallel sequencing, which uses simultaneous amplification of hundreds of millions of individual DNA fragments, which are imaged after each sequencing cycle to determine the order of nucleotides in each separate fragment simultaneously. Having taken several decades to generate the first draft of the human genome sequence in the years leading up to the millennium, in 2015 an entire individual human genome takes around a week to sequence, at a basic test cost not greatly exceeding $1000.

High-throughput sequencing generates huge volumes of data which require specialist computer hardware, software and informatics expertise to analyse. Bioinformaticians have developed many informatic techniques to map millions of sequence reads varying in length from 35 base pairs to around 700 base pairs to the genome, and to identify SNPs and structural rearrangements from the aligned reads (known as variant calling). Extensive testing of these algorithms has established the best parameters to maximise sensitivity of variant detection and minimise false positive variant calls. More recently, the increased body of experience in analysis of high-throughput sequence data has allowed these analysis pipelines to become more standardised and automatable.

Following the use of high-throughput sequencing for whole-genome sequencing, technologies for sequencing selected parts of the genome have been developed. These include automated multiplex polymerase chain reaction (PCR) systems, where multiple individual targets are amplified using the traditional PCR technique but at much higher throughput. The more widely adopted mechanism uses target enrichment either of selected custom DNA targets such as a panel of genes known to cause a particular condition, or generic targets such as the entire coding sequence of the genome, known as the exome. This works by shearing DNA from the whole genome into small pieces, then capturing the fragments covering the genome regions of interest, before washing off the unwanted fragments, and sequencing the enriched library of targeted sequences.

Using a targeted approach known as a 'panel test', sequence data can be generated in one test for anything from a handful of genes up to several hundred genes. For example, the Lynch syndrome genes can be tested all together in a clinically available panel of nine bowel cancer genes, which is quicker and cheaper than sequencing each gene individually one after the other, and may avoid the need for immunohistochemistry to direct where to start with single gene testing. Panel testing has been introduced fairly widely to clinical practice, particularly in the diagnosis of heterogeneous conditions, where mutations in a number of different genes cause the same phenotype.

Exome sequencing has been used with great success to identify the genes responsible for dozens of monogenic disorders since the first publication (Ng et al. 2009). More recently, exome sequencing has also been used as an extension of panel testing in the clinical diagnostic context. The challenge with panel testing is that new genes causing each heterogeneous phenotype are discovered each year, and adding new genes to an existing panel test involves a lengthy and expensive process of adaptation and revalidation of the test. As sequencing costs have fallen, it has been suggested that it is more cost-effective to carry out exome sequencing by a standardised protocol on every sample, and then select the relevant genes for analysis. This provides a very flexible approach, where 'virtual panels' for analysis can be changed swiftly in response to new gene discoveries, and data can be revisited retrospectively without repeating the laboratory element of the assay.

The large volume of sequence data which has been generated in the last decade has highlighted the extent of variation found in every individual genome. Every exome or genome sequence identifies many thousands of variants, the majority of which have no relevance to the phenotype in question, and the process of prioritising and filtering these variants is one of the greatest challenges currently facing geneticists. Individual variants are commonly categorised using a five-point system, as described in Box 2.

Assessing variant pathogenicity to place each variant into the categories given above is a highly technical and time-consuming process which needs to be done by experienced molecular geneticists, and which is not yet amenable to a high degree of automation. This therefore represents the most significant bottleneck in the high-throughput molecular diagnostic context at this time. A number of factors and techniques are commonly used to assess the pathogenicity of a variant; these are discussed in Box 3.

In silico prediction tools such as Polyphen (Adzhubei et al. 2010), SIFT (Kumar et al. 2009) and Condel (González-Pérez and López-Bigas 2011) can be used as screening tools for large data sets. These use a combination of information on amino acid structures, known protein structures and evolutionary conservation to provide a quick and simple way of testing large batches of variants, but their sensitivity and specificity are low. In future, it is likely to become possible to prioritise non-coding variants using *in silico* tools as well, using data from projects such as ENCODE (the Encyclopedia of DNA Elements), which aims to catalogue functional and regulatory elements in the human genome (The ENCODE Project Consortium 2011). At present, these tools can be used to give a consensus suggestion about a particular variant, but they cannot be relied upon as a mainstay of clinical diagnostic variant interpretation.

Whole-genome sequencing is also being investigated now as a clinical diagnostic tool, chiefly within the 100,000 Genomes Project in the UK, which is generating whole-genome sequences in thousands of patients with rare disease or cancer in the NHS. Whole-genome sequencing is more expensive and generates volumes of data which are difficult to store, but has a number of potential advantages over exome sequencing. Firstly, an unknown proportion of disease-causing variants may lie outside coding regions, either in introns affecting gene splicing, or in promoter or enhancer regions affecting gene expression, and these variants will always be missed by exome sequencing. Secondly, exome sequencing requires a step in the DNA preparation where the coding regions of DNA are captured for sequencing. Some genomic regions do not pull down well or are hard to map back to the genome, due to repetitive DNA sequences or variations in the ratio of AT: GC nucleotides. Some genes are therefore consistently difficult to capture with exome sequencing, but genome sequencing does not involve this capture step and therefore covers these difficult regions more completely. Thirdly, genome sequence data allows structural variations (deletions, duplications, inversions) to be detected reliably as well as small sequence variation, so it is possible that a genome sequence will mean that array CGH will not be needed as a separate test.

3 Translation of Research Findings into Clinically Useful Genetic Tests

As described above, the technological aspects of genetic testing have improved rapidly over the last decade. These advances have been driven by the requirements of research, often by extensive multinational collaborations such as the Human Genome Project and the many international GWAS consortia. Following closely behind these developments have been efforts to translate the technological advances into clinical practice, to provide immediate clinical benefit for patients. However, the requirements of genetic testing in the clinical context are different from the research context, as described in Table 2.

The ACCE framework (shown in Fig. 1) is a highly influential approach which has been designed to evaluate whether a test is appropriate to be used in clinical practice (Haddow and Palomaki 2003). This comprises a detailed assessment of the following:

Table 2 Comparison between research and clinical priorities

Test characteristic	Research priority	Clinical test priority
Accuracy	Global accuracy across the project is important	Individual accuracy for a clinical report for each patient is crucial
Throughput	Often needs to be very high	Healthcare system may not be able to afford high throughput
Cost	Moderate pressure to lower costs	High pressure to lower costs due to the requirement for cost-effectiveness evidence before implementation
Completeness	Some missing data will not significantly compromise the results	Missing data for an individual patient is a big problem
Time and labour required to perform test	High priority to minimise these, but no absolute deadline for results	Reliable turnaround time needed for clinical tests, including complex results

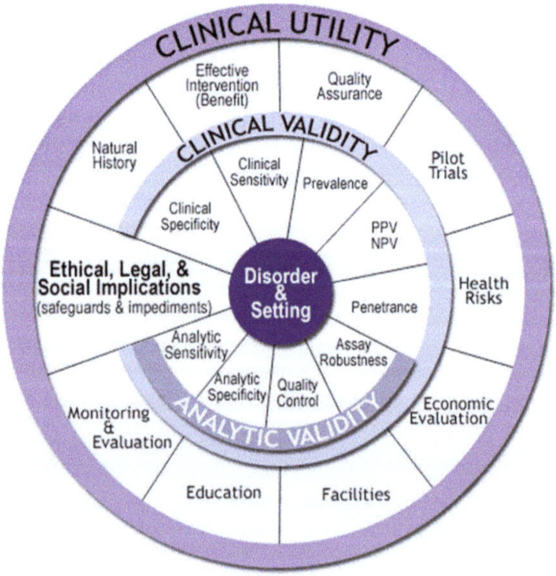

Fig. 1 The ACCE framework to assess the suitability of a genetic test for use in clinical practice, reproduced with permission from Haddow and Palomaki (2003)

- **A**nalytical validity,
- **C**linical validity,
- **C**linical utility and
- **E**thical, legal and social implications of the test.

Analytical validity refers to the performance of the test in accurately identifying DNA sequence variation in the gene(s) of interest and measures the aspects of the test which occur in the clinical laboratory. Ensuring and demonstrating analytical validity for a new technology requires labour-intensive validation, improving the reliability and completeness of the test, testing samples with known mutations to compare the test with current gold standard tests and finally piloting the test on prospective clinical samples.

Clinical validity is a measure of the ability of the test to predict the disease or phenotype in question. For example, many of the SNPs identified in genome-wide association studies are readily measurable in the laboratory, but it would not be appropriate to measure these as clinical assays because the increased risk of cancer associated with each of these SNPs is so low that knowing an individual's genotype has no value in predicting their chance of developing cancer or tailoring their treatment accordingly. Establishing clinical validity requires epidemiological data on the clinical sensitivity and specificity of the test in a particular population, and on the penetrance of the mutation; these data need to have been generated in the research context before the test can be adopted for clinical use.

Clinical utility defines whether carrying out the test will lead to an improved outcome for the patient receiving the test. This will depend on an accurate prediction of the cancer risks caused by a particular mutation and the availability and effectiveness of surveillance and cancer risk reducing measures, and also on less tangible benefits such as the relief which some patients experience from understanding the cause of their personal and family history of cancer.

The ethical, legal and social implications of genetic tests also need to be considered. In addition, genetic tests can be expensive due to their complexity, and cost-effectiveness analyses are therefore required to determine which tests to use in which groups of patients to maximise the health benefit from these technologies.

4 Interpretation of Genetic Test Reports

4.1 Variants of Unknown Clinical Significance (VUS)

The advances in genetic testing described here are leading to ever-increasing numbers of patients receiving a genetic diagnosis confirming a constitutional predisposition to cancer running in their family. This enables patients and family members to appreciate their risk of developing cancer in the future, and helps clinicians to focus screening and prevention strategies on those at highest risk, who stand to benefit the most from available interventions. Test results in cancer genetics must be accurate, robust and correctly interpreted to achieve these benefits. For example, if a variant is incorrectly designated as being the cause of a patient's cancer, relatives may undergo predictive testing which does not accurately reflect their future risk. This may lead to individuals being incorrectly informed that they are at high risk and using this information to access prophylactic surgery or inform reproductive decisions; it may also lead to inappropriate reassurance and removal of screening from individuals at high risk who go on to develop cancer.

In order to avoid these serious errors, the burden of proof required to designate a variant as pathogenic for diagnostic purposes is high. VUS results (see Box 2) are not used for diagnostic, predictive or reproductive purposes, and the family is managed as if no genetic diagnosis has been identified. As evidence accumulates, VUS can sometimes be reclassified as pathogenic or benign, and laboratories will revisit reports to assess this if requested.

4.2 Additional Unsought Genetic Findings

Traditional testing techniques only allowed one gene to be tested at a time, and therefore, genes were only tested in individuals with an associated phenotype predicted to have a high chance of being caused by a mutation in that gene. With the widening of testing to examine many genes simultaneously, a greater focus is needed on the relationship between mutations in a particular gene and the medical consequences of that mutation, in the context of an individual's lifestyle and environment (known as the phenotype). For example, a patient with bowel cancer who undergoes testing using the bowel cancer gene panel might be found to have a mutation in one of the Lynch syndrome genes, which would have a high likelihood of being pathogenic subject to the pathogenicity measures described above. However, if a mutation was found in the gene for Peutz-Jeghers syndrome (PJS), which is also on the panel because bowel cancer is part of this condition, the patient would need to be examined for the other clinical features of PJS, such as peri-oral pigmentation. If these features were found, the genotype and phenotype could be confirmed to match and the diagnosis would be clear.

If on the other hand a patient has a mutation in a gene for which they exhibit few or none of the classic clinical features, there are several possibilities which need to be distinguished:

1. The patient has a condition which is not the classic presentation of mutations in that particular gene, but the gene may be responsible for a more attenuated form of the phenotype and the result may therefore be relevant to the patient's presentation. This type of result occurs quite frequently, and our understanding of the spectrum of phenotypes which can be associated with mutations in each gene is increasing as a result.
2. The genetic variant is unrelated to the patient's presenting phenotype and is unlikely to be of medical relevance.

3. The genetic variant is unrelated to the patient's presenting phenotype but is likely to have consequences for their health in other ways.

This third category of genetic variants are known as **incidental findings** or additional findings, and they have been the subject of much debate in recent years. Incidental findings are a standard part of clinical practice, but their frequency is high in gene panel or exome tests because of the large number of variants found in every genome.

Predicting the clinical consequences of these variants is complex. For example, if a patient has their genome sequenced to diagnose their neurological condition, a full analysis of the genome may reveal a mutation in the *BRCA1* gene. If this patient has a strong family history of breast cancer, this family can be managed as any other *BRCA1* mutation-carrying family. However, if the patient has no personal or family history of breast or ovarian cancer, the significance of this mutation is less clear. Perhaps the patient is an only child whose parents died young, or the majority of close relatives are male; but it is also possible that the family carries other poorly understood genetic variation which counteracts the harmful effects of the *BRCA1* mutation (known as reduced penetrance of the mutation) and renders prophylactic mastectomy less beneficial.

The American College of Medical Genetics has issued guidelines recommending that additional findings are sought whenever a genomic test is used in a diagnostic context (Green et al. 2013; ACMG Board of Directors 2015), but European experts have urged caution due to an insufficient evidence base for this 'opportunistic screening' and its acceptability to patients (Burke et al. 2013). In general, when patients are asked if they wish to receive medically relevant additional findings, they indicate that they do, but research has not yet shown whether this preference persists once such a finding has actually been identified and returned (Bergner et al. 2014). Further data are being generated to address these uncertainties.

4.3 Interpreting Negative Test Results

In addition to appreciating the significance and management implications of positive genetic test results, it is equally important to understand the meaning of a negative test result. The relevant information should all be present in the diagnostic report, and if in doubt a clinical scientist can be consulted about what might have been missed by the test.

Some tests are very focused and specific, for example a test for the Ashkenazi Jewish founder mutations in the *BRCA1* and *BRCA2* genes. A negative result for this test will eliminate the population-specific risk of being a *BRCA1* or *BRCA2* carrier for a woman of Ashkenazi Jewish descent, but she will still have the same risk as a woman of any other ethnic origin of carrying a different *BRCA1* or *BRCA2* mutation, so it may be appropriate to continue to a full screen of these genes by full sequencing of all of the exons. It is important that a partial gene screen of this type is not over-interpreted to indicate the absence of a *BRCA1* or *BRCA2* mutation.

Capillary sequencing of a single gene is in general the most complete and authoritative test. If a complete gene sequence is negative, it is unlikely (although not impossible) that there is a pathogenic mutation in the coding region of the gene in that patient. However, there may still be a larger change such as one or more whole exons deleted or duplicated, and an additional test is required to look for this, commonly a multiplex ligation-dependent probe amplification test (MLPA).

A panel test or an exome sequence will study a much larger group of genes, and therefore in heterogeneous conditions (where a large number of genes could have caused the disease), these will have a higher overall detection rate. However, some genes may not be completely sequenced by these tests, and therefore, if there is one single gene of high importance for a particular phenotype, it may be more appropriate to request a single gene capillary sequencing test rather than a panel test. Some panel and exome tests have sufficient coverage to detect whole exon deletions or duplications reliably, while others do not. Some tests include additional capillary sequencing to cover the gaps in important genes on panel or exome tests, while others do not.

5 Direct-to-Consumer Genetic Testing

Developments in DNA analysis technology have also led to the emergence of commercial genetic tests offered direct to the consumer. Regulation of these tests varies widely around the world, and companies market the tests in different ways. Some tests are offered for primarily non-medical reasons such as ancestry tracking, while others are marketed as providing a health benefit. Because of the complexity of genetic testing, its analysis and interpretation, there is considerable anxiety amongst genetics health professionals that these direct-to-consumer tests may not prepare customers adequately for the possible outcomes of the test and may not provide appropriate information to patients about the significance of the results. As with all commercial sectors, it is likely that some providers will offer services in a responsible way which increases patients' options and autonomy, while others will offer inappropriate tests with insufficient or inaccurate information, and the regulatory context for these tests in many countries is aiming to address this.

6 Outlook

Genetic testing has made great advances in the last 15 years, and this is changing the way patients with a constitutional predisposition to cancer are managed. Genetic testing offers great benefits to cancer patients and their relatives in understanding their disease and their future risk of developing cancer. The newer genetic tests are technically complex, variable between diagnostic centres, and extensive in their remit. To ensure that all eligible patients receive appropriate genetic testing, these tests are increasingly being used in non-specialist mainstream clinics. This is essential, as clinical genetics services are unable to meet the increased demand for genetic testing which has come with the testing advances, but it is crucial that clinicians requesting the tests understand how they should be used, what the implications of a positive and negative result may be, and when to seek specialist advice.

Rapid genetic testing is now being introduced in some centres at the time of cancer diagnosis, for example to assist with decision-making regarding the extent of surgery for a primary tumour and to avoid the need for a second prophylactic procedure following a primary tumour resection if the patient is found to be at high genetic risk of developing a further cancer. In addition, treatment stratification according to the underlying genetic cause of the cancer is also now becoming a reality in some conditions, for example the use of poly ADP ribose polymerase (PARP) inhibitors in breast and ovarian cancers in *BRCA1* and *BRCA2* mutation carriers (Lee et al. 2014). More examples of treatment stratification by genetic testing are likely to come into practice as our understanding of the inherited basis of cancers increases, which will continue to increase the demand for rapid, reliable genetic testing to inform management.

Genetic testing of somatic variation in tumours is also used to guide management, both in terms of choosing the most appropriate chemotherapeutic agent and in determining the likely course of the disease, and therefore the degree of aggression required in selecting treatments. Many of the technologies described here are also used in examination of tumour DNA, both in research and clinical practice. These are not discussed here, but further information on this topic can be found in a recent review (Forbes et al. 2015).

Box 1: Nomenclature referring to changes in the DNA sequence as compared to the reference human genome

Variant: a position in the genome which is different from the reference human genome. There are approximately 4 million variants in each individual's genome.

Mutation: a variant for which evidence is available that it causes a disease phenotype. The word 'mutation' has negative associations for some people, and therefore, a term such as 'gene fault' is frequently used by health professionals when talking to patients.

Polymorphism: a variant which is known to be present in a proportion of the population (between 1 and 50 % of the population), which is not associated with a clinically significant risk of disease.

SNP (single nucleotide polymorphism): a common variant affecting a single DNA base which does not cause a clinically significant risk of disease.

Structural change (deletion, duplication, inversion): a larger section of DNA which is missing, duplicated or reversed compared to the reference human genome. These can cause disease or can be benign and present in many generations of a family.

Box 2: The classification system for assessing the likely effect of individual genetic variants and mutations

1. Definitely not pathogenic, for example a known common polymorphism.
2. No evidence that the variant is pathogenic.
3. Variant of unknown clinical significance (VUS or VUCS).
4. Expected to be pathogenic, for example a variant in a known gene where the precise variant has not been seen before but is likely to have a similar effect to known disease-causing variants.
5. Known pathogenic (disease-causing) variant in a known gene.

Box 3: Attributes of a genetic variant which are used to assign the variant to one of the categories of the classification system shown in Box 2

- Segregation of the variant with the phenotype within families—checking that the variant is present in people with the disease and absent in those without.
- Frequency of the variant in sequence data from control populations; there are several publically available control data sets which are frequently used for this purpose.
- Evidence in the literature and in locus-specific databases indicating whether the variant has been observed before, in individuals with or without a similar phenotype.
- The predicted effect of the variant on the protein, for example variants which prevent a complete protein from being produced (known as truncating or non-sense mutations) are more likely to be pathogenic.
- The degree of evolutionary conservation: variants affecting parts of the protein which have been highly conserved through evolution are more likely to be pathogenic.
- Knowledge of protein structure and function, for example mutations in functional domains of a particular protein may be known to have a significant functional impact.
- Animal studies of gene knockout or mutation may give an insight into potential functional effects of mutations.
- *In vitro* studies using cell cultures or other functional assays are valuable in determining the effect of a variant. However, these are beyond the capacity of a clinical laboratory and are time-consuming and expensive, and require expertise, so they are only available via interested research groups for a small minority of genes or pathways.

References

ACMG Board of Directors (2015) ACMG policy statement: updated recommendations regarding analysis and reporting of secondary findings in clinical genome-scale sequencing. Genet Med 17:68–69

Adzhubei IA, Schmidt S, Peshkin L et al (2010) A method and server for predicting damaging missense mutations. Nat Meth 7:248–249

Bentley DR, Balasubramanian S, Swerdlow HP et al (2008) Accurate whole human genome sequencing using reversible terminator chemistry. Nature 456:53–59

Bergner AL, Bollinger J, Raraigh KS et al (2014) Informed consent for exome sequencing research in families with genetic disease: the emerging issue of incidental findings. Am J Med Genet Part A 164:2745–2752

Burke W, Matheny Antommaria AH, Bennett R, et al (2013) Recommendations for returning genomic incidental findings? We need to talk! Genet Med 15:854–859

Forbes SA, Beare D, Gunasekaran P et al (2015) COSMIC: exploring the world's knowledge of somatic mutations in human cancer. Nucleic Acids Res 43:D805–D811

González-Pérez A, López-Bigas N (2011) Improving the assessment of the outcome of nonsynonymous SNVs with a consensus deleteriousness score, Condel. Am J Hum Genet 88:440–449

Green RC, Berg JS, Grody WW et al (2013) ACMG recommendations for reporting of incidental findings in clinical exome and genome sequencing. Genet Med 15:565–574

Haddow J, Palomaki G (2003) ACCE: a model process for evaluating data on emerging genetic tests. In: Khoury M, Little J, Burke W (eds) Human genome epidemiology: a scientific foundation for using genetic information to improve health and prevent disease. Oxford University Press, Oxford

Hirschhorn JN, Gajdos ZKZ (2011) Genome-wide association studies: results from the first few years and potential implications for clinical medicine. Annu Rev Med 62:11–24

Kumar P, Henikoff S, Ng PC (2009) Predicting the effects of coding non-synonymous variants on protein function using the SIFT algorithm. Nat Protocols 4:1073–1081

Lander ES, Linton LM, Birren B et al (2001) Initial sequencing and analysis of the human genome. Nature 409:860–921

Lee J-M, Ledermann JA, Kohn EC (2014) PARP inhibitors for BRCA1/2 mutation-associated and BRCA-like malignancies. Ann Oncol 25:32–40

Margulies M, Egholm M, Altman WE et al (2005) Genome sequencing in microfabricated high-density picolitre reactors. Nature 437:376–380

McKernan KJ, Peckham HE, Costa GL et al (2009) Sequence and structural variation in a human genome uncovered by short-read, massively parallel ligation sequencing using two-base encoding. Genome Res 19:1527–1541

Ng SB, Turner EH, Robertson PD et al (2009) Targeted capture and massively parallel sequencing of 12 human exomes. Nature 461:272–276

Peters BA, Kermani BG, Sparks AB et al (2012) Accurate whole-genome sequencing and haplotyping from 10 to 20 human cells. Nature 487:190–195

The Encode Project Consortium (2011) A user's guide to the encyclopedia of DNA elements (ENCODE). PLoS Biol 9:e1001046

The International HapMap Consortium (2005) A haplotype map of the human genome. Nature 437:1299–1320

References

Diagnosis and Management of Hereditary Meningioma and Vestibular Schwannoma

Adam Shaw

Abstract

Bilateral vestibular schwannomata and meningiomata are the tumours most commonly associated with neurofibromatosis type II (NF2). These tumours may also be seen in patients with schwannomatosis and familial meningioma, but these phenotypes are usually easy to distinguish. The main diagnostic challenge when managing these tumours is distinguishing between sporadic disease which carries low risk of subsequent tumours or NF2 with its associated morbidities and reduced life expectancy. This chapter outlines some of the diagnostic and management considerations along with associated evidence.

Keywords

Vestibular schwannoma · Meningioma · Neurofibromatosis type II · *NF2* · Schwannomatosis

Contents

A. Shaw (✉)
Department of Clinical Genetics, Guy's and St Thomas' NHS Foundation Trust, London, UK
e-mail: Adam.Shaw@gstt.nhs.uk

G. Pichert and C. Jacobs (eds.), *Rare Hereditary Cancers*,
Recent Results in Cancer Research 205, DOI 10.1007/978-3-319-29998-3_2

1 Introduction

The main focus of this chapter is neurofibromatosis type II (NF2). Other genetic conditions that can potentially cause meningioma or vestibular schwannoma (VS) are also discussed, but these are rare and the predominant diagnostic challenge faced by the clinician is distinguishing between sporadic occurrence of meningioma and/or VS, and NF2, particularly in its mosaic form where only a proportion of the body's cells are affected. NF2 is most appropriately managed in specialist centres with multidisciplinary input, due to the complex needs of the patients, high morbidity and multiple available treatment modalities, all with significant associated risk of complication. Suggestions for which patients with an apparently sporadic VS or meningioma should be investigated for NF2 are provided.

Meningiomata are typically benign tumours arising from arachnoidal cap cells of the meninges and are the most common primary brain tumour in adults accounting for a third of such. Around 90 % occur in the cranium, with the remainder affecting the spine. Malignant meningioma is rare, but occurs in around 2 % of cases. The incidence of meningioma in the USA is estimated to be 1.8 and 4.2 per 100,000 for men and women, respectively. True incidence may be higher due to under-reporting, and one Finnish study calculated the incidence to be 2.9 and 13.0 per 100,000 for men and women, respectively (Larjavaara 2008). Risk factors for sporadic meningioma include exposure to radiation, age and female gender. Meningioma is rare in childhood and can occur at any age in adulthood, but is most common over the age of 50 years.

Vestibular schwannomata (VS) are benign tumours arising from the eighth cranial nerve and account for 10 % of primary intracranial tumours in adults. Sporadic VS are typically very slow growing and may present as incidental findings on brain imaging. A retrospective review of over 46,000 brain MRI scans (requested for reasons other than to investigate auditory/vestibular symptoms) detected VS in 0.02 % (Lin 2005). Symptomatic VS are less common and are estimated to occur in 1–2 per 100,000 (Stangerup 2010). Sporadic VS are rare in childhood, and most occur over the age of 50 years with a median age of diagnosis of 59 years (Carlson 2015).

Hereditary phenotypes that can be associated with meningioma and/or VS include NF2 (OMIM 101000), meningioma, familial susceptibility to (OMIM 607174), and schwannomatosis (OMIM 162091). In diagnostic practice, the degree of overlap between these conditions is limited. Constitutional or mosaic mutations in *NF2* most commonly present with bilateral VS, with meningioma and/or ependymoma, an additional feature in up to 50 % of patients. In majority of families reported with a susceptibility to meningioma, the genetic aetiology is currently unknown. Although familial meningiomata are a feature of NF2, this diagnosis is extremely unlikely in the absence of VS. Of the two other genes associated with familial susceptibility to meningioma, mutations in *SUFU* have only been described in a single Finnish family, and mutations in *SMARCB1* are associated with spinal meningiomata rather than intracranial disease. Schwannomatosis is typically associated with multiple peripheral schwannomata development, with VS and meningioma occurring infrequently.

2 Risk Assessment

2.1 Meningioma

When assessing a patient with meningioma, consideration should be given to past medical history (previous meningioma, schwannoma, neuropathy, cataract, poor vision) and family history of neurological tumours (Table 1).

Although overt cataracts occur in NF2, milder posterior subcapsular lens opacities are more common and frequently asymptomatic. Vision may also be impaired in NF2 patients due to retinal hamartomata, epiretinal membrane and papilloedema from raised intracranial pressure. Detailed examination by an experienced ophthalmologist is therefore recommended.

A family history of hearing loss, balance disturbance, neurological tumours or unexplained neurology symptoms should be explored. A large proportion of cases of NF2 occur due to a *de novo* mutation in the *NF2* gene, and so the absence of a family history does not rule out the diagnosis if other criteria are met (Table 3).

Table 1 Differential diagnosis for patient presenting with meningioma

Potential diagnosis	Suggestive features
Sporadic meningioma	No significant family history or personal history of schwannomata
NF2	Other features include VS, ocular abnormalities[a], neuropathy, family history of NF2
Meningioma, familial susceptibility to	Significant family history of meningioma
Schwannomatosis	Multiple schwannomata

[a]Posterior subcapsular lens opacities, cataract, retinal hamartomata, epiretinal membrane and papilloedema from raised intracranial pressure

2.2 Vestibular Schwannoma

The presence of bilateral vestibular schwannomata is diagnostic for NF2. Some patients presenting with metachronous bilateral VS may not have NF2 but sporadic tumours occurring bilaterally, although this is likely to be rare. It should be considered in older patients and those in whom many years have passed before the development of the contralateral tumour.

Evaluation of the patient with unilateral VS should include consideration of the age at presentation, past history of VS, peripheral schwannoma, meningioma, ependymoma, ocular abnormalities (as per meningioma, above) and family history of hearing loss or neurological symptoms. The differential diagnosis is summarised in Table 2. Diagnostic criteria for NF2 have been published and are shown in Table 3. Genes known to be associated with genetic susceptibility to meningioma and VS are summarised in Tables 4 and 5, respectively.

Table 2 Differential diagnosis for patient presenting with vestibular schwannoma

Potential diagnosis	Suggestive features
Sporadic VS	No significant family history, unilateral VS, no history of meningioma, schwannoma, ependymoma, or ocular abnormalities[a]
NF2	Other features include meningioma, ocular abnormalities[a], neuropathy, family history of NF2 Consider mosaic NF2 in unilateral VS with other features
Schwannomatosis	Multiple peripheral schwannomata, bilateral Vestibular schwannoma rare

[a]Posterior subcapsular lens opacities, cataract, retinal hamartomata, epiretinal membrane and papilloedema from raised intracranial pressure

Table 3 Diagnostic criteria for NF2 (Baser 2002)

1	Bilateral vestibular schwannomata (VS) **or** family history of NF2 plus unilateral VS **or** any two of meningioma, glioma, neurofibroma, schwannoma, posterior subcapsular lenticular opacities
2	Unilateral VS **plus any two of** meningioma, glioma, neurofibroma, schwannoma, posterior subcapsular lenticular opacities
3	Two or more meningioma **plus** unilateral VS **or any two of** glioma, schwannoma and cataract

Table 4 Genes associated with susceptibility to meningioma

Gene	Penetrance	Comment
NF2	30–50 %	Neurofibromatosis type II Diagnosis unlikely in the absence of vestibular schwannoma
SUFU	Unknown	Single Finnish family reported (Aavikko 2012)
SMARCB1	5 %	Schwannomatosis Diagnosis unlikely in the absence of multiple peripheral schwannomata
SMARCE1	Unknown	Familial spinal meningioma

Table 5 Genes associated with susceptibility to vestibular schwannoma

Gene	Penetrance	Comment
NF2	Close to 100 %, lower for mosaic disease	Neurofibromatosis type II
SMARCB1	Low	Schwannomatosis Typically multiple peripheral schwannomata, Vestibular schwannoma rare

3 Differential Diagnosis

3.1 NF2 (OMIM 101000)

NF2 is a rare genetic condition with an estimated worldwide incidence of 1 in 33,000. It is inherited in an autosomal dominant fashion, but a high proportion of cases occur *de novo* due to an *NF2* mutation arising during meiosis. In addition, a significant number are either proven or assumed mosaic for an *NF2* mutation arising during postzygotic mitosis. In this situation, only a proportion of the patient's cells carry the mutation; these might be distributed throughout the body, restricted to an embryological tissue type, or an anatomical location. The *NF2* gene encodes the cell signalling protein neurofibromin 2 (also known as Merlin) which is expressed in all cells but has tissue-dependent function. In eighth cranial nerve Schwann cells, and in other neurological tissues, *NF2* acts as a tumour suppressor gene. Biallelic mutations can be demonstrated in DNA derived from sporadic VS tissue. Patients with NF2 have a constitutional loss-of-function mutation in the *NF2* gene, with a second-hit mutation deactivating the other allele in the tumour.

The hallmark of NF2 is the development of bilateral VS, typically becoming symptomatic between the ages of 17 and 24 years, but earlier or later presentation is common. Nearly all patients will develop symptoms before 30 years. Presentation during childhood is often due to other features such as ocular abnormalities, peripheral or spinal schwannoma, ependymoma or neuropathy. Approximately one-third of individuals suffer reduced visual acuity in either eye due to cataract, retinal hamartoma or epiretinal membrane. A mono- or polyneuropathy causing focal weakness is the initial presenting feature in 12 % of cases (Evans 1992).

One-third to one-half of individuals develop one or more meningiomata during their lifetime. Over one half of patients develop one or more non-vestibular schwannomata, most commonly in the spine, fifth, seventh, ninth or twelfth cranial nerves (Asthagiri 2009). Ependymomata are estimated to affect around one half of individuals but are frequently asymptomatic and do not require intervention (Plotkin 2011).

Age of first presentation of symptoms in NF2 is often remarkably consistent within families, suggesting a significant role of the specific mutation on tumour biology. Phenotype cannot be accurately predicted from the genotype of a particular individual, but associations are recognised.

Missense mutations tend to be associated with a later presentation, slower-growing VS and fewer other tumours. Nonsense and frameshift mutations (protein-truncating) are more likely to cause younger presentation and greater tumour load (Baser 2004). Mutations affecting donor or acceptor splice sites within the gene have been reported with a wide spectrum of severity. Mutations occurring towards the end of the gene and potentially producing a partially functional protein are more likely to result in milder disease with lower risk of meningioma (Smith 2011).

3.2 Meningioma, Familial Susceptibility to (OMIM 607174)

Multiple familial meningiomata is a rare entity with no recognised diagnostic criteria, or reliable estimates of incidence. The underlying molecular aetiology in the majority of families is unknown. Mutations in *SMARCE1* have been identified in four families with multiple spinal clear cell meningiomata (Smith 2013). No mutations in this gene were found in further 34 individuals with multiple cranial meningiomata. Mutations in *SUFU* were found in a single Finnish family with multiple cranial meningiomata, but no other cases with this association have been reported (Aavikko 2012). Although meningioma can occur in patients with NF2 and schwannomatosis caused by mutations in *SMARCB1*, schwannomata are more prevalent in these phenotypes (Bacci 2010). Insufficient data are currently available to draw reliable genotype–phenotype correlations.

4 Genetic Testing

When arranging genetic testing and interpreting the results, it is always necessary to consider which tissue the tested DNA is derived from and the likelihood of it being representative of the tissue affected by disease. Most routine genetic testing is performed on DNA derived from lymphocytes circulating in peripheral blood due to the ease of sampling, but this may miss mutations that are not present in all tissues. Mutations associated with intracranial tumour development may have occurred postconception and be restricted to neurological tissue which cannot be as readily sampled.

4.1 Bilateral Vestibular Schwannomata

DNA extracted from peripheral blood lymphocytes should be sent for analysis of the *NF2* gene. If this result is normal, then consider *NF2* analysis in tumour-derived DNA if available, and if possible, from two separate tumours. Most laboratories quote improved sensitivity and specificity with analysis from DNA extracted from tissue fresh frozen in liquid nitrogen at the time of biopsy. Analysis of DNA extracted from formalin-fixed, paraffin-embedded (FFPE) tissue may be possible, and discussion with the genetics laboratory is advised in advance.

The introduction of massively parallel sequencing techniques has improved the ability to detect low-level mosaicism for *NF2* mutations over traditional Sanger sequencing. Such techniques may detect mutations present in levels as low as 5–10 % in the DNA sample analysed. Nonetheless, a normal result of *NF2* testing on lymphocyte DNA, even by this methodology, does not exclude mosaic disease as many patients are likely to have mosaicism restricted to neural tissue.

Mosaicism for *NF2* mutations appears to be very common. Up to 50 % of patients meeting diagnostic criteria for NF2 have no *NF2* mutation detectable in lymphocyte-derived DNA. To date, no other genes have been associated with the NF2 phenotype, and it is most likely that most if not all such patients are either mosaic for *NF2* gene mutations or have constitutional *NF2* gene mutations that have not been detected by current analysis methods.

4.2 Unilateral Vestibular Schwannoma

Analysis of lymphocyte-derived DNA for the *NF2* gene should be considered in patients with young age of onset, personal or family history of meningioma, or other NF2-related pathology. If there is a history of peripheral schwannoma, then consideration should be given to the diagnosis of schwannomatosis with analysis of the *SMARCB1* gene if appropriate.

4.3 Meningioma

No genetic testing is indicated for a single sporadic meningioma diagnosed over the age of 50 years. In scenarios with a young age of diagnosis, multiple primary meningiomata or multiple first-degree relatives with meningiomata, genetic testing should be considered.

If predominantly intracranial disease, consider *NF2* gene testing in lymphocyte-derived DNA, followed by *SMARCB1* and *SUFU* if available. Mutations in any of these genes are relatively unlikely given current data.

If predominantly spinal meningiomata, then testing of *SMARCE1* in lymphocyte-derived DNA may be indicated if available.

5 Management

5.1 Surveillance

NF2 should be managed within specialised services with multidisciplinary input to ideally include neurosurgery, skull base surgery/ENT, neurology, ophthalmology, audiology, mental health and medical genetics.

Growth of VS in both sporadic and NF2-related disease is nonlinear, and longitudinal observation to demonstrate active growth is essential before intervention (Carlson 2015). Tumours can be very slow growing and exhibit reduction in size over time. Individuals presenting with bilateral VS may have had the tumours for many years with few or no symptoms. Surveillance interval should be decided based on tumour size, patient age, prior growth rate, symptoms and potential risk to hearing. Annual surveillance is common in adults under regular follow-up. Shorter intervals such as 3–6 months are common at initial presentation or in symptomatic paediatric patients. Older patients and those with evidence of static disease may only require reimaging every 3–5 years.

Surveillance should be by contrast enhanced brain MRI with internal auditory meatus protocols. Patients with cochlear or auditory brainstem implants with subcutaneous ferrous components require head-wrapping to reduce discomfort during MRI scanning. CT with contrast can be effective to monitor VS growth in patients unable to tolerate MRI or in whom it is contraindicated.

5.2 Therapeutic and Risk-Reducing Options

5.2.1 Vestibular Schwannoma

Surgical treatment for VS carries a high risk of profound hearing deficit, tinnitus and facial nerve damage. Other potential complications of skull base surgery include other cranial nerve damage, CSF leak, infection, headache and unexpected death. Nonetheless, surgical resection remains the treatment of choice for large VS that are unlikely to be amenable to other therapies and have already resulted in significant ipsilateral deafness.

Surgical approaches will depend on the tumour size, shape, relation to other structures, whether lobulated/multifocal, whether hearing is still present and whether a cochlear or auditory brainstem implant is to be sited. The most common surgical approach is translabyrinthine which results in the total loss of residual hearing, but provides optimal visualisation of the facial nerve, and allows siting of a cochlear implant during surgery (Moffat 2013). A retrosigmoid approach provides a more direct approach to expose VS tumours and can be used to preserve any residual hearing, but may be associated with an increased risk of facial nerve damage.

Radiotherapy (stereotactic radiosurgery/Gamma Knife) has been demonstrated to provide effective control of tumour growth with a reasonable side effect profile, although hearing outcomes are poor and the technique is most suitable for smaller tumours (Mallory 2014).

Bevacizumab, a monoclonal antibody to the vascular endothelial growth factor (VEGF), emerged as a potential treatment for NF2 due to VEGF receptor expression in VS tissue (Plotkin 2009). Ten patients were subsequently treated with 5 mg per 5 kg of body weight for a median of 12 months, with concomitant tumour shrinkage in 9. Further studies to validate these findings in larger populations are ongoing. Questions remain surrounding the optimum length of treatment and long-term effects. Proteinuria and hypertension are known associations, but in most patients, toxicity appears to be relatively mild (Slusarz 2014). Additional barriers to continuous treatment are that bevacizumab is contraindicated during pregnancy and perisurgery, and emerging evidence suggests that other tumours occurring in NF2 are unlikely to show a similar response (Nunes 2013).

Given the almost inevitable hearing loss seen in NF2, and the high risk of dual sensory impairment due to visual loss,hearing preservation or rehabilitation is a significant component of clinical management. Pre-emptive measures include presymptomatic learning of sign language and lip reading in patients known to be at risk. Similarly, restoration of limited or primitive auditory sensory input from cochlear implants and auditory brainstem implants, respectively, can potentially improve quality of life.

5.2.2 Meningioma

Meningioma management in NF2 is similar to that of sporadic meningioma except that additional complications from concurrent tumours and comorbidities may limit surgical options and outcomes. Meningiomata in NF2 may follow a saltatory growth pattern (Dirks 2012), so clear evidence of active tumour growth, attributable symptoms and likelihood of good neurological outcome is needed before surgical intervention. Radiotherapy may be considered when surgery is not considered suitable, but there are limited data on outcomes.

5.3 Ongoing Research and Future Developments

Much focus in NF2 research is currently given to trials of experimental medical treatments in the light of increasing understanding of the molecular pathophysiology and the initial studies of anti-VEGF therapy. Further trials of bevacizumab therapy are ongoing. Initial reports of everolimus therapy in NF2 are disappointing

(Karajannis 2014) but other studies are ongoing. Other novel chemotherapeutic agents such as lapatinib and axitinib are in trial (Karajannis 2015). The importance of inclusion of quality of life measures in research outcomes must be stressed, due to the complex symptom profile, progressive nature and reduced life expectancy (Ferner 2014).

6 Summary

The majority of meningiomata and vestibular schwannomata that present as single lesions are likely sporadic occurrences that do not appear to have a familial basis. Multiple primary tumours in the same individual or a family history of such tumours are suggestive of a genetic susceptibility. NF2, familial meningioma and schwannomatosis are the only genetic conditions currently recognised with these phenotypes. Management of these conditions is complex, requiring multidisciplinary input. Genetic testing can be a helpful component of management, but diagnosis and management are mostly dependent on clinical considerations.

References

Aavikko M, Li SP, Saarinen S, Alhopuro P, Kaasinen E, Morgunova E, Li Y, Vesanen K, Smith MJ, Evans DG, Pöyhönen M, Kiuru A, Auvinen A, Aaltonen LA, Taipale J, Vahteristo P (2012) Loss of SUFU function in familial multiple meningioma. Am J Hum Genet 91(3):520–526

Asthagiri AR1, Parry DM, Butman JA, Kim HJ, Tsilou ET, Zhuang Z, Lonser RR (2009) Neurofibromatosis type 2. Lancet 373(9679):1974–1986

Bacci C1, Sestini R, Provenzano A, Paganini I, Mancini I, Porfirio B, Vivarelli R, Genuardi M, Papi L (2010) Schwannomatosis associated with multiple meningiomas due to a familial SMARCB1 mutation. Neurogenetics 11(1):73–80

Baser ME, Friedman JM, Wallace AJ, Ramsden RT, Joe H, Evans DG (2002) Evaluation of clinical diagnostic criteria for neurofibromatosis 2. Neurology 59(11):1759–1765

Baser ME, Kuramoto L, Joe H, Friedman JM, Wallace AJ, Gillespie JE, Ramsden RT, Evans DG (2004) Genotype-phenotype correlations for nervous system tumors in neurofibromatosis 2: a population-based study. Am J Hum Genet 75:231–239

Carlson ML, Tveiten OV, Driscoll CL, Goplen FK, Neff BA, Pollock BE, Tombers NM, Castner ML, Finnkirk MK, Myrseth E, Pedersen PH, Lund-Johansen M, Link MJ (2015) Long-term quality of life in patients with vestibular schwannoma: an international multicenter cross-sectional study comparing microsurgery, stereotactic radiosurgery, observation, and nontumor controls. J Neurosurg 122(4):833–842

Dirks MS, Butman JA, Kim HJ, Wu T, Morgan K, Tran AP, Lonser RR, Asthagiri AR (2012) Long-term natural history of neurofibromatosis Type 2-associated intracranial tumors. J Neurosurg 117(1):109–117

Evans DG, Huson SM, Donnai D, Neary W, Blair V, Newton V, Harris R (1992) A clinical study of type 2 neurofibromatosis. Q J Med 84:603–618

Ferner RE, Shaw A, Evans DG, McAleer D, Halliday D, Parry A, Raymond FL, Durie-Gair J, Hanemann CO, Hornigold R, Axon P, Golding JF (2014) Longitudinal evaluation of quality of life in 288 patients with neurofibromatosis 2. J Neurol 261(5):963–969

Karajannis MA, Legault G, Hagiwara M, Giancotti FG, Filatov A, Derman A, Hochman T, Goldberg JD, Vega E, Wisoff JH, Golfinos JG, Merkelson A, Roland JT, Allen JC (2014) Phase II study of everolimus in children and adults with neurofibromatosis type 2 and progressive vestibular schwannomas. Neuro Oncol 16(2):292–297

Karajannis MA, Ferner RE (2015) Neurofibromatosis-related tumors: emerging biology and therapies. Curr Opin Pediatr 27(1):26–33

Larjavaara S, Haapasalo H, Sankila R, Helén P, Auvinen A (2008) Is the incidence of meningiomas underestimated? A regional survey. Br J Cancer 99(1):182–184

Lin D, Hegarty JL, Fischbein NJ, Jackler RK (2005) The prevalence of "incidental" acoustic neuroma. Arch Otolaryngol Head Neck Surg 131(3):241–244

Mallory GW, Pollock BE, Foote RL, Carlson ML, Driscoll CL, Link MJ (2014) Stereotactic radiosurgery for neurofibromatosis 2-associated vestibular schwannomas: toward dose optimization for tumor control and functional outcomes. Neurosurgery 74(3):292–300

Moffat DA, Lloyd SK, Macfarlane R, Mannion R, King A, Rutherford S, Axon PR, Donnelly N, Freeman S, Tysome JR, Evans DG, Ramsden RT (2013) Outcome of translabyrinthine surgery for vestibular schwannoma in neurofibromatosis type 2. Br J Neurosurg 27(4):446–453

Nunes FP, Merker VL, Jennings D, Caruso PA, di Tomaso E, Muzikansky A, Barker FG 2nd, Stemmer-Rachamimov A, Plotkin SR (2013) Bevacizumab treatment for meningiomas in NF2: a retrospective analysis of 15 patients. PLoS One 8(3):e59941

Plotkin SR, Stemmer-Rachamimov AO, Barker FG 2nd, Halpin C, Padera TP, Tyrrell A, Sorensen AG, Jain RK, di Tomaso E (2009) Hearing improvement after bevacizumab in patients with neurofibromatosis type 2. N Engl J Med 361(4):358–367

Plotkin SR, O'Donnell CC, Curry WT, Bove CM, MacCollin M, Nunes FP (2011) Spinal ependymomas in neurofibromatosis Type 2: a retrospective analysis of 55 patients. J Neurosurg Spine 14(4):543–547

Slusarz KM, Merker VL, Muzikansky A, Francis SA, Plotkin SR (2014) Long-term toxicity of bevacizumab therapy in neurofibromatosis 2 patients. Cancer Chemother Pharmacol 73 (6):1197–1204

Smith MJ, Higgs JE, Bowers NL, Halliday D, Patterson J, Gillespie J, Huson SM, Freeman SR, Lloyd S, Rutherford SA, King AT, Wallace AJ, Ramsden RT, Evans DG (2011) Cranial meningiomas in 411 NF2 patients with proven gene mutations: clear positional effect of mutations, but absence of female severity effect on age at onset. J Med Genet 48:261–265

Smith MJ, O'Sullivan J, Bhaskar SS, Hadfield KD, Poke G, Caird J, Sharif S, Eccles D, Fitzpatrick D, Rawluk D, du Plessis D, Newman WG, Evans DG (2013) Loss-of-function mutations in SMARCE1 cause an inherited disorder of multiple spinal meningiomas. Nature Genet 45:295–298

Stangerup SE, Tos M, Thomsen J, Caye-Thomasen P (2010) True incidence of vestibular schwannoma? Neurosurgery 67(5):1335–1340

Diagnosis and Management of Hereditary Thyroid Cancer

Gul Bano and Shirley Hodgson

Abstract

Thyroid cancers are largely divided into medullary (MTC) and non-medullary (NMTC) cancers, depending on the cell type of origin. Familial non-medullary thyroid cancer (FNMTC) comprises about 5–15 % of NMTC and is a heterogeneous group of diseases, including both non-syndromic and syndromic forms. Non-syndromic FNMTC tends to manifest papillary thyroid carcinoma, usually multifocal and bilateral. Several high-penetrance genes for FNMTC have been identified, but they are often confined to a few or single families, and other susceptibility loci appear to play a small part, conferring only small increments in risk. Familial susceptibility is likely to be due to a combination of genetic and environmental influences. The current focus of research in FNMTC is to characterise the susceptibility genes and their role in carcinogenesis. FNMTC can also occur as a part of multitumour genetic syndromes such as familial adenomatous polyposis, Cowden's disease, Werner's syndrome and Carney complex. These tend to present at an early age and are multicentric and bilateral with distinct pathology. The clinical evaluation of these patients is similar to that for most patients with a thyroid nodule. Medullary thyroid cancer (MTC) arises from the parafollicular cells of the thyroid which release calcitonin. The familial form of MTC accounts for 20–25 % of cases and presents as a part of the multiple endocrine neoplasia type 2 (MEN 2) syndromes or as a pure familial MTC (FMTC). They are caused by germline point mutations in the RET

G. Bano (✉)
Department of Endocrinology and Diabetes, Thomas Addison Unit,
St George's Healthcare NHS Trust, Blackshaw Road, Tooting, London, UK
e-mail: gbano@sgul.ac.uk

S. Hodgson
St. George's, University of London, London, UK

G. Pichert and C. Jacobs (eds.), *Rare Hereditary Cancers*,
Recent Results in Cancer Research 205, DOI 10.1007/978-3-319-29998-3_3

oncogene on chromosome 10q11.2. There is a clear genotype–phenotype correlation, and the aggressiveness of FMTC depends on the specific genetic mutation, which should determine the timing of surgery.

Keywords

Medullary Thyroid Cancer · Papillary Thyroid Cancer (non-medullary thyroid cancer) · Oncogenes · Tumour suppressor genes · Multiple Endocrine neoplasia · Genetic syndromes · Familial

Contents

1 Introduction

Thyroid cancer is the most prevalent endocrine malignancy. The incidence of primary epithelial cancer of the thyroid is 0.7 per 100,000 in males and 1.9 per 100,000 in females in the UK (Hodgson et al. 2014). The incidence of thyroid cancer today is 2.4 times what it was 3 decades ago. The rising incidence of thyroid cancer could be due to improved diagnostic procedures and advanced screening, but the increase in the diagnosis of significantly larger tumours cannot be attributed to improved screening alone (Davies and Welch 2006; Chen et al. 2009). Radiation is the most important environmental predisposing factor for epithelial thyroid cancer.

The cell line from which the cancer originates determines the subtype: parafollicular C cells for medullary thyroid cancer (MTC) and follicular cells for non-medullary thyroid cancer (NMTC). Differentiated thyroid carcinoma (DTC) comprises approximately 90 % of all cases of NMTC and consists of 2 distinct histological types: papillary thyroid cancer (PTC, 80–90 % of cases) and follicular (FTC, 10 %). Less frequent types are Hürthle cell carcinomas, anaplastic (undifferentiated) carcinomas and squamous cell carcinomas.

Other non-epithelial malignancies that may be observed in the thyroid include lymphomas and sarcomas. Rarely, thyroid paragangliomas have been reported, and germline mutations in *SDHA* and *SDHB* have been detected in confirmed thyroid paraganglioma cases (von Dobschuetz et al. 2015).

The aetiology of DTC is largely unknown and may vary according to histological type. The majority of PTC and FTC are sporadic, and familial tumours may account for 5–15 % of thyroid carcinoma cases. These can be syndromic or non-syndromic. A number of epidemiological studies have examined the risk of DTC in relation to family history of thyroid disease and cancer. Many reported familial clusters of thyroid cancer and several studies of families with clustering of thyroid cancer demonstrate a more aggressive clinical course (Pal et al. 2001; Frich et al. 2001; Hemminki and Dong 2000). Increased risk of DTC associated with a family history of thyroid cancer has been observed in most case–control and Cancer Registry studies, and thyroid cancer has one of the highest familial risks of all cancers. The reported excess risk in relatives of index cases ranges from twofold to tenfold. Individuals with a family history of PTC in first-degree relatives also have an increased risk of PTC, this excess risk being greater in subjects who report a family history of thyroid cancer in siblings (Xu et al. 2012). Additionally, among patients with PTC, those with a family history of thyroid cancer tend to develop multifocal primary tumours more frequently than those without a family history of thyroid cancer (Uchino et al. 2002).

2 Familial Non-medullary Thyroid Cancer (FNMTC)

FNMTC is defined as the presence of well-differentiated thyroid cancer (WDTC) of follicular cell origin in two or more first-degree relatives. FNMTC encompasses a heterogeneous group of diseases, including both non-syndromic and syndromic tumours (Sturgeon and Clark 2005).

The non-syndromic group of patients with FNMTC have familial follicular-derived NMTC in the absence of a specific genetic syndrome. However, most patients with FNMTC have familial papillary thyroid cancer (FPTC). Thyroid cancers in FNMTC have a well-documented predisposition to be multicentric, bilateral disease with early local invasion, extrathyroidal extension and lymph node metastases. These cancers have an increased risk of recurrence and have characteristic histology. The background thyroid may show lymphocytic thyroiditis, multinodular hyperplasia and multiple adenomatous nodules. Benign thyroid disease such as multinodular goitre, thyroiditis and other neoplasms occurs with increased frequency in this group of patients (Musholt et al. 2000). A large population-based study from five Nordic countries found the cumulative risk of WDTC by age 60 in relatives of FNMTC cases to be 46 times that of the general population (9.2 vs. 0.2 %), and 164 times in at-risk men (14.8 vs. 0.09 %). It is important to remember that even individuals with apparently sporadic WDTC may be part of unrecognised FNMTC kindred due to incomplete penetrance, incomplete family history or as yet unidentified disease in other family members.

Numerous somatic genetic abnormalities are detected in sporadic papillary thyroid cancers. *RET/PTC* rearrangements were the first genetic abnormalities to be associated with sporadic papillary thyroid cancers. *RET* rearrangements occur most often in papillary thyroid cancers associated with radiation exposure and in children. *RET/PTC1* and *PTC3* rearrangements are the most frequent alterations, and 15 *RET* rearrangements have been documented (Navas-Carrillo et al. 2014; Grogan et al. 2010). *RET/PTC* mutations have been reported both to be associated with more and with less aggressive thyroid cancers, so probably do not influence tumour behaviour (Giordano et al. 2005). A somatic *BRAF* point mutation is the most common abnormality in sporadic PTC and is found in about 50 % of these tumours. Most but not all reports suggest that *BRAF* mutations are more commonly associated with aggressive pathological parameters, radioiodine refractory, lymph node metastasis and increased cancer mortality. However, some reports suggest that up to 80 % of papillary thyroid cancers have a *BRAF* mutation, thus decreasing its prognostic value (Vasko et al. 2005; Xing et al. 2005). Somatic *RAS* mutations are reported to be more common in FTC than in PTC. *RAS* mutations are also found in some benign thyroid tumours. *TRK* mutations are found in about 5–15 % of PTCs (Grieco et al. 2009). *Pax 8/PPAR* gamma mutations are most often identified in follicular thyroid cancers but also occur in follicular adenomas (Krol et al. 2000). *p53* mutations are almost exclusively found in anaplastic thyroid cancers and in thyroid cancer cell lines. They may also be present in poorly differentiated thyroid cancers (Jossart et al. 1996).

3 Genetics of Non-syndromic FNMTC

The causative genes for FNMTC are largely unknown, though many candidates have been excluded, e.g. *RET*, *RAS*, *PTEN* and *BRAF* (Bonora et al. 2010). Several susceptibility loci have been identified by genetic linkage analysis in FNMTC families, including the *TCO* (thyroid cancer with oxyphilia) locus on chromosome 19p13.2 (Canzian et al. 1998), the *PRN1* locus on chromosome 1q21 (Malchoff et al. 2000) and the *NMTC1* locus on chromosome 2q21 (Mckay et al. 2001). There is also some evidence for the interaction of the *TCO* and *NMTC1* loci leading to increased risk in a small subset of FNMTC families. Other loci are being identified (see Table 1), but given that each has only been found in 1 or a few families, none accounts for the majority of FNMTC cases.

Germline mutations in *DICER* in man have been found to predispose to thyroid disease, notably multinodular goitre, and in mice, there is evidence of early neoplastic changes in the thyroid gland in mutation carriers, but there is no clear association with thyroid cancer in man (Slade et al. 2011). Germline alterations in the *ATM* gene may also be associated with increased papillary thyroid cancer risk (Gu et al. 2014). Some studies have revealed that common germline variants in the *RET* proto-oncogene, DNA repair genes *XRCC1*28 and *XRCC3*29 and xenobiotic metabolising genes *GSTT1* and *GSTM1* are significantly associated with DTC risk (Xu et al. 2012).

Table 1 Gene loci associated with thyroid cancer susceptibility

Tumour type	Gene	Chromosome	Inheritance
Familial multinodular goitre with progression to PTC	Unknown	14q31	[a]AD (Bignell et al. 1997)
PTC with papillary renal neoplasia	*PRN1* locus	1q21	Unknown (Malchoff et al. 2000)
Thyroid cancer with oxyphilia	Unknown/TCO/TIM44	19p13.2	[a]AD (Canzian et al. 1998)
Follicular variant of PTC (Ca type 1)	*NMTC1*	2q21	Unknown (Mckay et al. 2001)
Familial PTC	Unknown	8p23.1-p22	Unknown (Cavaco et al. 2008)
PTC	Unknown	1q21 and 6q22	Unknown (Suh et al. 2009)

[a]*AD* autosomal dominant

Some families have been reported with linkage to 14q, 19p, 2q, 1q, 8p, 6q and 12q, and many of these loci have been replicated by GWAS studies, but few candidate genes have yet been identified, and those that are being defined are usually regulatory (e.g. *SRGAP1* on 12q14), which regulates CDC42, which in turn acts as a signal convergence point in intracellular signalling networks). One family with multiple cases of NMTC showed linkage with a mutation in an enhancer region of 4q32 with binding sites for the POU2F1 and YY1 transcription factors.

Most highly penetrant mutations are only seen in isolated families, and the current evidence is for a few rare high-penetrance genes and a larger number of lower penetrance variants which contribute to thyroid cancer risk (Nagy and Ringel 2015; Nosé 2011).

4 Genetics of Syndromic FNMTC Cancers

Thyroid carcinomas may occur in several different multitumour genetic syndromes. These cancers are heterogeneous and tend to have an early age at diagnosis, and be multicentric and bilateral. The pathology of these tumours is distinct and should alert the clinician to the possibility of a familial cancer syndrome (Mazeh and Sippel 2013).

A number of syndromes are associated with an increased risk of NMTC. These include familial adenomatous polyposis (FAP), Cowden syndrome, Gardner's syndrome, Werner's syndrome and Carney complex.

Familial adenomatous polyposis (FAP) is an autosomal dominant disease characterised by gastrointestinal polyposis and colorectal cancers. It is caused by a germline mutation in the *APC* gene. Thyroid cancer is a rare manifestation (cumulative risk 2.8 % by age 60) and is usually multifocal and bilateral with a characteristic cribriform pattern which differentiates it from sporadic papillary cancer. Thyroid cancer mainly occurs with germline mutations between codons 1286 and 1513 of the *APC* gene. About 10 % of patients have metastases at the time of diagnosis. Mesodermal tumours (desmoids, osteomata of the skull) and congenital hypertrophy of the retinal pigment epithelium (CHRPE) may occur in addition to colonic polyposis (Xu et al. 2003). Gardner syndrome is characterised by colonic polyposis typical of FAP together with osteomas and soft tissue tumours. Screening by thyroid ultrasound examinations has been advocated.

Cowden syndrome is characterised by hamartomas, multiple papillomas, breast cancer, colonic polyps and thyroid disease. The underlying mutation is in *PTEN* although some cases are due to germline *KILLIN* methylation, and germline mutations in *SDHD* and *SDHB* may cause conditions mimicking some features of Cowden that is dominantly inherited (Bennett et al. 2010).

The thyroid cancer in Cowden syndrome, which is usually papillary, is often preceded by multinodular goitre, and early histology shows microscopic follicular adenomas. Thyroid disease both benign and malignant occurs in about two-thirds of subjects. Follicular thyroid cancer is more common in patients with germline *PTEN* mutations than those with *SDHX* and *KILLIN* alterations. *PTEN* frameshift mutations were found in 31 % of patients with thyroid cancer in Cowden syndrome compared to 17 % in those without thyroid cancer (Ngeow et al. 2011).

The autosomal recessive condition, Werner's syndrome, is caused by germline mutations in the *WRN* gene. Premature ageing begins in adolescence and early adulthood, and features include scleroderma-like skin changes, cataracts and a high incidence of neoplasia. Thyroid cancer, predominantly follicular, may occur (Ishikawa et al. 1999).

Carney complex is an autosomal dominant condition characterised by myxomas, pigmentation of the skin and mucosa and endocrine overactivity. The condition is caused by mutations in the *PRKAR1α* gene. Approximately 11 % of patients have thyroid pathology including adenomatous hyperplasia, follicular or papillary hyperplasia and PTC (Stratakis et al. 1997).

There are less well-established associations of non-medullary thyroid carcinoma with multiple endocrine neoplasia type 1 (MEN 1), McCune-Albright syndrome, Peutz–Jegher's syndrome and Ataxia–telangectasia (Harach 2001; Yang et al. 1999). Multiple endocrine neoplasia type 4 (MEN 4), a rare condition in individuals with germline mutations in p27Kip1 (*CDKN1B*), who present with endocrine lesions in the MEN 1 spectrum (commonly parathyroid and pituitary adenomas), is occasionally associated with papillary thyroid cancer (Molatore et al. 2010) (Table 2).

Table 2 Syndromes associated with an increased risk of thyroid cancer

Syndrome	Gene	Chromosome	Inheritance	Incidence of thyroid cancer	Type of thyroid cancer
Familial adenomatosis polyposis (FAP)	*APC*	5q21	AD	2–12 %	PTC cribriform-morular or classical variant
Gardner's syndrome	*APC*	5q21	AD	10 %	PTC cribriform or classical variant with sclerosis
Peutz–Jeghers' syndrome	*STK11/ LKB1*	19p13.3.	AD	Rare	PTC
Cowden's disease	*PTEN*	10q22-23	AD	>10 %	Follicular and occasional PTC
PTEN hamartoma tumour syndrome (PHTS)	*PTEN*	10q22-23.3	AD	5–10 %	Follicular, occasional PTC and anaplastic
Werner's syndrome (in Japanese)	*WRN*	8p11-21	AR	18 %	Follicular, anaplastic and PTC
Carney complex	*PKAR1A*	17q24	AD	4 and 60 %	Follicular and PTC
McCune-Albright syndrome	*GNAS1*	20q13.1-13.2	[a]Mosaic		Clear cell thyroid carcinoma

[a]Mosaic denotes the presence of two or more populations of cells with different genotypes in one individual who has developed from a single fertilised egg

5 Management of FNMTC

Despite common features, familial thyroid cancers are heterogeneous, show diverse natural histories and require better characterisation in distinguishing one type from another. The identification of hereditary cases and early diagnosis makes preventive surgery and adequate treatment possible, with improved outcomes for patients and their families.

The initial management of FNMTC includes a detailed family history and the exclusion of known syndromes. A history of radiation exposure is also important. The clinical evaluation of patients with FNMTC is similar to that for most patients with a thyroid nodule. Although there are no established guidelines for screening relatives of index cases with FNMTC, in those with a normal thyroid gland documented by physical examination, an ultrasound examination is recommended beginning at age 10. This could continue on an annual basis. When a suspicious nodule or nodules are identified, fine needle aspiration (FNA) for cytological examination is recommended. FNA may not be as accurate in these patients because of the multifocal nature of these tumours and coexisting benign thyroid nodules that are also more common than in patients with sporadic thyroid tumours. Metastatic disease may be the first presentation in these patients.

Given the aggressive nature of the disease and the low sensitivity of FNA cytology in FNMTC, the treatment of choice in a patient with a strong family history and a nodule is total thyroidectomy. Ipsilateral or bilateral central neck dissection and post-operative radioactive iodine ablative therapy along with thyroid stimulating hormone (TSH) suppression should be considered depending on the preoperative staging. The administration of radioiodine 1-131 is aimed at ablating any remnant thyroid tissue and potential microscopic residual tumour. This procedure decreases the risk of regional recurrence and facilitates the long-term surveillance based on serum thyroglobulin (Tg) measurement and diagnostic radioiodine whole-body scan (WBS). Thyroid hormone suppression therapy is an important part of the treatment of thyroid cancer. TSH suppressive treatment with levothyroxine (LT4) is of benefit in high-risk thyroid cancer patients. Treatment of regional disease is based on the combination of surgery and radioiodine therapy. External beam radiotherapy may be indicated when complete surgical excision is not possible or when there is no significant radioiodine uptake in the tumour. Distant metastases are more successfully cured if they take up radioiodine and are of small in size. Chemotherapy is not effective. Approximately 12 % of FNMTC has persistent disease and 44 % develops recurrences emphasising the importance of follow-up. Metastatic disease is managed as for sporadic cases (Mazeh and Sippel 2013; Rivkees et al. 2011).

6 Medullary Thyroid Carcinoma (MTC)

MTC is a well-differentiated rare thyroid tumour that arises from the parafollicular- or calcitonin (CT)-producing C cells derived from the neural crest. Its origin makes it a separate entity from the other DTC. It releases several neuroendocrine peptides, and these include calcitonin and carcinoembryonic antigen (CEA), which are useful tumour markers. It occurs in sporadic and familial forms.

Both sporadic and familial (F) MTC arise at the junctions of the upper and middle thirds of the lateral lobes, corresponding to the areas where C cells are present. The overall prevalence comprises 5–10 % of all thyroid malignancies and about 15 % of all thyroid cancer-related deaths. It is present in less than 1 % of thyroid glands at autopsy. The clinical presentation of MTC occurs mainly in the fourth and fifth decades, but a wide range of ages at diagnosis has been observed.

The familial form of MTC accounts for 20–25 % of cases and presents as a part of the MEN 2 syndromes or as a pure familial MTC (FMTC). MEN 2 syndrome consists of three variants: multiple endocrine neoplasia type 2a (MEN 2A), multiple endocrine neoplasia type 2b (MEN 2B) and FMTC . Genotype–phenotype correlations in MEN 2 and/or FTMC are well established.

7 Sporadic MTC

This accounts for about 80 % cases of MTC. These are typically unilateral and have no associated endocrinopathies. Peak age at diagnosis is between 40 and 60 years, with a mean age 50 years and more common in females. One-third of the patients will present with intractable diarrhoea due to increased gastrointestinal secretion and hypermotility that is caused by raised calcitonin levels.

8 Familial or Inherited Medullary Carcinoma Without Associated Endocrinopathies

This form is the least aggressive. It usually presents as a thyroid nodule. This group of MTC patients usually have no other clinical manifestations. The peak incidence is between the ages of 40 and 50 years (Mears and Diaz-Cano 2003).

9 MEN 2A (Sipple Syndrome)

MEN 2A syndrome patients tend to have bilateral medullary carcinoma or C-cell hyperplasia (CCH), pheochromocytoma and hyperparathyroidism. This syndrome is inherited as an autosomal dominant manner. Peak incidence of medullary carcinoma in these patients is in the 30s but can present in late adolescence or early adulthood. Males and females are equally affected. An association with cutaneous lichen amyloidosis (CLA), a characteristic pigmented and itchy skin lesion specifically localised in the interscapular region of the back, has been reported in less than 10 % of MEN 2A families and is associated with a specific *RET* 634 mutation. When present, CLA is almost invariably diagnostic of MEN 2A and may be considered pathognomonic.

10 MEN 2B

MEN 2B syndrome is characterised by young age at onset MTC and pheochromocytoma, but only rarely hyperparathyroidism. These patients have an unusual appearance, which is characterised by mucosal ganglioneuromas and a marfanoid habitus. Inheritance is autosomal dominant. MEN 2B patients usually develop medullary carcinoma early in life, diagnosed in infancy or early childhood, and males and females are equally affected.

MTC typically is the first abnormality observed in both MEN 2A and MEN 2B syndromes.

Thyroid pathology in FMTC cases usually is characterised by multiple and bilateral tumours, associated with neoplastic CCH and a tendency to early lymph node metastases (Metzgera and Milasb 2014; Ganeshan et al. 2013) (Table 3).

Table 3 Clinical features of the different forms of MTC

Clinical presentation	Inheritance	Features of MTC	Associations
Sporadic MTC	None	Unifocal	None
MEN 2A	Autosomal dominant	Multifocal, bilateral	Pheochromocytoma (42 %) Hyperparathyroidism (10–30 %) Cutaneous lichen planus amyloidosis (rare) Hirschsprung disease (rare)
MEN 2B	Autosomal dominant	Multifocal, bilateral	Pheochromocytoma (40 %) Multiple mucosal neuromata (>95 %) Marfanoid body habitus (80 %)
FMTC	Autosomal dominant	Multifocal, bilateral	None

Hereditary MTC is caused by a germline point mutation in the *RET* oncogene on chromosome 10q11.2. The *RET* oncogene has 21 exons distributed over 60 kb. About 85 % of all mutations responsible for FMTC are well known. In the majority of MEN 2A and FMTC patients, mutations are clustered in six cysteine residues (codons 609, 611, 618 and 620 in exon 10, and codons 630 and 634 in exon 11) in the *RET* cysteine-rich extracellular domain. These mutations have been detected in about 95 % of MEN 2A and 85 % of FMTC families. Somatic *RET* point mutations have been identified in the tumour in about 50 % of patients with sporadic MTC.

The clinical course and prognosis of MTC depend on whether it is hereditary or sporadic and the type of *RET* mutation present. Sporadic MTC can present at any age, and it is usually associated with a palpable mass and the presence of nodal metastases.

11 Genotype and Phenotype

Since the initial discovery of *RET* mutations responsible for MEN 2, more than 50 different point mutations across 7 exons (exons 8, 10, 11, 13–16) have been identified. Different mutations in the *RET* gene produce varying phenotypes of the disease, including age of onset and aggressiveness of MTC, and the presence or absence of other endocrine tumours. This should determine the timing and extent of surgery (Krampitz and Norton 2014).

Approximately 98 % of patients with MEN 2 have mutations in the cysteine-rich extracellular domain, especially codons 609, 611, 618, 620 and 634 of exons 10 and 11, and 85 % have a mutation of codon 634 of exon 11. Early aggressive behaviour and metastasis in MEN 2A and MEN 2B are particularly associated with *C634* and *M918T* mutations. This requires early intervention. The *883RET* mutation displays a more indolent form of MTC compared with the *M918T* mutation for MEN 2B. A polymorphism at codon 836 is associated with early metastases in patients with hereditary or sporadic MTC. A mutation at codon 918 is almost exclusively found in MEN 2B.

12 Genetic Testing and Risk Stratification

Genetic testing detects germline *RET* mutations in most individuals with MTC, and predictive testing is offered to all first-degree relatives of patients with newly diagnosed hereditary MTC. Due to the varying clinical effects of *RET* mutations, strategies based on clinical phenotype, age of onset and aggressiveness of MTC are used to guide the management.

In 2010, the North American Neuroendocrine Tumor Society (NANETS) published consensus guidelines for the diagnosis and management of MTC. These guidelines were developed by classifying *RET* mutations into 3 groups based on aggressiveness of MTC or levels of risk. Table 4 summarises the 3 groups of MTC risk levels and the recommendations for the timing of prophylactic thyroidectomy based on these risk levels (Wu et al. 2011; Elisei et al. 2012).

MTC patients with advanced disease have metastases to regional lymph nodes or distant sites such as brain, bone, lung and liver. In these patients, thyroidectomy with nodal clearance is rarely curative. Some patients undergo repeat operations to remove residual tumour. Distant metastases limited to a single organ can be considered for curative surgical resection or another treatment modality, such as radiofrequency ablation or external beam radiation therapy. Chemotherapy is ineffective in patients with MTC, and the responses that occur are short-lived. External beam radiotherapy may improve regional disease control, but survival is not increased.

Recently, several molecular-targeted therapeutics (MTTs) have been used in clinical trials of patients with locally advanced or metastatic MTC. The most effective agents are the multityrosine kinase inhibitors, vandetanib and

Table 4 NANETS classification of MTC risk levels and management recommendations

NANETS risk level for MTC	Most common codon mutations	Age at prophylactic thyroidectomy
Level 1	609 630 768 790 791 804 891	By 5–10 years of age By 5–10 years because of variability in onset of tumours in some families
Level 2	611 618 620 634	By 5 year of age By 5 years of age
Level 3	883 918 922	Within the first 6 months of life (preferably in the first month of life)

cabozantinib, approved by the US Food and Drug Administration (FDA) for patients with advanced MTC. Other multikinase inhibitors include sorafenib, axitinib and motesanib. Measurements of serum markers calcitonin (CT) and CEA are important in the post-surgical follow-up of patients with MTC because they reflect the presence of persistent or recurrent disease. After surgery, serum CT levels normalise (undetectable) in 60–90 % cases of patients with no lymph node involvement but only in 20 % of those with lymph node metastases (Sakorafas et al. 2008; Daumerie et al. 2013).

13 Ongoing Research

The field of the genetics of endocrinology is advancing rapidly. The main thrust of current research in FNMTC is to characterise the susceptibility genes which are being identified by linkage analysis and genome-wide association studies. The single nucleotide polymorphism (SNP) on 9q22-23, for instance, lies within the linkage disequilibrium region where the *FOXE1*, *XPA*, *HEMGN* and *C9orf156 genes* lie, and the association with *FOXE1* has also been shown by an independent candidate gene association study. The *FOXE1* and *NKX2-1* genes have prominent roles in thyroid development and differentiation and have altered expression in thyroid tumours. They may alter the levels of TSH, and free T3 and T4. The role of genes that regulate the expression of these genes is being studied. These genes are central to a regulatory network of transcription factors, and alterations in the genes involved may be related to thyroid cancer susceptibility (Kula et al. 2010). The SNP on 14q13.3 is located in the linkage disequilibrium region containing *BRMS1L*, *MBIP*, *SFTA3* and *NKX2-1*, the latter of which is also involved in thyroid development, and has altered levels in thyroid tumours. Variants in this gene appear to be associated with altered levels of serum TSH, and further work is required to elucidate the role of these genes in PTC development. Other genes that may play a part in NMTC susceptibility are microRNA genes, such as miR-221 and miR-222, and further work is underway to elucidate their role. Further areas of study are the part played in the aetiology of well-defined syndromes, by newly identified genes that cause already well-defined syndromes such as Cowden syndrome, with *KILLIN* and *SDHD* and *SDHB* (von Dobschuetz et al. 2015).

Studies of the somatic genetic changes that occur in the development of NMTC will allow further differentiation of these cancers into subtypes with different molecular and environmental causes and lead to the development of improved targeted treatments.

In the field of MTC, much work is being done to define the genotype/phenotype correlations, which are very helpful in guiding clinical management of germline mutation carriers.

14 Summary

Thyroid cancers are largely divided into medullary and non-medullary cancers, each with many subtypes. About 20–25 % of MTC cases occur in the context of inherited syndromes due to different germline *RET* mutations, which are well-defined entities with clear genotype–phenotype correlations and agreed management protocols. NMTC is often familial but as yet the genetic factors involved in susceptibility to NMTC are ill-understood. Several high-penetrance genes for these tumours have been identified in families with several cases of NMTC, but other loci appear to play a small part, conferring only small increments in risk, such that the familial component in NMTC susceptibility is likely to be due to a combination of genetic factors and environmental influences which currently makes genetic testing quite difficult

Key points

- Assessment of the possibility of a hereditary thyroid cancer syndrome should be a part of first clinical episode in a patient with benign or malignant thyroid disease.
- A history of papillary thyroid carcinoma in two or more first-degree relatives should raise the question of FNMTC and more aggressive cancer.
- The initial management of FNMTC should include a detailed family history and the exclusion of known syndromes. A history of radiation exposure is also important.
- Ultrasound-based screening for thyroid disease should be a part of long-term surveillance in patients with multitumour genetic syndromes causing a predisposition to thyroid cancer.
- Lifetime cancer risks, including thyroid cancer, have been defined for individuals with *PTEN* and other susceptibility gene mutations.
- Risk stratification by *RET* gene mutation, and new medical therapies, are available for patients with hereditary MTC.
- North American Neuroendocrine Tumor Society (NANETS) consensus guidelines are useful in the diagnosis and management of MTC.
- Measurements of serum markers calcitonin (CT) and carcinoembryonic antigen (CEA) are important in the post-surgical follow-up of patients with MTC because they reflect the presence of persistent or recurrent disease.
- Serum CT level normalises (undetectable) in 60–90 % cases of patients with no lymph node involvement but only in 20 % of those with lymph node metastases after surgery.

References

Bennett KL, Mester J, Eng C (2010) Germline epigenetic regulation of KILLIN in Cowden and Cowden-like syndrome. JAMA 304(24):2724–2731

Bignell GR, Canzian F, Shayeghi M, Stark M, Shugart YY, Biggs P et al (1997) Familial nontoxic multinodular thyroid goiter locus maps to chromosome 14q but does not account for familial nonmedullary thyroid cancer. Am J Hum Genet 61(5):1123–1130

Bonora E, Tallini G, Romeo G (2010) Genetic predisposition to familial nonmedullary thyroid cancer: an update of molecular findings and state-of-the-art studies. J Oncol 2010:1–7

Canzian F, Amati P, Harach HR, Kraimps JL, Lesueur F, Barbier J et al (1998) A gene predisposing to familial thyroid tumors with cell oxyphilia maps to chromosome 19p13.2. Am J Hum Genet 63(6):1743–1748

Cavaco BM, Batista LG, Sobrinho VL (2008) Mapping a new familial thyroid epithelial neoplasia susceptibility locus to chromosome 8p23. 1-p22 by high density single-nucleotide polymorphism genome-wide linkage analysis. J Clin Endocrinol Metab 93(11):4426–4430

Chen AY, Jemal A, Ward EM (2009) Increasing incidence of differentiated thyroid cancer in the United States, 1988–2005. Cancer 115(16):3801–3807

Daumerie C, Maiter D1, Gruson D (2013) Serum calcitonin estimation in medullary thyroid cancer: basal or stimulated levels? Thyroid Res 6(Suppl 1):S4

Davies L, Welch HG (2006) Increasing incidence of thyroid cancer in the United States, 1973–2002. JAMA 295(18):2164–2167

Elisei R, Alevizaki M, Conte-Devolx B, Frank-Raue K, Leite V, Williams GR (2012) European thyroid association guidelines for genetic testing and its clinical consequences in medullary thyroid cancer. Eur Thyroid J 1(4):216–231

Frich L, Glattre E, Akslen LA (2001) Familial occurrence of nonmedullary thyroid cancer: a population based study of 5673 first-degree relatives of thyroid cancer patients from Norway. Cancer Epidemiol Biomarkers Prev 10(2):113–117

Ganeshan D, Paulson E, Duran C, Cabanillas ME, Busaidy NL, Charnsangavej C (2013) Current update on medullary thyroid carcinoma. AJR 201(6):W867–W876

Giordano TJ, Kuick R, Thomas DG, Misek DE, Vinco M, Sanders D et al (2005) Molecular classification of papillary thyroid carcinoma: distinct BRAF, RAS, RET/PTC mutation-specific gene expression profiles discovered by DNA microarray analysis. Oncogene 24(44):6646–6656

Grieco A, Miranda C, Pierotti MA (2009) Rearrangements of NTRK 1 gene in papillary thyroid carcinoma. Mol Cell Endocrinol 321(1):44–49

Grogan RH, Mitmaker EJ, Clark OH (2010) The evolution of biomarkers in thyroid cancer—from mass screening to a personalized biosignature. Cancers V 2(2):885–912

Gu Y, Liu X, Yu Y, Shi J, Ai L, Sun H, Kanu JS, Wang C, Liu Y (2014) Association of ATM gene polymorphism with PTC Metastasis in female patients. Int J Endocr 2014:1–8

Harach HR (2001) Familial nonmedullary thyroid neoplasia. Endocr Pathol 12(2):97–112

Hemminki K, Dong C (2000) Familial relationships in thyroid cancer by histo-pathological type. Int J Cancer 85(2):201–205

Hodgson SV, Foulkes WD, Eng C, Maher ER (2014) A practical guide to human genetics, 4th edn. London, pp 31–46

Ishikawa Y, Sugano H, Matsumoto T, Furuichi Y, Miller RW, Goto M (1999) Unusual features of thyroid carcinomas in Japanese patients with Werner syndrome and possible genotype-phenotype relations to cell type and race. Cancer 85(6):1345–1352

Jossart GH, Epstein HD, Shaver JK, Weier HU, Greulich KM, Tezelman S et al (1996) Immunocytochemical detection of p53 in human thyroid carcinomas is associated with mutation and immortalization of cell lines. J Clin Endocrinol Metab 81(10):3498–3504

Krampitz GW, Norton JA (2014) Gene mutations (genotype and phenotype) of multiple endocrine neoplasia Type 2 and familial medullary thyroid carcinoma. Cancer 120(13):1920–1931

Krol TG, Sarraf P, Pecciarini L, Chen CJ, Mueller E, Spiegelman BM et al (2000) PAX8-PPARgamma fusion oncogene in human thyroid carcinoma. Science 289 (5483):1357–1360

Kula D, Kalemba M, Jurecka-Lubieniecka B, Puch Z, Kowalska M, Tyszkiewicz T, Kowal M, Handkiewicz-Junak D (2010) Genetic predisposition to papillary thyroid cancer. Endokrynol Pol 61(5):486–489

Malchoff CD, Sarfarazi M, Tendler B, Forouhar F, Whalen G, Joshi V et al (2000) Papillary thyroid carcinoma associated with papillary renal neoplasia: genetic linkage analysis of a distinct heritable tumor syndrome. J Clin Endocrinol Metab 85(5):1758–1764

Mazeh H, Sippel RS (2013) Familial nonmedullary thyroid carcinoma. Thyroid. 23(9):1049–1056

McKay JD, Lesueur F, Jonard L, Pastore A, Williamson J, Hoffman L et al (2001) Localization of a susceptibility gene for familial nonmedullary thyroid carcinoma to chromosome 2q21. Am J Hum Gene 69(2):440–446

Mears L, Diaz-Cano SJ (2003) Difference between familial and sporadic medullary thyroid carcinomas. Am J Surg Pathol 27(2):266–267

Metzgera R, Milasb M (2014) Inherited cancer syndromes and the thyroid: an update. Curr Opin Oncol 26(1):51–61

Molatore S, Marinoni I, Lee M, Pulz E, Ambrosio MR, Degli Uberti EC, Zatelli MC, Pellegata NS (2010) A novel germline CDKN1B mutation causing multiple endocrine tumors: clinical, genetic and functional characterization. Hum Mutat 31(11):E1825–E1835

Musholt TJ, Musholt PB, Petrich T et al (2000) Familial papillary thyroid carcinoma: genetics, criteria for diagnosis, clinical features, and surgical treatment. World J Surg 24(11):1409–1417

Nagy R, Ringel MD (2015) Genetic predisposition for nonmedullary thyroid cancer. Horm Cancer 6(1):13–20

Navas-Carrillo D, Ríos A, Rodríguez JM, Parrilla P, Orenes-Piñero E (2014) Familial nonmedullary thyroid cancer: screening, clinical, molecular and genetic findings. Biochim Biophys Acta 1846(2):468–76

Ngeow J, Mester J, Rybicki LA, Ni Y, Milas M, Eng C (2011) Incidence and clinical characteristics of thyroid cancer in prospective series of individuals with Cowden and Cowden-like syndrome characterized by germline PTEN, SDH, or KLLN alterations. J Clin Endocrinol Metab 96(12):E2063–E2071

Nosé V (2011) Familial thyroid cancer: a review. Mod Pathol 24:S19–S33

Pal T, Vogl FD, Chappuis PO et al (2001) Increased risk for nonmedullary thyroid cancer in the first degree relatives of prevalent cases of nonmedullary thyroid cancer: a hospital-based study. J Clin Endocrinol Metab 86(11):5307–5312

Rivkees SA, Mazzaferri EL, Verburg FA, Reiners C, Luster M, Breuer CK, Dinauer CA, Udelsman R (2011) The treatment of differentiated thyroid cancer in children: emphasis on surgical approach and radioactive iodine therapy. Endocr Rev 32(6):798–826

Sakorafas GH, Friess H, Peros G (2008) The genetic basis of hereditary medullary thyroid cancer: clinical implications for the surgeon, with a particular emphasis on the role of prophylactic thyroidectomy. Endocr Relat Cancer 15(4):871–884

Slade I, Bacchelli C, Davies H, Murray A, Rahman N et al (2011) DICER1 syndrome: clarifying the diagnosis, clinical features and management implications of a pleiotropic tumour predisposition syndrome. J Med Genet 48(4):273–278

Stratakis CA, Courcoutisakis NA, Abati A, Filie A, Doppman JL, Aidan Carney JA, Shawker T (1997) Thyroid gland abnormalities in patients with the syndrome of spotty skin pigmentation, myxomas, endocrine overactivity, and schwannomas (carney complex). J Clinical Endocr Metabol 82(7):2037–2043

Sturgeon C, Clark OH (2005) Familial nonmedullary thyroid cancer. Thyroid 15(6):588–593

Suh I, Filetti S, Vriens MR, Guerrero MA, Tumino S, Wong M et al (2009) Distinct loci on chromosome 1q21 and 6q22 predispose to familial nonmedullary thyroid cancer: a SNP array-based linkage analysis of 38 families. Surgery 146(6):1073–1080

Uchino S, Noguchi S, Kawamoto H et al (2002) Familial nonmedullary thyroid carcinoma characterized by multifocality and a high recurrence rate in a large study population. World J Surg 26(8):897–902

Vasko V, Hu S, Wu G, Xing JC, Larin A, Savchenko V et al (2005) High prevalence and possible de novo formation of BRAF mutation in metastasized papillary thyroid cancer in lymph nodes. J Clin Endocrinol Metab 90(9):5265–5269

von Dobschuetz E, Leijon H, Schalin-Jantti C, Schiavi F, Brauckhoff M, Peczkowska M et al (2015) A registry-based study of thyroid paraganglioma: histologic and genetic characteristics. Endocr Relat Cancer 22(2):191–204

Wu LS, Roman SA, Sosa JA (2011) Medullary thyroid cancer: an update of new guidelines and recent developments. Curr Opin Oncol 23(1):22–27

Xing M, Westra WH, Tufano RP, Cohen Y, Rosenbaum E, Rhoden KJ et al (2005) BRAF mutation predicts a poorer clinical prognosis for papillary thyroid cancer. J Clin Endocrinol Metab 90(12):6373–6379

Xu B, Yoshimoto K, Miyauchi A et al (2003) Cribriform-morular variant of papillary thyroid carcinoma: a pathological and molecular genetic study with evidence of frequent somatic mutations in exon 3 of the beta-catenin gene. J Pathol 199(1):58–67

Xu L, Li G, Wei Q, El-Naggar AK, Sturgis EM (2012) Family history of cancer and risk of sporadic differentiated thyroid carcinoma. Cancer 118(5):1228–1235

Yang GC, Yao JL, Feiner HD, Roses DF, Kumar A, Mulder JE (1999) Lipid rich follicular carcinoma of the thyroid in a patient with McCune—Albright syndrome. Mod Pathol 12 (10):969–973

Diagnosis and Management of Hereditary Gastric Cancer

Kevin John Monahan and Laura Hopkins

Abstract

A positive family history is consistently reported as a risk factor for gastric cancer (GC), but the molecular basis for the familial aggregation is largely unknown. The risk associated with having one first-degree relative (FDR) with GC is approximately 1.3–3.5 fold increased. Hereditary cancer syndromes have been relatively well characterised, but their rarity largely precludes the development of trials of surveillance. In hereditary diffuse gastric cancer (HDGC), patients have a *CDH1* mutation that results in a high penetrance of GC meaning that prophylactic gastrectomy is recommended, although this treatment results in significant psychosocial issues. The management of HDGC patients includes endoscopic surveillance, surgery and histological interpretation which require a high degree of selective expertise. Much of the remaining heritable risk of GC may be accounted for by low- and intermediate-penetrant genetic factors, i.e. common and rare variants, respectively. The advent of new methods such as next-generation sequencing has revealed a number of new candidate gene loci.

Keywords

Gastric adenocarcinoma · Hereditary diffuse gastric cancer · Endoscopy · Cancer genetics

K.J. Monahan (✉) · L. Hopkins
Family History of Bowel Cancer Clinic, Gastroenterology Department,
West Middlesex University Hospital, Chelsea and Westminster Hospitals NHS Trust,
London, UK
e-mail: k.monahan@imperial.ac.uk

G. Pichert and C. Jacobs (eds.), *Rare Hereditary Cancers*,
Recent Results in Cancer Research 205, DOI 10.1007/978-3-319-29998-3_4

Contents

1 Introduction

1.1 Epidemiology

Gastric cancer (GC) is the fifth most common cancer worldwide, and the third most common cause of cancer death (Ferlay 2012). In 2012, GLOBOCAN estimated 952,000 individuals were diagnosed with the condition with 723,000 recorded deaths. Significant variation between countries highlights the geographical impact on disease epidemiology. The incidence rates vary around the world, but 70 % of the cases occurred in developing countries with the highest rates in Eastern Asia, around half the world total, and lowest in Western Africa (Ferlay 2012). Eastern Asia also has the highest mortality rates with 24 per 100,000 in men and 9.8 per 100,000 in women (Ferlay 2012).

In Europe, 139,000 new cases of GC were diagnosed in 2012; however, the incidence rates are falling in most European countries. This can be explained by changes in lifestyle and environmental factors such as reduction in smoking and identification and treatment of helicobacter pylori (HP) (Ferlay et al. 2013). However, unlike other common adult cancers, the risk of GC in migrants is similar to that of the population of origin and does not approach that of the host population in the first-generation post-migration (Yaghoobi et al. 2010). Understanding the aetiology of this disease is essential to improve early detection and therefore survival.

The risk of GC significantly increases with age as around 9 out of 10 new cases occur in those over 55 years. The incidence rates significantly increase between the ages of 60–64 (Cancer Research UK 2015). GC is a multi-factorial disease so both genetic and environmental factors have a role in its aetiology. Environmental and lifestyle risks include smoking, diet and alcohol consumption. Other factors include HP infection, atrophic gastritis, exposure to ionising radiation, family history and genetic disorders.

1.2 Histological Classification of GC

GC is a solid tumour with complex genetic and environmental interactions that contribute to its initiation and progression. Most GCs are adenocarcinomas. Traditionally, GC is divided into two main subtypes on the basis of Lauren's classification—intestinal and diffuse (Hu et al. 2012). The relative frequencies are approximately 54 % for intestinal type, 32 % for the diffuse type and 15 % for the indeterminate type. These subtypes have different molecular profiles, and their development pathways are distinct. In 'high-incidence' areas, patients with *Helicobacter pylori*-associated chronic gastritis may develop atrophy followed by intestinal metaplasia which over time may culminate in neoplastic changes, especially adenocarcinoma of 'intestinal' type.

Diffuse gastric cancer (DGC) does not seem to arise from this stepwise neoplastic progression, arising instead from normal gastric mucosa with no definitive premalignant stage; DGC is associated with pathological characteristics such as loss of cell cohesion and signet-ring cells, and is often associated with a negative HP status. The histological phenotype of hereditary DGC (HDGC) in early stage includes patchy intramucosal signet-ring carcinoma cells in the lamina propria and its unique feature of carcinoma in situ associated with pagetoid (upward) spread of tumour cells along the preserved basement membrane. Over the past few decades, advances in technology and high-throughput analysis have enabled a greater appreciation of the molecular aspects of GC pathogenesis.

1.3 Screening and Surveillance for GC

The prognosis in unselected patients with cases of GC is poor, with an average 5-year survival rate of 20–25 % (Cancer Research UK 2015). This is because GC symptoms are often absent or nonspecific in early disease stages, and existence of symptoms, especially alarm symptoms, suggests that the GC is of very advanced stage, for which curative surgical resection is often impossible. Preventing GC can involve primary prevention and secondary prevention approaches. As a primary preventative strategy, HP treatment is theoretically promising, acting by reducing gastric inflammation and subsequent mucosal changes such as atrophy or intestinal metaplasia (IM). Regional guidelines recommend HP treatment for the purpose of GC prevention in countries with high-risk populations.

Several screening methods, including barium meal, upper GI gastroscopy and serum pepsinogen, have been proposed for the detection of early asymptomatic GCs. The latest report on GC screening from the UK National Screening Committee found that mass screening of the asymptomatic population is not recommended due to the low incidence of stomach cancer in the UK (Hillier and Fielder 2009). However, other countries with high incidence of GCs, such as Japan, have adapted population-based screening programmes. Although no randomised controlled trials have been reported, cohort and case-control studies generally showed a decreased risk of mortality from GC in the screened subjects (Tsubono and Hisamichi 2000).

In general, it is recognised that individuals with dyspepsia associated with chronic GI blood loss, progressive dysphagia, progressive unintentional weight loss, persistent vomiting, iron deficiency anaemia, epigastric mass and abnormal barium swallow should be referred for gastroscopy or upper GI cancer specialist. Specific screening recommendations are made later in this chapter for those with known hereditary syndromes who are at higher risk.

2 Family History, Heritability and GC Risk

About 10 % of gastric carcinomas show familial clustering, but only approximately 1–3 % of gastric carcinomas arise from inherited GC predisposition syndromes, such as HDGC, familial adenomatous polyposis (FAP), MUTYH-associated polyposis (MAP), Lynch syndrome, juvenile polyposis syndrome, Peutz–Jeghers syndrome, Li–Fraumeni syndrome and gastric hyperplastic polyposis (van der Post et al. 2015). The nature of heritable GC risk is not well understood outside the context of these well-characterised cancer syndromes. Thus, empirical associations based on family history may be drawn to determine those at increased lifetime risk.

Case-control studies consistently report that a family history of GC is an independent risk factor; particularly if it is a first-degree relative affected. However, the magnitude of the odds ratio (OR) associated with a positive family history varies with the ethnic group and with the geographic region. In published case-control studies, the OR varies from approximately 2 to 10, depending on the country. In the majority of studies, the OR was between 1.5-fold and 3.5-fold, but studies from Korea, Turkey and India reported higher OR. It is of interest that these three countries with the highest reported familial relative risks have very high or very low incidences of GC. Environmental risk factors, such as HP infection or diet, may contribute to familial clustering. However, in studies which adjusted for one or more of these risk factors, the impact of the relative risk associated with a positive family history remained essentially unchanged, which is in favour of genetic susceptibility underlying the observed familial clustering (Yaghoobi et al. 2010).

The relevant genes are so far largely unknown. It is hoped that molecular studies, including genome-wide association studies (GWAS), will illuminate the genetic factors underlying this important association.

Currently, there are no UK or international surveillance guidelines for these patients, although modification of lifestyle and environmental risk factors may have a role in risk reduction.

3 Gastric Cancer and Hereditary Syndromes

The highest lifetime risk of inherited GC is associated with HDGC; thus, the focus of this chapter is discussion of the management of HDGC.

3.1 Hereditary Diffuse Gastric Cancer (HDGC)

HDGC is an autosomal dominantly inherited cancer predisposition syndrome caused by germline mutations in the *CDH1* gene on chromosome 16q22. It comprises 16 exons transcribed into a 4.5-kb mRNA and encodes for the tumour suppressor protein E-cadherin. E-cadherin is a transmembrane calcium-dependent protein that is predominantly expressed at the basolateral membrane of epithelial cells, where it has a key role in cell adhesion. An acquired somatic mutation of *CDH1* results in impaired protein function and, therefore, is widely associated with cancers at many different sites.

GC will occur in 70–80 % of individuals with this mutation by 80 years. There is also an increased risk of lobular breast cancer (LBC) with a cumulative risk in women of 42 % by 80 years (van der Post et al. 2015).

For HDGC, there are established criteria to determine whether an individual is at risk of and requires genetic testing for the condition. In 2014, the recommendations were reviewed by van der Post et al. (2015), and their recent guidelines now include the following criteria (Table 1).

Table 1 Criteria for offering genetic testing to individuals at risk of HDGC (van der Post et al. 2015)

Requires genetic testing for HDGC	Consider genetic testing for HDGC
2 cases of GC (1 confirmed DGC) in first- and second-degree relatives	Family history of 2 or more cases of LBC diagnosed under the age of 50 years
1 case of DGC diagnosed under 40 years	History of bilateral LBC
Personal or family history of DGC and LBC, 1 diagnosed under 50 years	Personal or family history of cleft lip/palate in a patient with DGC
	Evidence of in situ signet-ring cells and/or pagetoid spread of signet-ring cells in the stomach

If any of these criteria are met, then the individual is referred for genetic counselling. Within this framework, a comprehensive family pedigree should be completed and histopathology results can be reviewed to confirm the diagnosis. The initial evaluation will often involve a multi-disciplinary team (MDT) including a geneticist with expertise in the field. Other members will include upper GI surgeons, gastroenterologists, pathologists, breast oncologist, psychologists and dieticians. This allows the patient to have open and detailed discussions about the implications of a positive result including gastric surgery and the alternatives of surveillance. If the patient is deemed high risk for carrying the mutation, they would be advised, at the age of consent (16–18 years), to undergo genetic testing for the *CDH1* gene.

Ideally, genetic testing should be carried out on the first family member affected with HDGC. If they are deceased, then enquires should be made as to whether frozen or formalin-fixed tissue is available for *CDH1* testing. If this is not possible, then it is appropriate to test the first-degree relative (FDR) unaffected by HDGC for the mutation. They would be expected to meet the screening criteria for the mutation and understand they only have a 50 % chance of having inherited the mutated *CDH1* allele.

3.2 HDGC: Genetic Testing

Genetic testing is performed on blood or tissue and should be done in a certified molecular diagnostics laboratory. The analysis for *CDH1* needs to include mutation analysis of the entire open reading frame and is performed by combining Sanger sequencing and multiplex ligation-dependent probe amplification (MLPA). This gene is also included on the Illumina Trusight© next-generation sequencing panel. Currently, there are >180 *CDH1* mutations identified; mostly, they are truncating mutations so produce a non-functioning protein, unable to carry out its function as a tumour suppressor. For tumour formation, the loss or inactivation of the second *CDH1* allele is also required.

In HDGC, the mutation in *CDH1* can take many forms (for example, a deletion, frameshift mutation, splice-site mutation or missense mutation) that can involve a variety of sites in the gene and is not only restricted to coding regions but could include the untranslated regions. A loss-of-function mutation in the remaining allele can be caused by a number of mechanisms, such as loss of heterozygosity or promoter hypermethylation, and can lead to GC (Barber et al. 2008). The identification of germline *CDH1* missense variants requires additional studies to assess their putative pathogenicity. A multidisciplinary approach combining familial and population data, in silico analysis and in vitro analysis is currently used to classify the variants as neutral, pathogenic or a variant of uncertain significance (VUS). Genetic parameters such as mutation frequency in healthy control population, co-segregation of the mutation within the pedigree and recurrence of the mutation in independent families may be considered as a first approach. However, the low number of individuals affected by the disease, the small size of the pedigrees and the absence of mutation hot spots (which prevents the establishment of any correlation between the mutation site and its functional consequence) make this approach challenging. Currently, there is no international database containing all germline *CDH1* mutations and variants identified to date.

3.3 HDGC Management: Surveillance

The Cambridge Protocol for Upper Gastrointestinal Surveillance in HDGC
Once a patient is confirmed as a *CDH1* mutation carrier, they will need a baseline oesophago-gastroduodenoscopy (OGD) to look for any gastric tumours that will change the long-term management plan. The OGD can also screen for other pathology such as Barrett's oesophagus as this may impact on the resection area. Following the procedure, most individuals would be advised to have a prophylactic gastrectomy. For many reasons, an individual may want to delay this procedure so in these cases endoscopic surveillance is warranted. In families that meet the criteria for developing HDGC but no mutation can be identified or in those individuals with a *CDH1* mutation of undetermined significance, it is recommended intensive endoscopic surveillance should be offered.

Ideally, the surveillance OGD should be carried out at centres of expertise annually. The endoscopy should be performed with white light definition with repeated inflation/deflation techniques and thorough washing of the mucosa with mucolytics and anti-foaming agents. Poor distension in any area is suggestive of a submucosal lesion and would be considered an area of concern requiring further investigation with a computerised tomography (CT) scan or endoscopic ultrasound (EUS).

HP infection does not have a direct link to HDGC but it is a recognised risk factor for sporadic GC. Therefore, at endoscopy, individuals should be tested for it and if positive should be treated with eradication therapy.

The disease starts as a microscopic focus of signet-ring cells not apparent macroscopically. By taking large numbers of random biopsies, the chance of identify an abnormal area is significantly increased. Current guidance advises biopsy of any visible lesions or 'pale areas' as well as random biopsies from the antrum, transitional zone, body, fundus and cardia. The 'Cambridge protocol' advises a minimum of 30 biopsies are taken equating to 6 samples from each area (van der Post et al. 2015).

3.4 Breast Cancer Surveillance

In 2000, the first reported association between breast cancer risk and HDGC was published (Pharoah et al. 2001). Genotype–phenotype correlations show not all families with HDGC have an increased risk of breast cancer, but it remains unclear as to who should be screened. Therefore, at present, all women with the *CDH1* mutation should be considered at risk and offered counselling on breast screening versus prophylactic mastectomy similar to the *BRCA* 1/2 guidance. Prophylactic mastectomy is not routinely offered for CDH1 mutation carriers but considered case by case.

HDGC is specifically associated with invasive LBC whereas *BRCA* 1/2 causes invasive ductal cancer (DBC). LBC associated with the *CDH1* mutation invades in sheets or chords of cells not forming a well-defined mass like in DBC. This means screening mammograms have a lower sensitivity so instead bilateral magnetic resonance imaging (MRI) scans should be part of the standard screening protocol. A breast MRI should be offered annually to women with the mutation from the age of 30 (van der Post et al. 2015).

3.5 Endoscopic Surveillance of Colorectal Cancer

Currently, there is not enough evidence to suggest the risk of colorectal cancer (CRC) in individuals with the *CDH1* mutation is increased above that of the general population. In HDGC families where there are confirmed cases of CRC, more information about age of onset, which family members have been affected, and histopathological characteristics should be collated. In these cases, colonoscopic surveillance should be thought about from 40 years of age [according to new international guidance (van der Post et al. 2015)]. In all other families, the national CRC surveillance guidelines would apply.

3.6 Prophylactic Gastrectomy

All individuals with a proven *CDH1* mutation should be offered a total gastrectomy. This is the only way to completely eradicate their risk of GC and prevent their death from invasive carcinoma. Most procedures are performed in early adulthood between the ages of 20 and 30 years, and current guidelines would advocate this (Blair et al. 2006). Due to the life-changing nature of the surgery, there needs to be very careful consideration in those over 75 years. At the time of surgery, individuals frequently have microscopic malignant changes in the removed stomach and are often found to have stage T1, N0 tumours (Norton et al. 2007). This pattern suggests there is likely to be dormant periods where the carcinoma does not spread (Barber et al. 2008). In individuals who have symptoms with invasive GC, only around 10 % have the chance of a cure (Koea et al. 2007).

The standard operation is a total gastrectomy with Roux-en-Y reconstruction and the jejuno-jejunal anastomosis placed at least 50 cm from the oesophageal–gastric anastomosis to reduce biliary reflux. The oesophageal resection line should be examined in the operating room to ensure it is passing through squamous mucosa and no gastric cardia remnants are left behind. Whether lymph nodes should be removed in a prophylactic gastrectomy remains a point of discussion. In early disease (T1a), the frequency of lymph node involvement is 2–5 %, but this increases to 17–28 % in submucosal invasion (T1b tumours) (Kang et al. 2010).

Therefore, because it is difficult to distinguish between these two with an OGD lymph node stations 1–7 are excised as part of the operation. The operation can be performed laparoscopically which is associated with shorter recovery and reduced morbidity.

3.7 Histopathology

The pathology of HDGC is unique but requires a high level of expertise in order to maximise recognition of specific findings. Multiple biopsies taken at endoscopy should be examined with haematoxylin and eosin (H&E) staining at three levels which facilitates easy detection of invasive DGC. The addition of the periodic acid-Schiff (PAS)-diastase staining detects neutral mucins and is used to identify or to confirm the presence of intramucosal lesions, helping to identify areas with a focus of signet-ring cells that have not infiltrated through the muscularis mucosae. There are two types of pre-invasive lesions in signet-ring cell carcinoma:

- In situ signet-ring cell carcinoma where the signet-ring cells in the basal membrane of the glands have hyperchromatic and depolarised nuclei.
- Pagetoid spread of a row of signet-ring cells below the preserved epithelium of the glands (Carneiro et al. 2012).

Following gastrectomy, the specimen should also be thoroughly examined by an experienced pathologist. Data from over 100 gastrectomies for HDGC have highlighted the majority already contain a tiny focus of signet-ring carcinoma or the pre-invasive lesions (van der Post et al. 2015). The pathologist should also comment on the surgical margins to confirm they are free of abnormal tissue (an 'R0' resection in the residual tumour classification).

The specimens with advanced HDGC often present as a linitis plastica, with diffuse infiltration of the stomach wall. The histology often shows an infiltrate of pleomorphic neoplastic cells with minimal cell differentiation. On occasions, the histology can show mainly or exclusively signet-ring cells. There is no specific histological appearance that suggests the cancer is hereditary in nature, although in situ lesions and pagetoid spread of signet-ring cells in the surrounding tissue do provide supportive evidence of HDGC.

3.8 Postsurgical Care and Survivorship

Surgical gastrectomy is associated with significant morbidity and survivorship issues, not only physiological but also psychological and social consequences. These include problems with eating, weight loss, abdominal pain and distorted body image. To support patients in this post-operative period, new guidelines suggest the establishment of 12-month recovery programmes guided by MDTs (van der Post et al. 2015).

After surgery, a 15–20 % loss of body weight is reported with most occurring in the first 6 months (Worster et al. 2014). Thus, dietary advice and specifically involvement of a dietician is pivotal. Patients should be advised to eat frequent small meals in order to avoid 'dumping syndrome' where the rapid entry of food into the small intestine leads to a shift in fluid from the blood into the intestine causing cardiovascular and abdominal symptoms that include nausea, vomiting, bloating diarrhoea, sweating and dizziness. Many of these symptoms arise from hypoglycaemia caused by the rapid transit of food into the small bowel stimulating the pancreas to release excess amounts of insulin into the blood stream. Other problems that are reported include lactose intolerance, steatorrhoea, small-bowel bacterial overgrowth, strictures and early satiety. It is important to monitor for iron, calcium and trace element deficiencies and ensure lifelong B12 injections due to the loss of intrinsic factor production in the stomach.

4 The Management of Other Hereditary Syndromes and GC Risk

Other syndromes that predispose to heritable gastric cancer risk include Lynch syndrome, and polyposis syndromes discussed below. Prophylactic gastrectomy is not recommended in these conditions; instead, an endoscopic surveillance protocol may be administered, although this surveillance is applied due to empirical rather than evidence from randomised controlled studies (Cairns et al. 2010). There are also no studies of the efficacy of chemoprophylaxis for the risk reduction of GC specifically in these syndromes, primarily because of the rarity of the GC phenotype thereof. Single gene testing as well as panel-based testing using the Illumina Trusight© provides comprehensive analysis of all of the syndromes discussed, as well as mutations in another candidate genes *CTNNA1*, *BRCA2* and *PALB2*.

4.1 Lynch Syndrome

Lynch syndrome is the most common hereditary CRC syndrome with an incidence of 1/3100 of the general population. It is autosomal dominant. The mutations accounting for Lynch syndrome are found in 5 mismatch repair genes: *MSH2, MLH1, MSH6, PMS2 and EPCAM2*. The diagnostic guidelines used to identify patients with lynch syndrome are the Amsterdam II or revised Bethesda criteria.

In Lynch syndrome, the penetrance for GC is 13–20 % (Hans et al. 1999). It has been demonstrated in two studies that the majority of GCs associated with Lynch syndrome are of the intestinal type (73–79 %). The goal of surveillance is to detect precancerous lesions that are at a curable stage. According to guidelines, families with two or more individuals with GC or mismatch repair gene carriers should have an OGD every two years after the age of 50 (Cairns et al. 2010).

Nevertheless, there is limited evidence for gastric screening or screening for other cancers is effective in Lynch syndrome and so instead it is suggested aspirin should be used to prevent extracolonic cancer following the CAPP2 study (Burn et al. 2011).

4.2 Familial Adenomatous Polyposis (FAP)

There is a risk of upper gastrointestinal malignancy in FAP but this is from duodenal polyps. Although individuals with this condition have multiple fundic gland polyps in the stomach, these polyps do not have malignant potential and so the OGD surveillance is mainly used to screen the duodenum. Gastric cancer arises from gastric adenomas (i.e. not from fundic gland polyps), although the incidence of GC in FAP is not known. The guidelines recommend 3-yearly OGDs from the age of 30 years unless there are very large numbers of duodenal polyps when it should be reduced to annual surveillance (Cairns et al. 2010).

4.3 *MUTYH*-Associated Polyposis (MAP)

MAP is an inherited autosomal recessive condition where the individual affected develops multiple adenomatous polyps throughout the colon. The lifetime risk in a homozygous person developing CRC is 100 % at 60 years (Cairns et al. 2010). It accounts for around 0.4–3 % of all CRCs. The MutY human homologue (*MUTYH*) gene, located on chromosome 1p, encodes for MUTYH glycosylase which is involved in DNA damage repair. Rarely, this condition results in upper gastrointestinal polyps in the duodenum and fundus of the stomach. Therefore, it is recommended the OGD surveillance is carried out from the age of 30 and then every 3–5 years (Cairns et al. 2010). Genetic screening should be offered to the partner and FDRs of a homozygote individual.

4.4 Peutz–Jeghers Syndrome (PJS)

PJS is an autosomal dominant syndrome with high penetrance and characterised by the association of gastrointestinal polyposis and mucocutaneous pigmentation. A germline mutation within *STK11* results in dysregulated signal transduction and inhibition of the mTOR pathway. The gastrointestinal cancer risk includes gastro-oesophageal, small-bowel, pancreatic and CRCs with a cumulative risk of 57 % by the age of 70 (Beggs et al. 2010). Guidelines recommend 2-yearly OGD and colonoscopy from the age of 25 years (Cairns et al. 2010).

Table 2 Summary of inherited conditions associated with gastric cancer

Syndrome	Gene mutation	Mode of inheritance	Phenotype
HDGC	*CDH1, CTNNA1*	Autosomal dominant	Gastric, breast, colorectal, thyroid cancer
Lynch syndrome	*MSH2, MLH1, MSH6, PMS2, and EPCAM2*	Autosomal dominant	Colorectal, gynaecological cancers predominantly and some other sites including gastric
FAP	*APC*	Autosomal dominant	Colorectal and small-bowel tumours, benign fundic gland polyps predominantly and rarely gastric cancer arising from adenomas
MAP	*MUTYH*	Autosomal recessive	Similar to FAP but milder phenotype typically
JPS/PJS	*BMPR1A, SMAD4/STK11*	Autosomal dominant	Small and large bowel neoplasia predominantly
Li–Fraumeni Syndrome	*TP53*	Autosomal dominant	Multiple sarcomas

4.5 Juvenile Polyposis Syndrome (JPS)

JPS is a rare autosomal dominant disorder with prevalence between 1/50,000 and 1/120,000 of the population. The germline mutations occur in 3 genes *SMAD4*, *BMPR1A* and *ENG1*. It is defined by the presence of multiple hamartomatous polyps throughout the gastrointestinal tract but predominantly in the colon and rectum. The GC risk is around 21 %, and OGD surveillance should be performed 1–2 yearly from the age of 25 years (Cairns et al. 2010).

4.6 Li–Fraumeni Syndrome

Li–Fraumeni syndrome is a rare hereditary cancer syndrome associated with germline mutations in the *TP53* gene. Although sarcomas, brain tumours, leukaemias, breast and adrenal cortical carcinomas are typically recognised as Li–Fraumeni syndrome-associated tumours, the occurrence of GC is also recognised in up to 4.9 % of families (Masciari et al. 2011). Surveillance guidelines do not currently exist for these patients however (Table 2).

5 Ongoing and Future Research

5.1 Other Genes Involved in HDGC Predisposition

The molecular background of HDGC patients without *CDH1* mutations remains to be clarified, including any specific morphological features of GC in the setting of other hereditary cancer syndromes. Additional molecular mechanisms might be involved in the pathogenesis of HDGC that are not currently fully understood. A truncating allele of *CTNNA1* (which encodes catenin α-1) was identified by exome sequencing in a family with multiple cases of GC over four generations, as well as other family members who had premalignant gastric changes visible on histology, but had no *CDH1* germline mutation (Zang et al. 2012). This suggests either that the pathogenicity of *CTNNA1* mutations may be mediated through loss of CDH1 function or that the cancer-initiating potential of *CDH1* mutations is imparted through α-catenin-associated pathways. More research is needed to understand the role and mutation detection rate of *CTNNA1* mutations.

Other families have recently been described with *BRCA2* and *PALB2* mutations. It is likely that other HDGC-associated genes will be discovered through whole exome/genome- or other unbiased next-generation sequencing-empowered methodologies.

The use of hypothesis-free genome-wide association studies (GWAS) has identified variation in novel susceptibility loci which confer lower penetrance risk. A statistically significant association has been identified in a large Japanese population between diffuse GC and a polymorphic genetic variation (rs2294008 and rs2976392) within exon 1 of the *PSCA* gene (which encodes prostate stem cell antigen [PSCA]).

5.2 Data from High-Throughput Studies

Advances in technology, such as next-generation sequencing, have enabled the emergence of new, exciting molecular profiling in the context of GC and other solid tumours. Examples include exome-wide (DNA sequencing) and transcriptome-wide (RNA sequencing) analysis. For instance, exome-wide sequencing of 15 gastric adenocarcinomas and matched normal DNA identified a cell adhesion pathway with molecular abnormalities that was associated with GC; *FAT4*, a member of the cadherin family, was mutated in 5 % of the cancer cases (Zang et al. 2012). Functionally, the study showed that *FAT4* is a tumour suppressor and that inactivation of the gene leads to cancer progression. Genes with products involved in chromatin remodelling, such as *ARID1A*, were also prominent in the cancer profile in this study. In addition, another group identified *ARID1A* as an important gene in the development of GC, with a high mutation frequency (Zang et al. 2012). Thus, high-throughput approaches have identified new driver gene targets. However, fairly little is known about the function of these novel genes; thus, the development of new targeted therapies may not be feasible currently.

The Cancer Genome Atlas Research (TGCA) Network performed extensive molecular profiling of nearly 300-GC tissue samples using six discrete platforms with the aim of identifying novel molecular characterisation of GC (The Cancer Genome Atlas 2014). They identified four defined subtypes: tumours positive for Epstein–Barr virus; tumours showing chromosomal instability; tumours with a stable genome; and tumours with microsatellite instability. This molecular classification could be central to the development of novel targeted therapeutic strategies.

5.3 Future Research on Gastric and Breast Surveillance

Multiple chromo-endoscopic technologies have emerged in the past 15 years, such as autofluorescence imaging, narrow band imaging (NBI) and dye spray chromoendoscopy; however, the role for these methods for endoscopic monitoring of individuals at risk for diffuse GC has not yet been elucidated. It is likely that the Cambridge protocol where multiple biopsies are taken leads to scarring which can masquerade as pale areas and therefore it would be valuable to compare the yield of this technique and a more targeted biopsy approach offered by these new technologies. Such studies could also inform on the interobserver variation in the identification of pale areas and help define features indicative of a signet-ring cell focus.

There are no studies specifically addressing screening for LBC. Trials on breast screening in the general population and MRI screening in high-risk groups or *BRCA1/2* are informative but do not directly extrapolate to the screening scenario in HDGC. The outcomes of the above-stated recommendations of breast surveillance in HDGC women should be further prospectively investigated.

6 Conclusions

Gastric cancer is a common disease worldwide with important environmental risk factors such as HP status. HP infection is associated with one of the histological subtypes, intestinal, but not with diffuse-type GC. Thus, HP does not appear to have a role in GC pathogenesis in patients with HDGC.

A positive family history is a strong and consistently reported risk factor for GC, but the molecular basis for the familial aggregation is largely unknown. A single FDR with GC is associated with a 2- to 3-fold increased risk of GC.

The known cancer syndromes do not account for a large part of the familial clustering. Unlike the situation for other common cancers, guidelines have not been developed for the assessment of the family history of individuals with GC.

Although these hereditary cancer syndromes have been relatively well characterised, the rarity of the GC phenotype precludes the development of trials of surveillance. On the other hand, the high penetrance of GC in HDGC patients with proven *CDH1* mutations means that prophylactic gastrectomy is recommended, although this treatment results in significant 'survivorship' issues; therefore, this is not for other patients than this specific group.

New international guidelines for surveillance and management of HDGC have been presented in this chapter. Surveillance of at-risk HDGC individuals requires a high level of expertise both endoscopic and histological evaluation. The risk associated with other inherited syndromes is managed by testing of at-risk individuals with regular endoscopic surveillance.

Not all families who fulfil clinical criteria for HDGC have identifiable mutations in *CDH1*. Other genes found to have germline predisposition to this syndrome include *CTNNA1, BRCA2* and *PALB2*. Carcinogenesis in many of these families may be delivered through aberrantly activated α-catenin pathways.

Much of the remaining heritable risk may be accounted for by low- and intermediate-penetrant genetic factors, i.e. common and rare variants, respectively. The heritability of GC is poorly understood although advances in this field have been forthcoming in recent years with the advent of new investigative technologies including GWAS and whole-exomic sequencing.

Acknowledgements Prof. Rebecca Fitzgerald, Cambridge, kindly provided an advance copy of the updated international guidelines for the management of HDGC (Published online http://www.ncbi.nlm.nih.gov/pubmed/25979631).

References

Barber M, Murral A, Ito Y et al (2008) Mechanisms and sequelae of E-cadherin silencing in hereditary diffuse gastric cancer. J Pathol 216(3):295–306

Beggs AD, Latchford AR et al (2010) Peutz-Jeghers syndrome: a systematic review and recommendations for management. Gut 59:975–986

Blair V, Martin I, Shaw D et al (2006) Hereditary diffuse gastric cancer: diagnosis and management. Clin Gastroenterol Hepatol 4(3):262–275

Burn J et al (2011) Long-term effect of aspirin on cancer risk in carriers of hereditary colorectal cancer: an analysis from CAPP2 randomised controlled trial. Lancet 378:2081–2087

Cairns SR et al (2010) BSG guidelines for colorectal cancer screening and surveillance in moderate and high risk groups (update from 2002). Gut 59:666–690

Cancer research UK (2015) http://www.cancerresearchuk.org/cancerinfo/cancerstats/types/stomach/incidence/. Accessed July 2015

Carneiro F, Charlton A, Huntsman D (2012) Hereditary diffuse gastric cancer. In: Bosman FT (ed) WHO classification of tumours of the digestive system. 4th edn: IARC

Ferlay J (2012) GLOBOCAN 2012 v1.0 cancer incidence and mortality worldwide. IARC CancerBase

Ferlay J, Steliarova-Foucher E, Lortet-Tieulent J et al (2013) Cancer incidence and mortality patterns in Europe: estimates for 40 countries in 2012. Eur J Cancer 49:1374–1403

Hillier SH, Fielder H (2009) Screening for stomach cancer: a report for the National Screening Committee. Accessed July 2015.http://legacy.screening.nhs.uk/policydb_download.php?doc=49

Hu B et al (2012) Gastric cancer: classification, histology and application of molecular pathology. J Gastrointest Oncol 3(3):251–261

Kang HJ, Kim DH, Jeon TY et al (2010) Lymph node metastasis from intestinal-type early gastric cancer: experience in a single institution and reassessment of the extended criteria for endoscopic mucosal resection. Gastrointest Endosc 72(3):508–515

Koea JB, Karpeh MS, Brennan MF (2007) Gastric cancer in young patients: demographic, clinicopathological and prognostic factors in 92 patients. Ann Surg Oncol 7(5):346–351

Masciari S et al (2011) Gastric cancer in individuals with Li-Fraumeni syndrome. Genet Med 13:651–657

Norton JA, Ham CM, Van Dam J et al (2007) CDH1 truncating mutations in the E-cadherin gene: an indication for total gastrectomy to treat hereditary diffuse gastric cancer. Ann Surg 245 (6):837–839

Pharoah PD, Guilford P et al (2001) Incidence of gastric and breast cancer in CDH1 (E-cadherin) mutation carriers from hereditary diffuse gastric cancer families. Gastroenterology 121:1348–1353

The Cancer Genome Atlas (2015) http://cancergenome.nih.gov/newsevents/newsannouncements/TCGA_STAD_press_release_2014. Accessed July 2015

Tsubono Y, Hisamichi S (2000) Screening for gastric cancer in Japan. Gastric Cancer 3:9–18 (November 7)

van der Post RS, Vogelaar IP, Carneiro F et al (2015) Hereditary diffuse gastric cancer: updated clinical guidelines with an emphasis on germline *CDH1* mutation carriers. J Med Genet. 52(6):361–74

Vasen HFA et al (1999) New clinical criteria for hereditary non-polyposis colorectal cancer. Gastroenterology 116(6):1453–1456

Worster E, Liu X et al (2014) The impact of prophylactic total gastrectomy on health related quality of life: a prospective cohort study. Ann Surg 464:673–679

Yaghoobi M et al (2010) Family history and the risk of gastric cancer. Br J Cancer, 102:237–242. http://www.nature.com/bjc/journal/v102/n2/full/6605380a.html

Zang ZJ et al (2012) Exome sequencing of gastric adenocarcinoma identifies recurrent somatic mutations in cell adhesion and chromatin remodelling genes. Nat Genet 44:570–574

Diagnosis and Management of Hereditary Pancreatic Cancer

Jeremy L. Humphris and Andrew V. Biankin

Abstract
Hereditary pancreatic cancer can be diagnosed through family history and/or a personal history of pancreatitis or clinical features suggesting one of the known pancreatic cancer predisposition syndromes. This chapter describes the currently known hereditary pancreatic cancer predisposition syndromes, including Peutz–Jeghers syndrome, familial atypical multiple mole melanoma, hereditary breast and ovarian cancer, Li–Fraumeni syndrome, hereditary non-polyposis colon cancer and familial adenomatous polyposis. Strategies for genetic testing for hereditary pancreatic cancer and the appropriate options for surveillance and cancer risk reduction are discussed. Finally, ongoing research and future directions in the diagnosis and management of hereditary pancreatic cancer will be considered.

Keywords
Pancreatic cancer · Inherited · Screening

J.L. Humphris (✉) · A.V. Biankin
The Kinghorn Cancer Centre, Cancer Research Program, 370 Victoria St., Darlinghurst, NSW 2010, Australia
e-mail: j.humphris@garvan.org.au

A.V. Biankin
Wolfson Wohl Cancer Research Centre, Institute of Cancer Sciences, University of Glasgow, Garscube Estate, Switchback Road, Glasgow Bearsden G61 1BD, United Kingdom

G. Pichert and C. Jacobs (eds.), *Rare Hereditary Cancers*,
Recent Results in Cancer Research 205, DOI 10.1007/978-3-319-29998-3_5

Contents

1 Introduction

Up to 10 % of pancreatic cancers (PCs) have a hereditary component, but the underlying genetic cause has only been identified in a minority. Genetic counselling and testing are important in suspected inherited PC cases, to disseminate information regarding genetic testing and disease risk. Screening trials are available for high-risk individuals (i.e. >5–10 % lifetime risk), although more long-term data are required to determine the risks, benefits and optimal approaches to PC surveillance. Novel approaches are needed to define the missing heritability in PCs and to incorporate this into clinical practice.

2 Epidemiology

2.1 Demographics

2.1.1 Age

PC is largely a disease of advancing age with mean age at diagnosis of 71 years and is rarely diagnosed before 40 years of age (Ryan et al. 2014). Only 5–10 % of cases are diagnosed before 50 years, but this cohort may be enriched with individuals with an inherited genetic predisposition (Raimondi et al. 2009). The incidence increases exponentially in both sexes after age 40 from 2.3 cases per 100,000 for 40–44 year olds to 57 cases per 100,000 in those 70–74 years (AIHW 2014). Reports of younger age at diagnosis in familial PC cases are inconclusive (Barton et al. 2011), but some studies suggest earlier onset by 5 years and a higher proportion (≈16 %) of young-onset disease (Petersen et al. 2006). In familial pancreatic cancer (FPC) families with identified mutations, the median age of diagnosis was

60–62.8 years for BRCA2 and 66.7 years for PALB2 (Hahn et al. 2003a; Jones et al. 2009a). Anticipation has been reported in 32–85 % of FPC families with successive generations developing PC 10–20 years earlier (McFaul et al. 2006).

2.1.2 Ethnicity

The worldwide incidence of PC shows significant variability with the highest rates seen in the more developed regions of North America, Western and Central/Eastern Europe and Australia/New Zealand. The lowest rates are seen on less developed regions in Africa and South Asia. Subpopulation stratification shows variability with higher risk in people of African American and Ashkenazi Jewish heritage compare to those of Caucasian, Hispanic and Asian descent (Eldridge et al. 2011; Raimondi et al. 2009). This is likely the culmination of both genetic and non-genetic risk factors (Fig. 1).

2.1.3 Gender

In comparison with ethnicity, there are only small gender differences in the risk of developing PC. The lifetime risk of developing PC before age 75 for males is 0.9 and 0.6 % for females (AIHW 2014) which has been attributed to higher cigarette smoking rates in men (Raimondi et al. 2009).

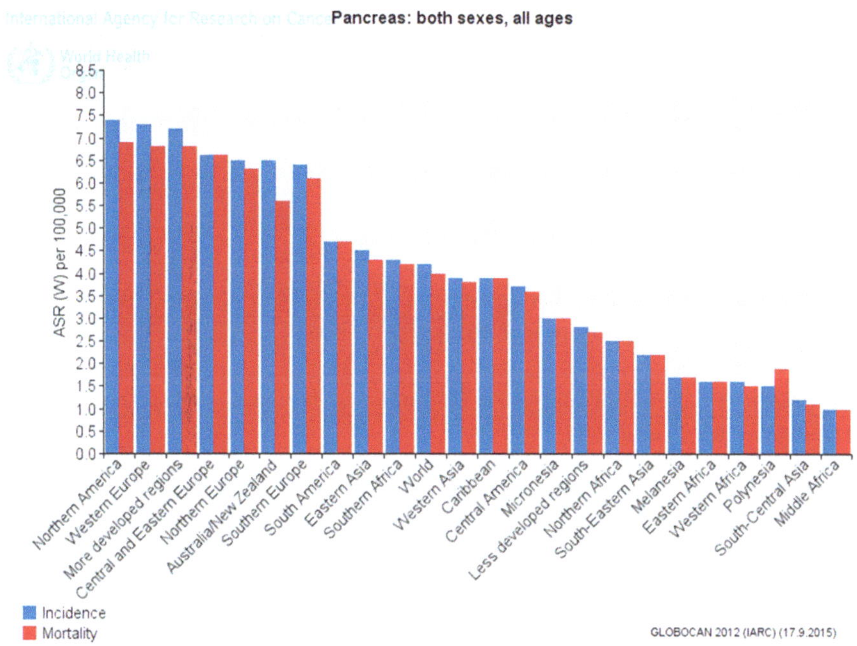

Fig. 1 Age-specific pancreatic cancer incidence and mortality in worldwide populations. The incidence to mortality ratio approaches 1 in all populations. Reproduced with permission (Ferlay J)

2.2 Non-genetic Risk Factors

Epidemiologic studies have identified several environmental and lifestyle risk factors for PC which frequently coexist and are likely to interact (Raimondi et al. 2009). These are summarised in Table 1.

2.2.1 Genetic Risk Factors

The conventional paradigm based on case–control and cohort studies is that 5–10 % of patients diagnosed with PC have a hereditary component based on family history of the disease (Ghadirian et al. 1991). Studies requiring histological confirmation have shown lower rates (1.9–2.7 %) of familial aggregation (Bartsch et al. 2004; Hemminki and Li 2003). The 5–10 % figure may be correct but as large sequence cohorts are beginning to show germline mutations in cancer predisposition genes frequently occur in the absence of family history, showing that while family history is predictive of carrier status, it is imperfect (Grant et al. 2014). Inherited predisposition to PC manifests as 3 distinct clinical scenarios (Bartsch et al. 2012): (1) hereditary tumour predisposition syndromes including hereditary breast–ovarian cancer (HBOC), Peutz–Jeghers Syndrome (PJS), familial atypical multiple mole melanoma (FAMMM), Li–Fraumeni, hereditary nonpolyposis colorectal cancer (HNPCC) and familial adenomatous polyposis (FAP) which account for 15–20 % of the burden of inherited disease (Hruban et al. 2010) (2) hereditary pancreatitis due to mutations in *PRSS1* and 3. Familial PC (FPC) which is defined as a family with at least 2 first-degree relatives with PC, which do not fulfil the diagnostic criteria for an inherited tumour syndrome (Brand et al. 2007). The majority (80 %) of hereditary PC is attributed to FPC with a pattern consistent with autosomal dominant inheritance in 50–80 % of families (Lynch et al. 1990; McFaul et al. 2006) (Table 2).

Table 1 Non-genetic risk factors for PC

Risk factor	Estimated risk (95 % CI)
Active cigarette smoking (Bosetti et al. 2012)	OR 2.20 (1.71–2.83)
Ceased cigarette smoking (Bosetti et al. 2012)	
>1 but <10 years	OR 1.64 (1.36–1.97)
>10 years	OR 1.12 (0.86–1.44)
Diabetes mellitus (Li et al. 2011)	
<2 years duration	RR 7.94 (4.70–12.55)
>10 years duration	OR 1.51 (1.16–1.96)
BMI (>35 vs. <25) (Arslan et al. 2010)	OR 1.55 (1.16–2.07)
Heavy alcohol (≥6 drinks/day) (Genkinger et al. 2009; Anderson et al. 2012)	OR 1.46 (1.16–1.83)
Chronic pancreatitis (>2 years) (Duell et al. 2012)	OR 2.71 (1.96–3.74)
Allergy (hay fever and animal allergy) (Olson and Kurtz 2013; Cotterchio et al. 2014)	OR 0.73 (0.64–0.74)

Table 2 Genetic risk factors for PC–hereditary cancer syndrome and moderate- to high-penetrance genes

Clinical risk group	Syndrome	Relative risk (95 % CI)	Estimated lifetime PC risk (70–80 years)	Other associated tumours	Prevalence in FPC kindreds
General population	NA	1	0.96		
1 FDR PC	NA	4.6 (0.5–16.4)			
2 FDR PC	FPC	6.4 (1.8–16.4)			
≥3 FDR PC	FPC	32 (10.2–74.7)			
Genetic risk group					
BRCA2 (Grant et al. 2014; Couch et al. 2007a; Zhen et al. 2014)	HBOC/FPC	3.51	3.36 %	Breast, ovarian	0.7–6 %
PALB2 (Schneider et al. 2011a; Jones et al. 2009; Zhen et al. 2014)	FPC	Elevated but not defined	Elevated but not defined	Breast	0–3 %
BRCA1	HBOC	2.26	2.16 %	Breast, ovarian	0.3–1.2 %
MSH2, MLH1, MSH6, PMS2, 5′ EPCAM deletion (Grant et al. 2014)	HNPCC	8.6	3.68 % (1.45–5.88 %)	Colon, endometrial	Each <1 %
PRSS1	Hereditary pancreatitis	58	30–40 % in smokers, 20 % in non-smokers	Pancreas only	NA
STK11 (Grant et al. 2014; Schneider et al. 2011b)	Peutz–Jeghers syndrome	132	11–32 %	Gastrointestinal, breast, gynaecologic, pancreas	0 %
CDKN2A (Zhen et al. 2014; Grant et al. 2014)	FAMMM	38	17 %	Melanoma	0–2.5 %[a]
ATM (monoallelic) (Roberts et al. 2012b)	Ataxia telangiectasia (bi-allelic)	Elevated but not defined	Elevated but not defined	Breast, colon	2.4 %
TP53	Li–Fraumeni syndrome	Elevated but not defined	Elevated but not defined	Sarcoma, breast, brain, adrenocortical	NA

[a]Higher prevalence in some populations, e.g. Italian (up to 30 % of FPC) (Ghiorzo et al. 2012)

3 Main Section

3.1 Hereditary Tumour Predisposition Syndromes

3.1.1 Hereditary Breast–Ovarian Cancer

Inherited pathogenic germline *BRCA2* mutations place carriers at increased risk of cancers of the pancreas, prostate, gallbladder, bile duct, stomach and melanoma in addition to breast and ovarian cancer (The Breast Cancer Linkage Consortium 1999; Moran et al. 2012). The prevalence of germline *BRCA2* mutations in patients with PC depends on the ethnic ancestry of the population studied and is higher in groups with founder mutations such as those of Ashkenazi Jewish descent. In an early report, Goggins et al. (1996) found *BRCA2* mutations in 7 % of patients with apparent sporadic PC (3 of 41) of which one was the Ashkenazi founder mutation. Studies have shown *BRCA2* mutations in 5–10 % of Ashkenazi Jews with PC (Ozcelik et al. 1997; Ferrone et al. 2009). In familial PC, the mutation prevalence increases with rising number of affected relatives: 6–12 % in families with two or more with PC and 16 % from families in which 3 or more have PC (Murphy et al. 2002; Couch et al. 2007b). The relative risk of developing PC in *BRCA2* mutation carriers is approximately 3.5–6 (The Breast Cancer Linkage Consortium 1999; Risch et al. 2006). A substantial proportion of mutation-positive PC patients report neither a history of PC nor breast–ovarian cancer (Goggins et al. 1996; Murphy et al. 2002). This is likely due to reduced penetrance for PC rather than there being PC-specific genotype–phenotype correlation for BRCA2 mutations as has been seen in some breast–ovarian cancers (Thompson and Easton 2001).

In contrast, the role of *BRCA1* mutations in predisposition to PC is less well established. Overall studies in *BRCA*1 kindreds with young-onset breast or ovarian cancer suggested a 2.26-fold (95 % CI = 1.26–4.06) increased risk of pancreatic cancer (Brose et al. 2002; Iqbal et al. 2012). *BRCA1* mutations are uncommon without a history of breast cancer (Skudra et al. 2007) or Ashkenazi heritage (Shi et al. 2009; Lucas et al. 2013). Other studies have found no increase in the prevalence of *BRCA1* mutations in patients with pancreatic cancer (Ferrone et al. 2009; Axilbund et al. 2009).

3.1.2 Familial Atypical Multiple Mole Melanoma

Familial atypical multiple mole melanoma (FAMMM) is a syndrome characterised by predisposition to melanoma and PC. Clinical diagnostic features include family history of melanoma in at least one close relative, multiple melanocytic naevi (often >50) some of which show visible atypical and characteristic microscopic features. FAMMM is caused by germline mutations in *CDKN2A* (p16), which encodes the tumour suppressors ARF and INK4A. Individuals with FAMMM have a 38-fold increased risk of developing PC compared to the general population, contributing to a lifetime risk of 17 % by age 75 (Rutter et al. 2004; Vasen et al. 2000).

3.1.3 Peutz–Jeghers Syndrome

Peutz–Jeghers syndrome is an autosomal dominant disorder characterised by gastrointestinal tract hamartomatous polyps and mucocutaneous pigmentation (Beggs et al. 2010). In 80–94 % of individuals who meet the clinical criteria, pathogenic mutations (two-thirds single nucleotide variants and one-third large deletions) in *STK11* are identified (McGarrity et al. 2013). These individuals have a 132-fold increased risk of pancreatic cancer compared with the general population, and the lifetime risk of pancreatic cancer in these individuals has been estimated to be 11–32 % (Hearle et al. 2006; Korsse et al. 2013).

3.1.4 Hereditary Nonpolyposis Colorectal Cancer

Hereditary nonpolyposis colorectal cancer (HNPCC or Lynch syndrome) is the result of germline mutations in the DNA mismatch repair genes *MSH2*, *MLH1*, *MSH6*, and *PMS2*. Recently, heritable somatic methylation of MSH2 has been described due to germline deletion of the last two exons of EPCAM which produces silencing of the adjacent gene, MSH2 (Ligtenberg et al. 2009; Kuiper et al. 2011). Patients are at increased lifetime risk for a wide range of tumour types, but the predominant malignancies are colonic and endometrial cancer. The other associated tumour types are lower risk with <5 % lifetime risk and include PC, gastric, small bowel, ureteric and skin tumours. A recent study of 147 families containing a mutation in a mismatch gene reported a 8.6-fold (95 % CI, 4.7–15.7) increased risk of pancreatic cancer compared with the general population (Kastrinos et al. 2009). This corresponds to a 3.68 % (95 % CI, 1.45–5.88 %) lifetime (by age 70) risk of pancreatic cancer (Kastrinos et al. 2009).

3.1.5 Familial Adenomatous Polyposis

Familial adenomatous polyposis (FAP) is an autosomal dominant disorder characterised by the early development of hundreds to thousands of colonic adenomatous polyps. The natural history is that untreated nearly all affected patients will develop colorectal carcinoma by age 40 (Vasen et al. 2009). In more than 70 % of patients who meet the clinical criteria, a germline mutation in the *APC* can be identified (Vasen et al. 2009; Groden et al. 1991). Patients with FAP are at increased risk for other neoplasms, including thyroid tumours, gastric, duodenal and ampullary adenocarcinoma. The relative risk for the development of PC is 4.46, and some evidence suggests precursor lesions progress through the intraductal papillary mucinous neoplasm (IPMN) pathway (Chetty et al. 2005).

3.1.6 Li–Fraumeni Syndrome

Li–Fraumeni syndrome (LFS) is an autosomal dominant highly penetrant cancer predisposition syndrome characterised by a variety of early onset tumours. The syndrome, described in 1969 by Li and Fraumeni based on a retrospective analysis of families with childhood rhabdomyosarcoma(Li and Fraumeni 1969), was characterised by the presence of five cancers: sarcoma, adrenocortical carcinoma, breast cancer, leukemia, and brain tumours (Li et al. 1988; Garber et al. 1991). Several different clinical classification systems exist, but these tumour types form the core clinical features. Li–Fraumeni Syndrome is caused by germline mutations in the *TP53* gene and is inherited in an autosomal dominant pattern. The risk of PC is increased but has not been quantified (Birch et al. 2001; Ruijs et al. 2010).

3.1.7 Hereditary Pancreatitis

Hereditary pancreatitis is a rare autosomal dominant form of inherited pancreatitis. This typically manifests as recurrent acute pancreatitis by age 10, chronic pancreatitis by age 20 and increased risk of PC after age 40 (Howes et al. 2004). In families, meeting the clinical criteria gain-of-function mutations (missense and rarely duplications or triplications) in the cationic trypsinogen gene (*PRSS1*) are found in around 80 % (Whitcomb et al. 1996). Patients with hereditary pancreatitis have a 58-fold (95 % CI 23–105) increased risk of developing pancreatic cancer and a lifetime risk (by age 70) of 30–40 % (Lowenfels et al. 1997). Cigarette smoking increases the risk by twofold and brings the age at diagnosis forward 20 years (Lowenfels et al. 2001). The lifetime risk in non-smokers is estimated to be <20 % (Rebours et al. 2009).

3.1.8 Familial Pancreatic Cancer

In FPC kindreds, the relative risk of developing PC escalates with increasing number of affected first-degree relatives (FDR) from twofold with one affected FDR to sixfold and 14–32-fold (up to 57-fold) with 2 and 3 affected FDRs, respectively (Klein et al. 2004; Tersmette et al. 2001). FPC is likely to be a heterogeneous syndrome with phenotype determined by the underlying genetic predisposition and modified by environmental risk factors. Familial clustering can also occur through phenocopying as a result of shared or common environmental exposures within families, as suggested by a non-significant in FPC kindred's spouses (Klein 2013a, b). FPC kindreds also appear to be at increased risk of developing malignancy of the breast, ovary, colorectum and melanoma, particularly if the proband developed young-onset (<50 years) PC (Wang et al. 2009b; Brune et al. 2010). This finding is consistent with previous reports where in 40 % of FPC families PC was the sole tumour entity and in the remaining 60 % other tumour types, namely breast, colon and lung, were seen (Schneider et al. 2011a). Defining the precise organotypic distribution of tumours which cluster with PC is important because it (a) supports an underlying genetic predisposition or common environmental factor potentially even in the absence of multiple PC cases in the family, (b) allows a more precise definition and clinical recognition of the syndrome and (c) facilitates broader and more precise risk assessment and employment of risk reduction strategies in at-risk family members (Wang et al. 2009a). These results highlight the importance of complete family history of all cancer types in clinical assessment of FPC pedigrees (Cote et al. 2007). The underlying genetic basis of PC predisposition has been identified in less than 25 % of such families (Roberts et al. 2012a), despite 50–80 % of families demonstrating an autosomal dominant inheritance pattern (Lynch et al. 1990; McFaul et al. 2006). Overall, 0.6 % of the general population is estimated to carry a mutation in a moderate- to high-risk pancreatic cancer predisposition gene with an attendant lifetime risk of developing pancreatic cancer (by the age of 85) of 32 % (Klein et al. 2002).

Studies to date have delineated the underlying genetic basis in at best 25 % of these families with mutations in *BRCA2*, *PALB2* (Partner And Localizer of BRCA2) and *ATM* (Ataxia telangiectasia) mutated accounting for 3.7–19 % (Hahn et al. 2003; Couch et al. 2007a), 4.2 % (Jones et al. 2009) and 3.6 % (Roberts et al. 2012a), respectively (Lal et al. 2000). The prevalence of *BRCA2* mutations in FPC as discussed above depends in part on enrichment with family history of other related cancers and ancestry particularly Ashkenazi Jewish heritage. *PALB2* and *ATM* are recently implicated as PC predisposition genes and demonstrate the capability of next-generation sequencing of PC cohorts to identify new risk genes. *PALB2* binds to *BRCA2* and stabilises it in the nucleus, truncating mutations are found in 0.6–3 % of familial PC probands particularly those families with an additional case(s) of breast cancer (Jones et al. 2009; Tischkowitz et al. 2009). Truncating *ATM* mutations segregated with disease 2 FPC kindreds and were subsequently identified in 2.5 % of FPC probands (Roberts et al. 2012b). The risk of developing PC due to pathogenic germline *PALB2* or *ATM* mutations and their contribution to sporadic disease has not been defined.

Palladin (*PALLD*) a cytoskeletal protein when mutated is overexpressed in non-neoplastic stromal cells where it facilitates tumour invasion and metastasis (Brentnall et al. 2012). A missense mutation (p.P239S) in the palladin (*PALLD*) gene was identified in a large FPC kindred which segregated with disease (Pogue-Geile et al. 2006), but subsequent studies have failed to replicate this finding in other FPC probands (Zogopoulos et al. 2007).

3.1.9 Low-Penetrance Susceptibility Variants

Seven PC genome-wide association studies have identified several relatively common but low-penetrant loci associated with PC risk, including the ABO locus. For a complete list of loci, see www.ebi.ac.uk/gwas.

4 Precursor Lesions and Progression to PC

Pancreatic cancer develops from solid and cystic precursor neoplasms through the serial acquisition of mutations, which provide a selective advantage to the cells. The evolution of PC progresses through several stages from non-invasive precursor lesions such as pancreatic intraepithelial neoplasia (PanIN) or cystic neoplasms in particular mucin-producing intraductal papillary mucinous neoplasm (IPMN) and mucinous cystadenoma (Hruban et al. 2000). Based on the genetic evolution of PC, it is estimated that it takes 10 years from the initiating mutation to the establishment of the founder non-metastatic cancer cell and a further 5 years for the development of metastatic potential (Yachida et al. 2010). The detection of PC precursors depends on the underlying lesion, PanINs arise in the smaller pancreatic ducts and the vast majority measure less than 5 mm, as such they are difficult to detect with current imaging techniques (Hruban et al. 2008). In contrast, mucinous cyst adenomas (MCNs) and the duct obstruction and upstream dilatation produced by IPMN are typically detectable on imaging studies (Hruban et al. 2004).

5 PC Risk Assessment

The primary goal of developing PC risk prediction models is to be able to personalise PC risk and in doing so inform genetic testing and potential screening options (Klein 2013b). Multiple risk factors for PC have been identified, after increasing age the next major risk factor is a family history of the disease (Lennon et al. 2014). In those with a known mutation efforts have been made to quantitate this risk, but the majority of individuals at increased genetic risk do not have a known mutation and in effect each person presents with a unique risk factor profile. PancPro is a Bayesian model developed from pedigree data from the National Familial Pancreas Tumour Registry (NFPTR) and calculates the risk that a person carries a high-penetrance PC gene and their risk by age of developing PC (Klein 2013b). The input variables required from each at-risk individual include personal and family history of cancer, current age and age at cancer diagnosis. The model has been validated in an independent cohort and shown an observed to predicted pancreatic cancer ratio of 0.83 (95 % CI, 0.52–1.20) (Wang et al. 2007). PancPRO may be a useful strategy to rank families based on their PC risk and suitability for a screening programme (Leonardi et al. 2012).

6 Genetic Testing for Hereditary Pancreatic Cancer

6.1 Initial Approach

The initial assessment in the index patient should begin with a thorough personal and family history of malignancy. This should include the presence and type of cancer diagnoses in first- and second-degree relatives (±third-degree), age at diagnosis and maternal or paternal lineage (Lu et al. 2014, Network, Version 2.2015). Using this information, a comprehensive, three-generation pedigree should be generated and used to develop a preliminary determination of the risk of a familial predisposition to cancer (Lu et al. 2014). Hallmark features suggestive of an inherited predisposition include (a) personal history: early age at PC diagnosis (<50 years) and previous cancer or premalignant diagnoses with unusual quantity or histological appearance and (b) family history: kindreds with early onset cancer diagnoses (<50 years), members with multiple synchronous or metachronous primary tumours, rare tumours, ancestry with established founder mutations, e.g. Ashkenazi Jewish, and family history of multiple close relatives from the same lineage with PC or spectrum of genetically related cancers (Whitcomb et al. 2015; Syngal et al. 2015). Table 3 summarises the genes to consider for testing based on clinical criteria.

Table 3 Indications for cancer predisposition assessment and consideration of genetic testing (Whitcomb et al. 2015; Syngal et al. 2015; Network, version 2.2015; Hampel et al. 2014)

Clinical criteria	Syndrome to consider	Gene(s) to consider
1. PC diagnosed any age, if any of the following criteria are met – ≥2 cases PC in close relative (1st and 2nd degree)[a] – ≥2 cases breast, ovarian or aggressive prostate cancer in close relatives – Ashkenazi Jewish ancestry	FPC HBOC	*BRCA2* *BRCA1*, *BRCA2*, *PALB2* *BRCA1*, *BRCA2*
2. PC and ≥1 PJ polyp	PJS	*STK11*
3. PC and ≥2 additional cases of any Lynch syndrome-associated cancer in the same person or close relative (LS tumour: CRC, EC, urothelial, gastric, ovarian, SB cancer, glioblastoma, sebaceous adenocarcinoma, biliary tract and PC)	Lynch syndrome	*MSH2*, *MLH1*, *PMS2*, *MSH6*, *5′ EPCAM deletion*
4. ≥3 cases of PC and/or melanoma in close relatives or PC and melanoma in the same person	FAMMM	*CDKN2A*
5. Personal history of ≥2 attacks of acute pancreatitis of unknown aetiology, a family history of pancreatitis, or early age of onset of chronic pancreatitis	HP	*PRSS1*

[a]*BRCA1*, *PALB2* and *ATM* mutation testing has also been suggested for FPC but the clinical utility in this setting is not well established (Syngal et al. 2015)

The potential benefits of genetic testing to the proband, although not typically applicable in the PC setting, include provision of the risk estimation of developing another cancer and implementation of risk reduction and preventative options (Whitcomb et al. 2015). The result can also impact treatment with consideration of a more extensive pancreatic resection as patients with inherited predisposition frequently show multi-focal disease, and patients may benefit from a precision or personalised treatment regimen, for example DNA damaging agent and/or PARP inhibitor chemotherapy if a BRCA1/2 or PALB2 mutation is identified. Genes with established clinical utility can be tested in family members and if found to carry the mutation can be considered for early detection strategies for PC as part of a research protocol and for other at-risk organs undergo surveillance and consider preventative intervention in accordance with published guidelines.

The increasing access to and performance of genomic sequencing in clinical and research settings has shown that a significant proportion of individuals with germline cancer predisposing mutations do not fulfil the classic clinical diagnostic criteria (Holter et al. 2015). This results from variability in the clinical genotype–phenotype correlation and incomplete penetrance leading to limited sensitivity and specificity of the classic diagnostic criteria. It is therefore imperative that the clinical features and guidelines undergo revision and modification and incorporate new findings as they arise. One approach is to integrate family history with specific genomic feature in the tumour (Carnevale and Ashworth 2015), for example, somatic hypermutation as a marker of microsatellite instability (The Cancer

Genome Atlas Network 2012) or somatic genomic instability as a marker of defective homologous recombination (Waddell et al. 2015). This approach may optimise identification of individuals with genetic predisposition to cancer and provide information on effective therapies, for example DNA damaging agents or PARP inhibitors in BRCA deficient tumours and immune checkpoint inhibitors in MMR-deficient tumours (Kaufman et al. 2015).

6.2 Surveillance and Management

The current evidence supporting PC surveillance strategies is at this time limited to observational studies (Syngal et al. 2015). Although screening has intuitive appeal with the potential benefit of early diagnosis and as a consequence improved treatment and prognosis, it has not been demonstrated that this translates into better outcome for patients. Demonstrating a reduction in mortality in a rare disease like hereditary PC will take several years and a large number of patients (Syngal et al. 2015). Screening can be associated with lead-time and length bias, which can lead to false conclusions of benefit (Grimes and Schulz 2002; Barratt et al. 2002). PCs diagnosed in screening trials have predominantly but not universally been resectable. However as with sporadic disease, resected patients often progress to metastatic disease due to subclinical metastatic disease at diagnosis (Al-Sukhni et al. 2012).

Expert opinion has recommended that individuals with a relative risk of 5–10-fold compared to the general population should be considered for PC surveillance (Canto et al. 2013b; Del Chiaro et al. 2010) as summarised in Table 4. The majority of significant lesions are found in older patients (>65 years); in view of this, recent guidelines suggest screening begin at 50 years of age, or 10 years younger than the earliest age of PC diagnosis in kindreds. Patients with PJS should start surveillance at 35 years (Syngal et al. 2015). The majority of significant lesions are found in older patients in particular >65 years (Canto et al. 2013a).

Table 4 Summary of the Cancer of the Pancreas Screening (CAPS) consortium consensus statement of criteria for consideration of screening (Canto et al. 2013a)

Familial PC group
Individuals with three affected kindreds, of which at least one is an FDR
Individuals with at least two affected FDRs with PC
Individuals with two or more affected blood relatives with PC, with at least one affected FDR
Germline mutation carrier group
STK11 mutation carriers, regardless of family history of PC
CDKN2A carriers with one affected FDR
BRCA2 mutation carriers with one affected FDR
BRCA2 mutation carriers with two affected family members, neither of which is a FDR
PALB2 mutation carriers with one affected FDR
Mismatch repair gene mutation carriers with one affected FDR

Current PC screening trials are predominantly imaging based, which provides limited or no information on the biology of the lesion. Biomarkers, of which carbohydrate antigen 19.9 (CA19.9) is the only currently clinically used, have a poor sensitivity for small pancreatic tumours with only 50 % of tumours <3 cm having an elevated level (Steinberg 1990). As PC spreads outside the pancreas abnormalities that are not produced by or specific to PC cells accumulate such as inflammatory markers (Goggins 2011). These represent epiphenomena and are unlikely to provide prognostic or predictive value. In view of recent large-scale sequencing studies of PC, which highlight the significant heterogeneity of tumours, it brings into question whether it is possible to identify a "one-size-fits-all" biomarker of early PC. Other biomarkers in blood ((e.g. PAM4-based immunoassay) (Gold et al. 2010), MIC-1 (Koopmann et al. 2006), circulating-free DNA (Mulcahy et al. 1998) and microRNA (Liu et al. 2012)), pancreatic juice (Berthelemy et al. 1995) and cyst fluid (Jabbar et al. 2014), either alone or in combination require further prospective validation to determine their clinical utility.

In recent years, multiple PC surveillance programmes have been established and initial findings reported (as shown in Table 5). The primary modalities used include endoscopic ultrasound (EUS) and magnetic resonance imaging with/without magnetic resonance cholangiopancreatography (MRI/MRCP) as they do not involve radiation exposure. The sensitivity of these modalities to detect cystic pancreatic lesions is 93 % with EUS, 81 % with MRCP and 27 % by Computerised Tomography (CT) (Canto et al. 2012). The ability to detect PanIN is unknown but likely to be much lower due to the aforementioned limitations. Overall, the studies demonstrate that precursor lesions or invasive cancers can be demonstrated in a variable but significant proportion of at-risk individuals but no study has shown better outcomes for patients (Schneider et al. 2011b; Canto et al. 2012). The variable yield (1–50 %) is partly dependent on the definition of the target lesions, which range from early cancer and high-grade dysplastic precursor lesions to IPMN with low–intermediate dysplasia to PanIN with any grade of dysplasia. The prevalence of detectable neoplasia is also dependent on the risk in the population being studied, the modalities used, the duration of follow-up and the number that undergo definitive pathological assessment, i.e. surgical resection.

Therapeutic intervention if undertaken for precursor lesions in current clinical practice constitutes a pancreatic resection. Pancreatectomy for a precursor lesion with a low probability of progression is associated with significant morbidity and unlikely to change the outcome for the patient. Typically, the long-term survivors, after pancreatectomy for PC, are those with early-stage tumours (<2 cm and confined to the pancreas) and lymph node-negative cancers (Agarwal et al. 2008). However, even in this small group a high rate of nodal metastases and poor prognosis has been described (Franko et al. 2013). Currently, early-stage cancers along with the high-grade precursor lesions (IPMN, MCN and PanIN 3 and CIS), represent the best opportunity to reduce mortality from PC as they are likely to progress and are potentially curable. Improving our understanding of the inherited predisposition to PC will lead to more precise risk assessment and potentially better selection of candidates who will benefit from screening. Screening brings with it the

Table 5 Summary of PC screening trials using a predominantly imaging-based approach in high-risk individuals

Study	Risk category	Patients (n)	Follow-up (months)	Imaging modality	Findings				
					Yield	PC	IPMN	PanIN 2–3	Other
Brentnall et al. (1999) Ann Int Med	FPC	14	15	CT, EUS, ERCP ± KRAS analysis in pancreatic juice	50 %	–	–	7[a]	–
Kimmey et al. (2002) Gastrointest Endosc	FPC	46		EUS, ERCP	26 %	–	–	12[a]	–
Canto et al. (2004) Clin Gastro Hepatol	FPC, PJS	38	22	EUS	5 %	1	1	–	–
Canto et al. (2006) Clin Gastro Hepatol	FPC, PJS	78	12	EUS, CT	10 %	1	6	1	–
Poley et al. (2009) Am J Gastro	FPC, PJS, Other syndromes with ≥2 affected (BRCA, p16, p53, HP)	44	Initial finding	EUS	23 %	3	7	–	–
Langer et al. (2009) Gut	FPC, BRCA2	76		EUS, MR/MRCP	0.76 %	–	1	–	–
Verna et al. (2010) Clin Cancer Res	FPC, BRCA2, CDKN2A	51	Initial finding	EUS, MRI	12 %	2	4	–	4 EPM[c]
Ludwig et al. (2011) Am J Gastro	FPC, BRCA	109		MRCP followed by EUS	8.30 %	1	5	2	–
Vasen et al. (2011) Gastroenterology	CDKN2A	79	48	MRI/MRCP	20 %	7	9	–	–
Al-Sukhni et al. (2011) J Gastrointest Surg	FPC, BRCA, PJS, CDKN2A, HP	262	50	MRI/MRCP	7.30 %	3	15	–	1 PNET
Schneider et al. (2011) Familial Cancer	FPC, BRCA, PALB2	72	44	EUS, MR/MRCP	13 %	1	7	2	–
Canto et al. (2012) Gastroenterology	FPC, BRCA2, PJS	216	29	EUS, CT, MRI	43 %	0	82	5[b]	3 PNET

[a]Widespread dysplasia; [b]5 pancreatic resection and all had multi-focal IPMN and PanIN; [c]EPM extrapancreatic malignancies—2 ovarian cancers (in BRCA-1/2 mutation carriers), 1 retroperitoneal carcinoid, 1 papillary thyroid cancer

risk of overtreatment and additional controlled trials are needed to determine the risks, benefits and optimal approaches to PC screening. Most would agree that a solid mass or cyst meeting current clinical guidelines should be resected, but patients frequently have widespread abnormalities on EUS complicating this decision.

7 Ongoing Research and Future Developments

Our traditional approach to understanding cancer predisposition emerged because of limitations in our ability to sequence individual genes, let alone exomes or genomes. The pragmatic reality of only testing those with a high risk of developing a malignancy based on clinical history of malignancy has generated an acquisition bias to our understanding of cancer predisposition today. This approach has been successful and allowed definition of several highly penetrant cancer predisposition genes and corresponding syndromes associated with PC, but most are predominantly characterised by malignancy in other organs. In some cases, e.g. BRCA mutations, this has led to significant improvements in clinical management. This "forward genetics" approach has served us well for many years, yet has instilled a dogma that may limit progress in the emerging "reverse genetics" era. Now that the challenges have completely shifted from the technological limitations of DNA sequencing, to the far greater challenge of understanding the biological basis of cancer predisposition and defining clinical validity and clinical utility, and then delivering an appropriate and viable benefit to the community.

Several challenges and knowledge gaps materialised by the broader availability and lower threshold for genomic sequencing. These include the following: (1) our current knowledge allows us to accurately predict the relative risk of developing a cancer in the setting of a family history. What we do not know is the risk of carriers without a family history. The interpretation of deleterious variants and estimation of risk in the absence of a related phenotype or family history is currently unknown, and there is little evidence to guide counselling and clinical decision making. Even in the presence of a potentially related phenotype, it may be difficult to assign causality to a deleterious variant and additional evidence may be required (MacArthur et al. 2014). (2) Current disease models propose a complex genetic predisposition pattern for most PC, which results from the convergence of several inherited and acquired (genetic and non-genetic) risk factors which interact and increment leading to progression from precursor lesion to invasive cancer (Whitcomb et al. 2015). Another challenge will be unravelling the contribution of multiple loci, including combinations of different genes, coexistent variants within genes and gene-environment interactions (Walsh et al. 2011; Couch et al. 2014). (3) Approximately 80 % of the heritability of PC remains unexplained, this has been termed the "missing heritability" which may lie in common but low-penetrant variants identified in genome-wide association studies, structural variants and epigenetics (Manolio et al. 2009). (4) Currently, we only utilise limited endpoints to assess for cancer predisposition: increased incidence and young age of onset. Some inherited deleterious variants may not substantially lower the age of onset, or dramatically increase the incidence of a particular cancer, but may lead to a poor prognosis cancer since the initiating mutation is still environmentally determined, but "progressor" mutations may already be present. To circumvent these hurdles, we need to identify other ways to gather the evidence required to impact on clinical management (MacArthur et al. 2014). We also need to define the role of other measures such as functional readouts, or surrogate measures of the consequences of specific genomic variants, an example is using whole-genome sequences to identify surrogates of genetic defects in tumours. Such examples include microsatellite instability and mutational signatures associated with defects in DNA maintenance. The latter is a specific signature of point mutations that are associated with defects in *BRCA1* and *BRCA2* function (Alexandrov et al. 2013). Variants associated with such surrogate measures can then focus experimental approaches to demonstrate the functional significance of these variants.

To circumvent these hurdles along with the substantial diversity of the human genome and the complexity of cancer genomes, infer that our traditional approach to identifying predisposition genes and quantifying relative risk will require even larger numbers. As we accumulate more cancer genomes through large-scale international efforts such as the International Cancer Genome Consortium (ICGC) (Hudson et al. 2010) and The Cancer Genome Atlas (TCGA), the germline sequences that accompany these genomes will provide insights into the prevalence of known predisposition loci in the germ line and perhaps point to novel candidates (Stadler et al. 2014). In addition, familial tumour registries such as the National Familial Pancreas Tumour Registry (NFPTR) (Klein 2013b) with detailed data and biospecimen acquisition provide an important resource for identification of candidate risk genes, clustering of related tumour types, the estimation of risk and the assessment of early detection strategies. Follow-up and biospecimen acquisition (germ line DNA, and where appropriate, tumour DNA) of patients and their families for index cases with variants of unknown significance may also bear fruit in the longer term. The concept of healthy controls of advanced age may be helpful and requires assessment; however, it is likely that only large-scale "knowledge bank" approaches that track generations over time with well-documented clinical histories will begin to unravel this complexity.

8 Summary and Key Points

- A total of 5–10 % of PCs have a heritable component based on family history.
- The majority (80 %) of the heritability is currently unexplained by known predisposition genes.
- Hereditary PC can occur in the setting of well-established inherited tumour predisposition syndromes, but the majority do not fulfil these criteria.

- Clinical genetic testing in probands fulfiling clinical criteria for genes with current direct clinical utility.
- Screening can be considered if >5 % lifetime risk in a ethically approved peer-reviewed research study.
- Improved genomic sequencing technology has led to greater throughput (cancer gene panels or exome/genome sequencing) with increased availability and lowering of testing thresholds. This posits several challenges and highlights knowledge gaps and advocated for new approaches to cancer predisposition assessment and incorporation into clinical care.

References

(AIHW) A. I. O. H. A. W. (2014) Australian cancer incidence and mortality (ACIM) books: pancreatic cancer. AIHW, Canberra. http://www.aihw.gov.au/acim-books%3E

Al-Sukhni W, Borgida A, Rothenmund H, Holter S, Semotiuk K, Grant R et al (2012). Screening for pancreatic cancer in a high-risk cohort: an eight-year experience. J Gastrointest Surg: official J Soc Surg Aliment Tract 16(4):771–783

Agarwal B, Correa AM, Ho L (2008) Survival in pancreatic carcinoma based on tumor size. Pancreas 36:e15–e20

Alexandrov LB, Nik-Zainal S, Wedge DC, Campbell PJ, Stratton MR (2013) Deciphering signatures of mutational processes operative in human cancer. Cell Rep 3:246–259

Anderson M, Zolotarevsky E, Cooper K et al (2012) Alcohol and tobacco lower the age of presentation in sporadic pancreatic cancer in a dose-dependent manner: a multicenter study. Am J Gastroenterol 107:1730–1739. doi:10.1038/ajg.2012.288 Epub 2012 Aug 28

Arslan AA, Helzlsouer KJ, Kooperberg C et al (2010) Anthropometric measures, body mass index, and pancreatic cancer: a pooled analysis from the Pancreatic Cancer Cohort Consortium (PanScan). Arch Intern Med 170:791–802

Axilbund JE, Argani P, Kamiyama M et al (2009) Absence of germline BRCA1 mutations in familial pancreatic cancer patients. Cancer Biol Ther 8:131–135

Barratt A, Mannes P, Irwig L, Trevena L, Craig J, Rychetnik L (2002) Cancer screening. J Epidemiol Commun Health 56:899–902

Barton J, Schnelldorfer T, Lohse C et al (2011) Patterns of pancreatic resection differ between patients with familial and sporadic pancreatic cancer. J Gastrointest Surg 15:836–842. doi:10.1007/s11605-011-1417-x Epub 2011 Feb 26

Bartsch D, Kress R, Sina-Frey M et al (2004) Prevalence of familial pancreatic cancer in Germany. Int J Cancer 110:902–906

Bartsch D, Gress T, Langer P (2012) Familial pancreatic cancer–current knowledge. Nat Rev Gastroenterol Hepatol 9:445–453. doi:10.1038/nrgastro.2012.111 Epub 2012 Jun 5

Beggs AD, Latchford AR, Vasen HFA et al (2010) Peutz-Jeghers syndrome: a systematic review and recommendations for management. Gut 59:975–986

Berthelemy P, Bouisson M, Escourrou J et al (1995) Identification of K-ras mutations in pancreatic juice in the early diagnosis of pancreatic cancer. Ann Intern Med 123:188–191

Birch JM, Alston RD, McNally R et al (2001) Relative frequency and morphology of cancers in carriers of germline TP53 mutations. Oncogene 20:4621–4628

Bosetti C, Lucenteforte E, Silverman DT et al (2012) Cigarette smoking and pancreatic cancer: an analysis from the International Pancreatic Cancer Case-Control Consortium (Panc4). Ann Oncol 23:1880–1888

Brand RE, Lerch MM, Rubinstein WS et al (2007) Advances in counselling and surveillance of patients at risk for pancreatic cancer. Gut 56:1460–1469

Breast Cancer Linkage Consortimu (1999) Cancer risks in BRCA2 mutation carriers. J Natl Cancer Inst 91:1310–1316

Brentnall T, Bronner M, Byrd D, Haggitt R, Kimmey M (1999). Early diagnosis and treatment of pancreatic dysplasia in patients with a family history of pancreatic cancer. Ann Intern Med 131 (4):247–255

Brentnall TA, Lai LA, Coleman J et al (2012) Arousal of cancer-associated stroma: overexpression of palladin activates fibroblasts to promote tumor invasion. PLoS ONE 7:e30219

Brose MS, Rebbeck TR, Calzone KA et al (2002) Cancer risk estimates for BRCA1 mutation carriers identified in a risk evaluation program. J Natl Cancer Inst 94:1365–1372

Brune K, Lau B, Palmisano E, Canto M, Goggins M, Hruban R et al (2010). Importance of age of onset in pancreatic cancer kindreds. J Natl Cancer Inst 102(2):119–26. doi: 10.1093/jnci/djp466. Epub 2010 Jan 12

Canto M, Goggins M, Hruban R, Petersen G, Giardiello F, Yeo C et al (2006). Screening for early pancreatic neoplasia in high-risk individuals: a prospective controlled study. Clin Gastroenterol Hepatol 4(6):766–781; quiz 665. Epub 2006 May 6

Canto M, Goggins M, Yeo C, Griffin C, Axilbund J, Brune K, et al (2004). Screening for pancreatic neoplasia in high-risk individuals: an EUS-based approach. Clin Gastroenterol Hepatol 2(7):606–621

Canto M, Hruban R, Fishman E, Kamel I, Schulick R, Zhang Z et al (2012). Frequent detection of pancreatic lesions in asymptomatic high-risk individuals. Gastroenterology 142(4):796–804; quiz e14-5. doi: 10.1053/j.gastro.2012.01.005. Epub Jan 12.

Canto MI, Harinck F, Hruban RH et al (2013a) International Cancer of the Pancreas Screening (CAPS) consortium summit on the management of patients with increased risk for familial pancreatic cancer. Gut 62:339–347

Canto MI, Harinck F, Hruban RH et al (2013b) International Cancer of the Pancreas Screening (CAPS) consortium summit on the management of patients with increased risk for familial pancreatic cancer. Gut 62:339–347

Carnevale J, Ashworth A (2015) Assessing the Significance of BRCA1 and BRCA2 mutations in pancreatic cancer. J Clin Oncol JCO 2015 OCT 1; 33(28):3080–3081

Chetty R, Salahshor S, Bapat B et al (2005) Intraductal papillary mucinous neoplasm of the pancreas in a patient with attenuated familial adenomatous polyposis. J Clin Pathol 58:97–101

Cote M, Schenk M, Schwartz A et al (2007) Risk of other cancers in individuals with a family history of pancreas cancer. J Gastrointest Cancer. 38:119–126. doi:10.1007/s12029-008-9022-2

Cotterchio M, Lowcock E, Hudson TJ et al (2014) Association between allergies and risk of pancreatic cancer. Cancer Epidemiol Biomarkers Prev

Couch F, Johnson M, Rabe K et al (2007a) The prevalence of BRCA2 mutations in familial pancreatic cancer. Cancer Epidemiol Biomarkers Prev 16:342–346

Couch FJ, Johnson MR, Rabe KG et al (2007b) The prevalence of BRCA2 mutations in familial pancreatic cancer. Cancer Epidemiol Biomarkers Prev 16:342–346

Couch FJ, Hart SN, Sharma P et al (2014) Inherited mutations in 17 breast cancer susceptibility genes among a large triple-negative breast cancer cohort unselected for family history of breast cancer. J Clin Oncol

del Chiaro M, Zerbi A, Capurso G et al (2010) Familial pancreatic cancer in Italy. Risk assessment, screening programs and clinical approach: a position paper from the Italian Registry. Dig Liver Dis 42:597–605

Duell EJ, Lucenteforte E, Olson SH et al (2012) Pancreatitis and pancreatic cancer risk: a pooled analysis in the International Pancreatic Cancer Case-Control Consortium (PanC4). Ann Oncol 23:2964–2970

Eldridge RC, Gapstur SM, Newton CC et al (2011) Jewish ethnicity and pancreatic cancer mortality in a large U.S. Cohort Cancer Epidemiol Biomarkers Prev 20:691–698

Ferlay JSI, Ervik M, Dikshit R et al (2013) Globocan 2012 v1.0, cancer incidence and mortality worldwide: IARC cancerbase no. 11 [Internet]. International Agency for Research on Cancer, Lyon, France. Available from: http://globocan.iarc.fr. Accessed on 14 Dec 2015

Ferrone CR, Levine DA, Tang LH et al (2009) BRCA germline mutations in Jewish patients with pancreatic adenocarcinoma. J Clin Oncol 27:433–438

Franko J, Hugec V, Lopes T, Goldman C (2013) Survival Among Pancreaticoduodenectomy Patients Treated for Pancreatic Head Cancer <1 or 2 cm. Ann Surg Oncol 20:357–361

Garber JE, Goldstein AM, Kantor AF et al (1991) Follow-up study of twenty-four families with Li-Fraumeni syndrome. Cancer Res 51:6094–6097

Genkinger JM, Spiegelman D, Anderson KE et al (2009) Alcohol intake and pancreatic cancer risk: a pooled analysis of fourteen cohort studies. Cancer Epidemiol Biomarkers Prev 18:765–776

Ghadirian P, Boyle P, Simard A et al (1991) Reported family aggregation of pancreatic cancer within a population-based case-control study in the Francophone community in Montreal. Can Int J Pancreatol 10:183–196

Ghiorzo P, Fornarini G, Sciallero S et al (2012) CDKN2A is the main susceptibility gene in Italian pancreatic cancer families. J Med Genet 49:164–170

Giardiello FM, Offerhaus GJ, Lee DH, Krush AJ, Tersmette AC, Booker SV, Kelley NC, Hamilton SR (1993) Increased risk of thyroid and pancreatic carcinoma in familial adenomatous polyposis. Gut 34:1394–1396

Goggins M (2011) Markers of pancreatic cancer: working toward early detection. Clin Cancer Res 17:635–637

Goggins M, Schutte M, Lu J et al (1996) Germline BRCA2 gene mutations in patients with apparently sporadic pancreatic carcinomas. Cancer Res 56:5360–5364

Gold DV, Goggins M, Modrak DE et al (2010) Detection of early-stage pancreatic adenocarcinoma. Cancer Epidemiol Biomarkers Prev 19:2786–2794

Grant RC, Selander I, Connor AA et al (2014) Prevalence of germline mutations in cancer predisposition genes in patients with pancreatic cancer. Gastroenterology

Grimes DA, Schulz KF (2002) Uses and abuses of screening tests. Lancet 359:881–884

Groden J, Thliveris A, Samowitz W et al (1991) Identification and characterization of the familial adenomatous polyposis coli gene. Cell 66:589–600

Hahn S, Greenhalf B, Ellis I et al (2003) BRCA2 germline mutations in familial pancreatic carcinoma. J Natl Cancer Inst 95:214–221

Hampel H, Bennett RL, Buchanan A et al (2014) A practice guideline from the American College of Medical Genetics and Genomics and the National Society of Genetic Counselors: referral indications for cancer predisposition assessment. Genet Med

Hearle N, Schumacher V, Menko FH et al (2006) Frequency and spectrum of cancers in the Peutz-Jeghers syndrome. Clin Cancer Res 12:3209–3215

Hemminki K, Li X (2003) Familial and second primary pancreatic cancers: a nationwide epidemiologic study from Sweden. Int J Cancer 103:525–530

Holter S, Borgida A, Dodd A et al (2015) Germline BRCA mutations in a large clinic-based cohort of patients with pancreatic adenocarcinoma. J Clin Oncol

Howes N, Lerch MM, Greenhalf W et al (2004) Clinical and genetic characteristics of hereditary pancreatitis in Europe. Clin Gastroenterol Hepatol 2:252–261

Hruban RH, Goggins M, Parsons J, Kern SE (2000) Progression model for pancreatic cancer. Clin Cancer Res 6:2969–2972

Hruban RH, Takaori K, Klimstra DS et al (2004) An illustrated consensus on the classification of pancreatic intraepithelial neoplasia and intraductal papillary mucinous neoplasms. Am J Surg Pathol 28:977–987

Hruban RH, Maitra A, Goggins M (2008) Update on pancreatic intraepithelial neoplasia. Int J Clin Experimen Pathol 1:306

Hruban R, Canto M, Goggins M, Schulick R, Klein A (2010) Update on familial pancreatic cancer. Adv Surg 44:293–311

Hudson TJ, Anderson W, Artez A et al (2010) International network of cancer genome projects. Nature 464:993–998
Iqbal J, Ragone A, Lubinski J et al (2012) The incidence of pancreatic cancer in BRCA1 and BRCA2 mutation carriers. Br J Cancer 107:2005–2009
Jabbar KS, Verbeke C, Hyltander AG et al (2014) Proteomic mucin profiling for the identification of cystic precursors of pancreatic cancer J National Cancer Institute 106
Jones S, Hruban RH, Kamiyama M et al (2009) Exomic sequencing identifies PALB2 as a pancreatic cancer susceptibility gene. Science 324:217
Kastrinos F, Mukherjee B, Tayob N et al (2009) Risk of pancreatic cancer in families with Lynch syndrome. JAMA 302:1790–1795
Kaufman B, Shapira-Frommer R, Schmutzler RK et al (2015) Olaparib Monotherapy in Patients With Advanced Cancer and a Germline BRCA1/2 Mutation. J Clin Oncol 33:244–250
Kimmey M, Bronner M, Byrd D, Brentnall T (2002). Screening and surveillance for hereditary pancreatic cancer. Gastrointest Endosc 56(4 Suppl):S82–6
Klein A (2013a) Identifying people at a high risk of developing pancreatic cancer. Nat Rev Cancer 13:66–74. doi:10.1038/nrc3420 Epub 2012 Dec 6
Klein AP (2013b) Identifying people at a high risk of developing pancreatic cancer. Nat Rev Cancer 13:66–74
Klein AP, Beaty TH, Bailey-Wilson JE et al (2002) Evidence for a major gene influencing risk of pancreatic cancer. Genet Epidemiol 23:133–149
Klein AP, Brune KA, Petersen GM et al (2004) Prospective risk of pancreatic cancer in familial pancreatic cancer kindreds. Cancer Res 64:2634–2638
Koopmann J, Rosenzweig CNW, Zhang Z et al (2006) Serum markers in patients with resectable pancreatic adenocarcinoma: macrophage inhibitory cytokine 1 versus CA19-9. Clin Cancer Res 12:442–446
Korsse SE, Harinck F, van Lier MGF et al (2013) Pancreatic cancer risk in Peutz-Jeghers syndrome patients: a large cohort study and implications for surveillance. J Med Genet 50:59–64
Kuiper RP, Vissers LE, Venkatachalam R et al (2011) Recurrence and variability of germline EPCAM deletions in Lynch syndrome. Hum Mutat 32:407–414
Lal G, Liu G, Schmocker B et al (2000) Inherited predisposition to pancreatic adenocarcinoma: role of family history and germ-line p16, BRCA1, and BRCA2 mutations. Cancer Res 60:409–416
Langer P, Kann PH, Fendrich V, Habbe N, Schneider M, Sina M et al (2009). Five years of prospective screening of high-risk individuals from families with familial pancreatic cancer. Gut 58(10):1410–1418
Lennon AM, Wolfgang CL, Canto MI et al (2014) The early detection of pancreatic cancer: what will it take to diagnose and treat curable pancreatic neoplasia? Cancer Res 74:3381–3389
Leonardi G, Marchi S, Falconi M et al (2012) "PancPro" as a tool for selecting families eligible for pancreatic cancer screening: an Italian study of incident cases. Dig Liver Dis 44:585–588
Li FP, Fraumeni JJF (1969) Soft-tissue sarcomas, breast cancer, and other neoplasmsa familial syndrome? Ann Intern Med 71:747–752
Li FP, Fraumeni JF Jr., Mulvihill JJ et al (1988) A cancer family syndrome in twenty-four kindreds. Cancer Res 48:5358–5362
Li D, Tang H, Hassan MM et al (2011) Diabetes and risk of pancreatic cancer: a pooled analysis of three large case-control studies. Cancer Causes Control 22:189–197
Ligtenberg MJ, Kuiper RP, Chan TL et al (2009) Heritable somatic methylation and inactivation of MSH2 in families with Lynch syndrome due to deletion of the 3' exons of TACSTD1. Nat Genet 41:112–117
Liu R, Chen X, Du Y et al (2012) Serum microRNA expression profile as a biomarker in the diagnosis and prognosis of pancreatic cancer. Clin Chem 58:610–618

Lowenfels AB, Maisonneuve P, Dimagno EP et al (1997) Hereditary pancreatitis and the risk of pancreatic cancer. International Hereditary Pancreatitis Study Group. J Natl Cancer Inst 89:442–446

Lowenfels AB, Maisonneuve P, Whitcomb DC et al (2001) Cigarette smoking as a risk factor for pancreatic cancer in patients with hereditary pancreatitis. JAMA 286:169–170

Lu KH, Wood ME, Daniels M et al (2014) American society of clinical oncology expert statement: collection and use of a cancer family history for oncology providers. J Clin Oncol 32:833–840

Lucas AL, Shakya R, Lipsyc MD et al (2013) High prevalence of BRCA1 and BRCA2 germline mutations with loss of heterozygosity in a series of resected pancreatic adenocarcinoma and other neoplastic lesions. Clin Cancer Res 19:3396–3403

Ludwig E, Olson SH, Bayuga S, Simon J, Schattner MA, Gerdes H et al (2011). Feasibility and yield of screening in relatives from familial pancreatic cancer families. Am J Gastroenterol 106 (5):946–954

Lynch H, Fitzsimmons M, Smyrk T et al (1990) Familial pancreatic cancer: clinicopathologic study of 18 nuclear families. Am J Gastroenterol 85:54–60

Macarthur DG, Manolio TA, Dimmock DP et al (2014) Guidelines for investigating causality of sequence variants in human disease. Nature 508:469–476

Manolio TA, Collins FS, Cox NJ et al (2009) Finding the missing heritability of complex diseases. Nature 461:747–753

McFaul C, Greenhalf W, Earl J et al (2006) Anticipation in familial pancreatic cancer. Gut. 55:252–258 Epub 2005 Jun 21

McGarrity TJ, Amos C, Frazier ML et al (2013) Peutz-Jeghers Syndrome. 2001 Feb 23 (Updated 2013 Jul 25). In: Pagon RA, Adam MP, Ardinger HH et al (eds) GeneReviews® [Internet]. University of Washington, Seattle (WA), 1993–2014. Available from: http://www.ncbi.nlm.nih.gov/books/NBK1266/

Moran A, O'Hara C, Khan S et al (2012) Risk of cancer other than breast or ovarian in individuals with BRCA1 and BRCA2 mutations. Fam Cancer 11:235–242. doi:10.1007/s10689-011-9506-2

Mulcahy HE, Lyautey J, Lederrey C et al (1998) A prospective study of K-ras mutations in the plasma of pancreatic cancer patients. Clin Cancer Res 4:271–275

Murphy KM, Brune KA, Griffin C et al (2002) Evaluation of candidate genes MAP2K4, MADH4, ACVR1B, and BRCA2 in familial pancreatic cancer: deleterious BRCA2 mutations in 17 %. Cancer Res 62:3789–3793

National Comprehensive Cancer Network guidelines for prevention, detection and risk reduction. Genetic/familial high-risk assessment: Breast and ovarian version 2.2015.www.nccn.org/professionals/physician_gls/f_guidelines.asp. Accessed 15th December 2015

Olson S, Kurtz R (2013) Epidemiology of pancreatic cancer and the role of family history. J Surg Oncol 107:1–7. doi:10.1002/jso.23149 Epub 2012 May 15

Ozcelik H, Schmocker B, di Nicola N et al (1997) Germline BRCA2 6174delT mutations in Ashkenazi Jewish pancreatic cancer patients. Nat Genet 16:17–18

Petersen GM, de Andrade M, Goggins M et al (2006) Pancreatic cancer genetic epidemiology consortium. Cancer Epidemiol Biomarkers Prev 15:704–710

Pogue-Geile KL, Chen R, Bronner MP et al (2006) Palladin mutation causes familial pancreatic cancer and suggests a new cancer mechanism. PLoS Med 3:e516

Poley JW, Kluijt I, Gouma DJ, Harinck F, Wagner A, Aalfs C et al (2009). The Yield of First-Time Endoscopic Ultrasonography in Screening Individuals at a High Risk of Developing Pancreatic Cancer. Am J Gastroenterol 104(9):2175–2181

Raimondi S, Maisonneuve P, Lowenfels A (2009) Epidemiology of pancreatic cancer: an overview. Nat Rev Gastroenterol Hepatol. 6:699–708. doi:10.1038/nrgastro.2009.177 Epub 2009 Oct 6

Rebours V, Boutron-Ruault MC, Schnee M et al (2009) The natural history of hereditary pancreatitis: a national series. Gut 58:97–103

Risch HA, McLaughlin JR, Cole DE et al (2006) Population BRCA1 and BRCA2 mutation frequencies and cancer penetrances: a kin-cohort study in Ontario, Canada. J Natl Cancer Inst 98:1694–1706

Roberts N, Jiao Y, Yu J et al (2012a) ATM mutations in patients with hereditary pancreatic cancer. Cancer Discov 2:41–46. doi:10.1158/2159-8290.CD-11-0194 Epub 2011 Dec 29

Roberts NJ, Jiao Y, Yu J et al (2012b) ATM mutations in patients with hereditary pancreatic cancer. Cancer Discov 2:41–46

Ruijs MW, Verhoef S, Rookus MA et al (2010) TP53 germline mutation testing in 180 families suspected of Li–Fraumeni syndrome: mutation detection rate and relative frequency of cancers in different familial phenotypes. J Med Genet 47:421–428

Rutter JL, Bromley CM, Goldstein AM et al (2004) Heterogeneity of risk for melanoma and pancreatic and digestive malignancies. Cancer 101:2809–2816

Ryan DP, Hong TS, Bardeesy N (2014) Pancreatic adenocarcinoma. N Engl J Med 371:1039–1049

Schneider R, Slater E, Sina M et al (2011a) German national case collection for familial pancreatic cancer (FaPaCa): ten years experience. Fam Cancer 10:323–330. doi:10.1007/s10689-010-9414-x

Schneider R, Slater EP, Sina M et al (2011b) German national case collection for familial pancreatic cancer (FaPaCa): ten years experience. Fam Cancer 10:323–330

Shi C, Hruban RH, Klein AP (2009) Familial pancreatic cancer. Arch Pathol Lab Med 133:365–374

Skudra S, Staka A, Pukitis A et al (2007) Association of genetic variants with pancreatic cancer. Cancer Genet Cytogenet 179:76–78

Stadler ZK, Schrader KA, Vijai J, Robson ME, Offit K (2014) Cancer genomics and inherited risk. J Clin Oncol 32:687–698

Steinberg W (1990) The clinical utility of the CA 19-9 tumor-associated antigen. Am J Gastroenterol 85:350–355

Syngal S, Brand RE, Church JM et al (2015) ACG clinical guideline: genetic testing and management of hereditary gastrointestinal cancer syndromes. Am J Gastroenterol 110:223–262

Tersmette A, Petersen G, Offerhaus G et al (2001) Increased risk of incident pancreatic cancer among first-degree relatives of patients with familial pancreatic cancer. Clin Cancer Res 7:738–744

The Cancer Genome Atlas Network (2012). Comprehensive molecular characterization of human colon and rectal cancer. Nature 487(7407):330–337

Thompson D, Easton D (2001) Variation in cancer risks, by mutation position, in BRCA2 mutation carriers. Am J Hum Genet 68:410–419

Tischkowitz MD, Sabbaghian N, Hamel N et al (2009) Analysis of the gene coding for the BRCA2-interacting protein PALB2 in familial and sporadic pancreatic cancer. Gastroenterology 137:1183–1186

Vasen HFA, Gruis NA, Frants RR et al (2000) Risk of developing pancreatic cancer in families with familial atypical multiple mole melanoma associated with a specific 19 deletion of p16 (p16-Leiden). Int J Cancer 87:809–811

Vasen HFA, van der Meulen–de Jong AE, de vos tot Nederveen Cappel WH, Oliveira J (2009) GROUP, O. B. O. T. E. G. W. 2009 Familial colorectal cancer risk: ESMO Clinical Recommendations. Annals of Oncology 20:iv51–iv53

Verna EC, Hwang C, Stevens PD, Rotterdam H, Stavropoulos SN, Sy CD et al (2010). Pancreatic cancer screening in a prospective cohort of high-risk patients: a comprehensive strategy of imaging and genetics. Clinical cancer research 16(20):5028–5037

Vasen HF, Wasser M, van Mil A, Tollenaar RA, Konstantinovski M, Gruis NA et al (2011). Magnetic resonance imaging surveillance detects early-stage pancreatic cancer in carriers of a p16-Leiden mutation. Gastroenterology 140(3):850–856

Waddell N, Pajic M, Patch A-M et al (2015) Whole genomes redefine the mutational landscape of pancreatic cancer. Nature 518:495–501

Walsh T, Casadei S, Lee MK et al (2011) Mutations in 12 genes for inherited ovarian, fallopian tube, and peritoneal carcinoma identified by massively parallel sequencing. Proc Natl Acad Sci 108:18032–18037

Wang W, Chen S, Brune KA et al (2007) PancPRO: risk assessment for individuals with a family history of pancreatic cancer. J Clin Oncol 25:1417–1422

Wang L, Brune K, Visvanathan K et al (2009a) Elevated cancer mortality in the relatives of patients with pancreatic cancer. Cancer Epidemiol Biomarkers Prev 18:2829–2834. doi:10.1158/1055-9965.EPI-09-0557 Epub 2009 Oct 20

Wang L, Brune KA, Visvanathan K et al (2009b) Elevated cancer mortality in the relatives of patients with pancreatic cancer. Cancer Epidemiol Biomark Prev 18:2829–2834

Whitcomb DC, Gorry MC, Preston RA et al (1996) Hereditary pancreatitis is caused by a mutation in the cationic trypsinogen gene. Nat Genet 14:141–145

Whitcomb DC, Shelton C, Brand RE (2015) Genetics and genetic testing in pancreatic cancer. Gastroenterology

Yachida S, Jones S, Bozic I et al (2010) Distant metastasis occurs late during the genetic evolution of pancreatic cancer. Nature 467:1114–1117

Zhen DB, Rabe KG, Gallinger S et al (2014) BRCA1, BRCA2, PALB2, and CDKN2A mutations in familial pancreatic cancer: a PACGENE study. Genet Med

Zogopoulos G, Rothenmund H, Eppel A et al (2007) The P239S palladin variant does not account for a significant fraction of hereditary or early onset pancreas cancer. Hum Genet 121:635–637

Diagnosis and Management of Hereditary Renal Cell Cancer

Fred H. Menko and Eamonn R. Maher

Abstract

Renal cell cancer (RCC) is the common denominator for a heterogeneous group of diseases. The subclassification of these tumours is based on histological type and molecular pathogenesis. Insight into molecular pathogenesis has led to the development of targeted systemic therapies. Genetic susceptibility is the principal cause of RCC in about 2–4 % of cases. Hereditary RCC is the umbrella term for about a dozen different conditions, the most frequent of which is von Hippel–Lindau disease. Here, we describe the main hereditary RCC syndromes, consider criteria for referral of RCC patients for clinical genetic assessment and discuss management options for patients with hereditary RCC and their at-risk relatives.

Keywords

Renal cell cancer · Hereditary · Molecular pathogenesis · Management

Contents

F.H. Menko (✉)
Antoni van Leeuwenhoek Hospital, The Netherlands Cancer Institute, Amsterdam, The Netherlands
e-mail: f.menko@nki.nl

E.R. Maher (✉)
Department of Medical Genetics, University of Cambridge, Cambridge, UK
e-mail: erm1000@medschl.cam.ac.uk

G. Pichert and C. Jacobs (eds.), *Rare Hereditary Cancers*,
Recent Results in Cancer Research 205, DOI 10.1007/978-3-319-29998-3_6

1 Introduction

The kidneys are composed of a parenchyma and collecting system. In this chapter, malignancies in adults that originate in the renal parenchyma are described. These are adenocarcinomas, referred to as renal cell carcinomas (RCCs). The incidence of renal cell cancer is variable across the world and even across Europe. A typical age distribution is given in Fig. 1. Mean renal cell cancer risk until the age of 80 years is about 1.2 for men and 0.7 for women.

Important risk factors for RCC are smoking, obesity and hypertension (Chow et al. 2010). RCC risk is increased for first-degree relatives of patients, and this reflects genetic predisposition factors (Clague et al. 2009). RCC is in fact the common denominator for a heterogeneous group of conditions, and aetiology differs for the various subgroups. RCC may be subclassified according to histology

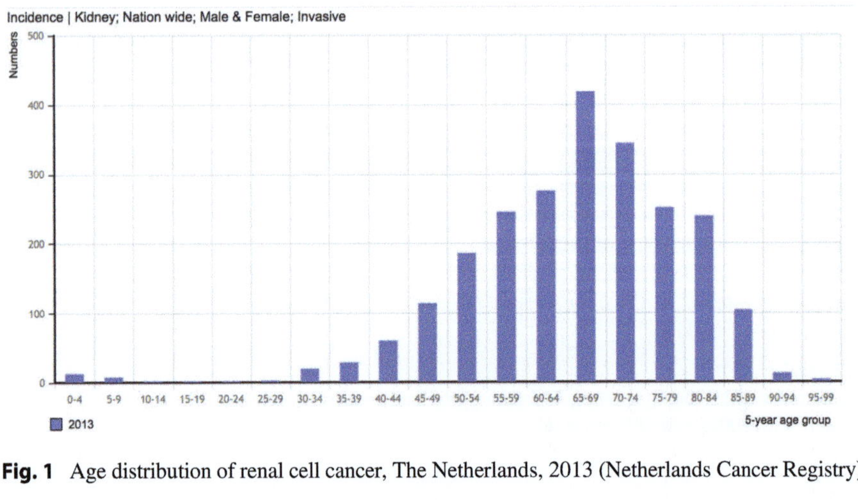

Fig. 1 Age distribution of renal cell cancer, The Netherlands, 2013 (Netherlands Cancer Registry)

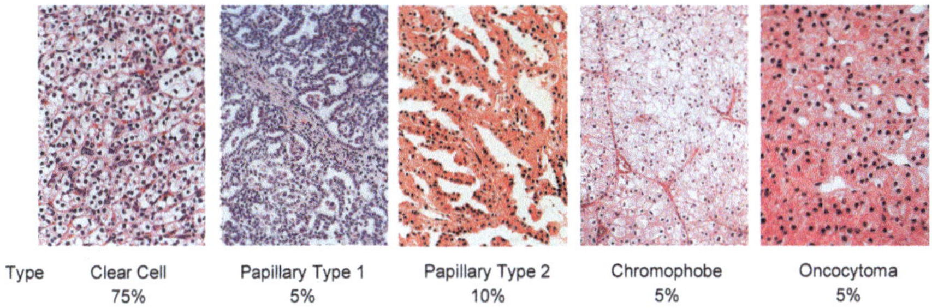

Fig. 2 The main histological subtypes of renal cell cancer and their frequencies (Linehan et al. 2003)

and molecular pathogenesis (Srigley et al. 2013; Shuch et al. 2015), and the current classification is a refinement of the WHO classification established in 2004 (Eble et al. 2004).

In Fig. 2, the main histological subtypes of RCC and their frequencies are depicted (in which oncocytoma is a benign tumour). Clear cell renal cell cancer (ccRCC) is the most common subtype.

In the past, almost all RCCs were diagnosed after clinical symptoms had developed. At present, however, many renal tumours are found coincidentally on abdominal imaging. About 80 % of small (≤4 cm) solid tumours found coincidentally are malignant and about 20 % are benign (Frank et al. 2003; Gill et al. 2010). The hereditary RCC syndromes were originally defined on the basis of clinical characteristics. From about 1990 onward, the development of DNA technology allowed the identification of the underlying genetic basis. Characteristics of hereditary RCC include early age at onset (Shuch et al. 2014; Fig. 3), bilateral and multifocal disease (Fig. 4), a typical histological pattern for each syndrome and other manifestations of the syndrome involved.

A classical study on hereditary RCC (Cohen et al.) in 1979 identified a chromosomal translocation involving chromosomes 3 and 8 in a kindred in which 10 patients in successive generations had renal cell cancer. Many years later, studies of families with von Hippel–Lindau (VHL) disease led to the identification of the *VHL* gene on the short arm of chromosome 3 (Latif et al. 1993). Subsequently, it was shown that somatic mutations in the *VHL* gene were involved in most sporadic clear cell RCCs. The VHL story has been outlined in detail by Richard et al. (2013) and Gossage et al. (2015). It illustrates how the study of rare hereditary tumour syndromes is important, not only for the families involved, but also for the clarification of signalling pathways in sporadic cancer.

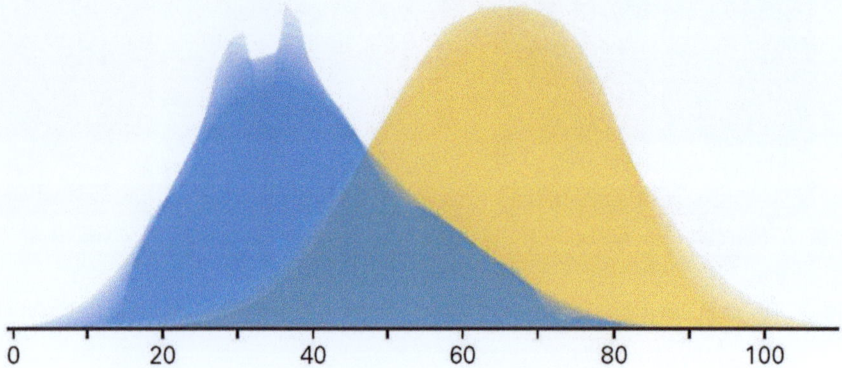

Fig. 3 Age distribution of RCC in hereditary syndromes (*left*) in comparison with the age distribution in the general population (*right*) (Shuch et al. 2014)

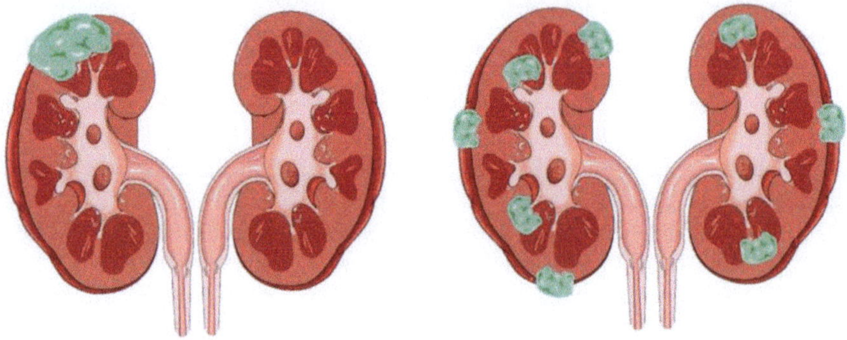

Fig. 4 *Left* A unilateral and unifocal sporadic renal cell cancer. *Right* Bilateral and multifocal hereditary renal cell cancers (Linehan et al. 2003)

2 Risk Assessment and Differential Diagnosis

About 2–4 % of RCC is due to high-penetrance germline mutations. The inheritance patterns of these syndromes are autosomal dominant with high penetrance, i.e. inherited from parent to child with a 50 % risk for children of affected individuals to inherit the causative gene defect and a high risk of clinical manifestations in mutation carriers. De novo germline mutations may also occur in which patients have unaffected parents. The main hereditary renal cell cancer syndromes are summarised in Table 1 (Maher 2011; Bausch et al. 2013).

Table 1 Hereditary renal cell cancer syndromes: an overview[a]

Syndrome	Inheritance	Gene	RCC risk	Histological subtype of renal tumour
von Hippel–Lindau disease	AD	*VHL*	70 %	Clear cell RCC
Birt–Hogg–Dubé syndrome	AD	*FLCN*	15 %	Chromophobe RCC, chromophobe RCC and oncocytoma, clear cell RCC
Hereditary leiomyomatosis and renal cell cancer	AD	*FH*	15 %	Aggressive form of papillary type 2 RCC
Hereditary papillary renal cell carcinoma	AD	*MET*	Increased	Papillary type 1 RCC
Paraganglioma-related disorders	AD	*SDHB* *SDHD*[b] *SDHC* *TMEM127*	15 %	Various types of RCC
Chromosome 3 translocations	Chromosomal	Chromosome 3	Increased (up to 70 %)	Clear cell RCC
PTEN hamartoma tumour syndrome	AD	*PTEN*	5–35 %	Mostly papillary RCC
Tuberous sclerosis complex	AD	*TSC1/TSC2*	2–4 %	Angiomyolipoma, clear cell RCC
Hereditary *BAP1* tumour syndrome	AD	*BAP1*	Increased	Clear cell RCC

[a]Based on Maher (2011) and Bausch et al. (2013)
[b]Inheritance is characterised by maternal imprinting: the syndrome will only become clinically manifest when the mutation is inherited from the father

2.1 von Hippel–Lindau Disease

In 1904, the ophthalmologist von Hippel examined a patient named Otto Mayer who had retinal haemangioblastoma (von Hippel 1904). Lindau, in 1926, noted that retinal haemangioblastomas occurred in combination with cerebellar haemangioblastomas (Lindau 1926). VHL disease is now defined as an autosomal dominant predisposition for haemangioblastomas of the retina and cerebellum, renal cell cancer, phaeochromocytoma, non-functioning pancreatic islet cell tumours and endolymphatic sac tumours. Renal, pancreatic and epididymal cysts also occur and can be useful clinical indicators to the diagnosis (e.g. in a patient with cerebellar haemangioblastoma) (Maher et al. 1990; Lonser et al. 2003; Maher et al. 2011). The full spectrum of clinical features in VHL is depicted in Fig. 5.

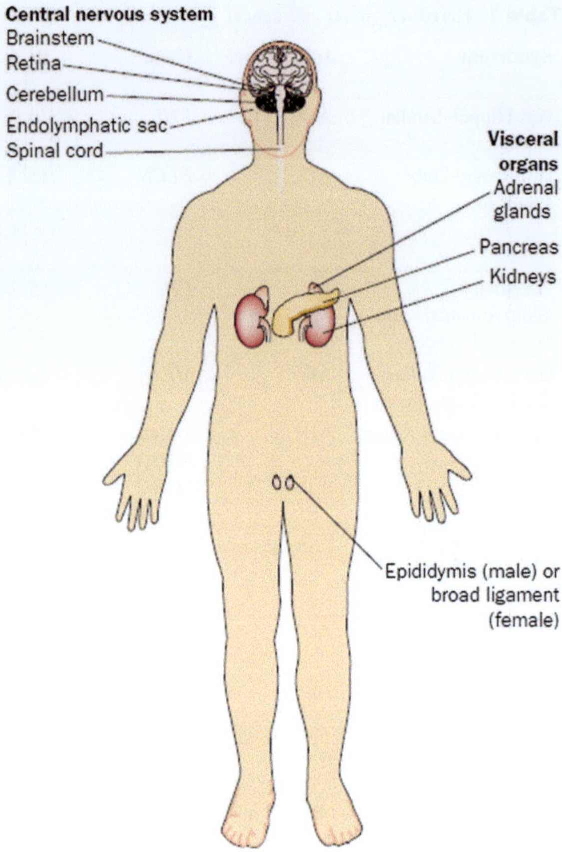

Fig. 5 Organs involved in von Hippel–Lindau disease (Lonser et al. 2003)

Renal cell cancer is a major complication of VHL with a risk of about 70 % by the age of 60 years and is characterised by early age at onset, bilateral occurrence, cystic appearance and clear cell histology.

2.2 Birt–Hogg–Dubé (BHD) Syndrome

In 1977, Birt, dermatologist, together with his colleagues Hogg, pathologist, and Dubé, internist, described a large family with characteristic benign skin pathology, now classified as fibrofolliculomas (Birt et al. 1977). In later years, lung cysts, spontaneous pneumothorax and RCC were recognised as core features of BHD, and in 2002, causative germline defects in the folliculin (*FLCN*) gene on chromosome 17p11.2 were identified (Nickerson et al. 2002; Schmidt 2013). Clinical expression is variable, and the lesions may remain unnoticed at medical examination (Leter et al. 2008; Menko et al. 2009) (Fig. 6).

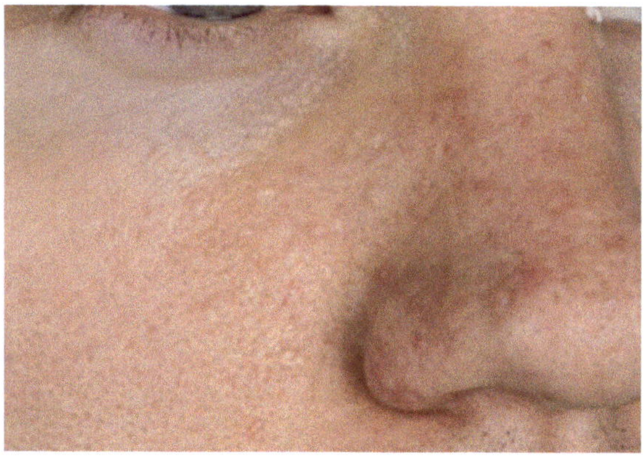

Fig. 6 Clinical appearance of inconspicuous fibrofolliculomas in a patient with BHD who also had spontaneous pneumothorax and renal cell cancer (Menko et al. 2013)

In 2009, the European BHD Consortium proposed clinical diagnostic criteria in which multiple fibrofolliculomas or a combination of characteristic pulmonary and renal features was considered to be diagnostic (Menko et al. 2009). In BHD, renal cancer risk is about 15 % (5–25 %) (Houweling et al. 2011). Based on four studies with a total number of 84 patients, most symptomatic RCCs are diagnosed between 35 and 55 years (range 20–83 years) (Pavlovich et al. 2002; Maffé et al. 2011; Houweling et al. 2011; Benusiglio et al. 2014). Many investigators found a typical RCC histology in BHD, consisting of a mixed type combining chromophobe with oncocytic elements, but other subtypes including ccRCC do occur.

Any association between BHD and cancers other than RCC is controversial. In some families, BHD may be associated with an increased colorectal cancer risk (Nahorski et al. 2010). Facial angiofibromas may resemble fibrofolliculomas, and therefore, tuberous sclerosis complex which also features lung and renal pathology should be considered in the differential diagnosis of BHD.

2.3 Hereditary Leiomyomatosis and Renal Cell Cancer

Hereditary leiomyomatosis and renal cell cancer [sometimes called Reed's syndrome, Reed et al. (1973)] is characterised by multiple cutaneous leiomyomas (histologically confirmed in at least one lesion), severe symptoms due to early-onset multiple uterine leiomyomas and early-onset type 2 papillary renal cell cancer (Alam et al. 2005; Smit et al. 2011; Gardie et al. 2011; Lehtonen 2011; Schmidt and Linehan 2014). The skin leiomyomas are illustrated in Fig. 7.

Recently, phaeochromocytoma/paraganglioma was identified as part of the HLRCC phenotype (Castro-Vega et al. 2014; Clark et al. 2014), and almost 8 % of patients with HLRCC show nodular adrenal hyperplasia (Shuch et al. 2013a). Among 103 published cases with HLRCC-associated renal cell cancer, mean age at diagnosis was 41 years with a wide range of 10–91 years. In 7 % of cases, RCC was diagnosed before the age of 20 years (Menko et al. 2014). In HLRCC type 2

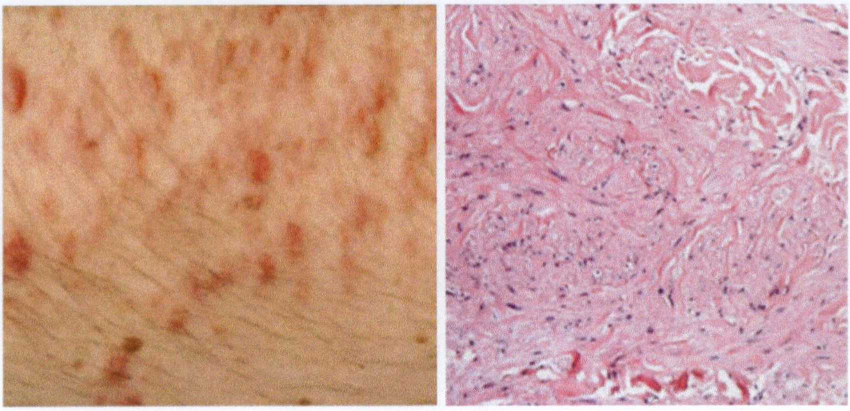

Fig. 7 HLRCC: the clinical and histological appearance of cutaneous leiomyomas (Menko et al. 2014)

papillary renal cancer shows typical cytological features and an aggressive biological behaviour. It is presently classified as a separate entity, "HLRCC-associated renal cell cancer" (Srigley et al. 2013).

HLRCC is due to germline mutations in the *FH* (*fumarate hydratase*) gene on chromosome 1q which encodes one of the enzymes of the mitochondrial tricarboxylic acid (TCA) or Krebs cycle (Tomlinson et al. 2002). The accumulation of succinated proteins in tissues due to increased fumarate can be demonstrated by an immunohistochemical assay and this can be applied for diagnostic purposes (Bardella et al. 2011).

2.4 Hereditary Papillary Renal Cell Carcinoma

In 1994, Zbar et al. described a family with autosomal dominant predisposition for papillary renal cell cancer, and subsequently, nine additional families with HPRCC were identified (Zbar et al. 1995). The underlying gene defect was localised on chromosome 7q, and activating germline mutations in the *MET* (mesenchymal–epithelial transition factor) proto-oncogene were identified (Schmidt et al. 1997). Papillary renal cell cancer is subdivided into two main histological subtypes, types 1 and 2, based on the description by Delahunt and Eble (1997). In HPRCC, the papillary renal cancer is usually of the type 1 subtype.

At present, several dozen HPRCC families associated with *MET* mutations have been reported (Olivero et al. 1999; Schmidt et al. 2004; Salvi et al. 2008; Wadt et al. 2012).

2.5 Paraganglioma-Related Disorders

A number of disorders are characterised by the development of RCC and paraganglioma. In addition to VHL disease and HLRCC (see above) they include conditions with mutations in genes encoding subunits of succinate dehydrogenase (an enzyme that is upstream of fumarate hydratase in the Krebs/TCA cycle). Thus, *SDHB* mutation carriers are at increased risk for renal cell cancer (Ricketts et al. 2008), and RCC has also been described in carriers of *SDHC* and *SDHD* mutations (Ricketts et al. 2008, 2010, 2012; Evenepoel et al. 2015). Oncocytoma may also be associated with *SDHB* (Henderson et al. 2009). In the current classification of RCC, *SDHB*-associated RCC is classified as a separate entity (Srigley et al. 2013; Gill et al. 2014). Immunohistochemistry for SDHB expression is a sensitive investigation for identifying tumours likely to be associated with a germline *SDH* mutation (Van Nederveen et al. 2009; Gill et al. 2011; Papathomas et al. 2014). Recently, *TMEM127* mutations have been added to the list of causative gene defects (Qin et al. 2014).

2.6 Chromosome 3 Translocations

Since the report by Cohen et al. in 1979, a series of reports have confirmed the association between translocations involving chromosome 3 and renal cell cancer (Valle et al. 2005; McKay et al. 2011). Age at diagnosis varied widely, and tumours were often multifocal and bilateral. An association with thyroid cancer has been suggested by Li et al. (1993). However, in the absence of a family history of RCC or evidence of disruption of a specific tumour suppressor gene, chromosome 3 translocation carriers are not at high risk of developing RCC and do not need renal surveillance (Woodward et al. 2010).

Familial RCC has also been described in a family with a chromosomal translocation not involving chromosome 3, i.e. a chromosome 5;19 translocation (Wake et al. 2013).

2.7 *PTEN* Hamartoma Tumour Syndrome

In 1963, Lloyd and Dennis described a patient named Rachel Cowden, with a remarkable complex of clinical features, including mucocutaneous lesions, breast pathology and a multinodular goitre, and they named the condition Cowden's disease. After identification, in 1996, of underlying mutations in the *PTEN* gene localised on chromosome 10q23, it became clear that *PTEN* mutations could also be found in associated conditions presenting in childhood: Bannayan–Riley–Ruvalcaba syndrome (BRRS), Proteus-like syndrome and macrocephaly with autism and/or learning disability. In addition, these different syndromes could be present in one and the same family in which a germline *PTEN* mutation had been identified (Lachlan et al. 2007).

Therefore, these syndromes are now grouped together as *PTEN* hamartoma tumour syndrome (PHTS) (Mester and Eng 2015). PHTS is characterised by mucocutaneous features, macrocephaly and an increased risk for various malignancies including breast, non-medullary thyroid, endometrial, colorectal and renal cell cancers.

The reported renal cell cancer risk in PHTS has varied between <10 and >30 %, and this variation is probably due to differences in the ascertainment of families (Tan et al. 2012; Daniels et al. 2012; Bubien et al. 2013; Nieuwenhuis et al. 2014). Various histological RCC subtypes, mostly papillary, but also clear cell and chromophobe tumours, have been observed (Mester et al. 2012; Shuch et al. 2013b).

2.8 Tuberous Sclerosis Complex

Tuberous sclerosis complex (TSC) is a multisystem autosomal dominant syndrome, caused by germline mutations in the *TSC1* or *TSC2* gene. From childhood onward, clinical symptoms may involve the skin, eyes, brain, heart, lungs and kidneys. Characteristic lesions are facial angiofibromas, retinal hamartomas, hypomelanotic macules, cerebral tubers, cardiac rhabdomyomas in childhood and lymphangioleiomyomatosis (LAM) of the lungs. The main renal features include angiomyolipomas, renal cysts, polycystic renal disease and, infrequently, renal cell cancer. The RCC risk is about 2–4 % with a mean age at diagnosis of around 30 years. A variation of histological subtypes has been reported including mixed chromophobe oncocytic lesions. Less often other tumour types may occur (Crino et al. 2006; Curatolo et al. 2008; Yang et al. 2014).

For revised diagnostic criteria, surveillance and management options, the reader is referred to Northrup and Krueger (2013) and Krueger and Northrup (2013).

2.9 Hereditary *BAP1* Tumour Syndrome

Germline *BAP1* (BRCA1-associated protein 1) mutations lead to uveal melanoma, skin melanoma, atypical melanocytic tumours and mesothelioma. Recently, *BAP1* has been added to the list of renal cell cancer predisposition genes (Popova et al. 2013), and a family with a *BAP1* mutation and renal cell cancer as the only clinical manifestation has been described (Farley et al. 2013).

2.10 Other Hereditary Syndromes

Hyperparathyroidism jaw tumour syndrome (HPT-JT) is a rare autosomal dominant predisposition for hyperparathyroidism, due to germline mutations in the *HRPT2* (*CDC73*) gene (Jackson et al. 1990; Carpten et al. 2002). Various renal abnormalities have been reported in HPT-JT including renal cysts and hamartomas and a single case of papillary renal cell carcinoma. In addition, Wilms' tumour has been observed in HPT-JT (Teh et al. 1996; Haven et al. 2000; Bricaire et al. 2013). Germline mutations in *CDKN2B* have been associated with renal cell cancer in several families (Jafri et al. 2015). Finally, a hereditary predisposition for thyroid cancer and papillary renal cell cancer has been proposed (Malchoff et al. 2000).

2.11 Familial Non-syndromic RCC (FRCC)

FRCC refers to those patients and families with clinical characteristics of hereditary RCC (early age at diagnosis, bilateral disease, a positive family history) but without a known underlying syndrome. Tollefson et al. (2010) defined FRCC as the occurrence of RCC in a proband and a first- or second-degree family member, whereas Woodward et al. (2008) described clear cell FRCC as the occurrence of RCC in at least two close relatives with a confirmed history of clear cell RCC in at least one of these patients. The inheritance pattern of FRCC has not been established. Whereas autosomal recessive inheritance has been proposed (Hemminki and Li 2004), most kindreds show an autosomal dominant pattern (Woodward et al. 2008). FRCC is a diagnosis made by exclusion of a known hereditary syndrome, and most probably, FRCC represents a heterogeneous group of conditions. Notably, germline mutations in *FLCN* (the Birt–Hogg–Dubé syndrome gene), *SDHB* and *CDKN2B* have each been reported in patients with features of non-syndromic inherited RCC susceptibility such as familial, multicentric or early-onset RCC (Ricketts et al. 2008; Woodward et al. 2008; Jafri et al. 2015).

3 Genetic Testing

Until recently, genetic testing was based on a specific clinical diagnosis. For example, in a patient with a clinical diagnosis of VHL, the identification of a pathogenic *VHL* germline mutation would confirm the clinical diagnosis and would allow presymptomatic testing of at-risk relatives. However, a problem in diagnostic genetic testing is the variability of clinical phenotypes, and therefore, the possibility of a syndrome diagnosis in patients with RCC may be overlooked if some clinical features are absent. Features suggestive of a hereditary renal cell cancer syndrome and suggested referral criteria for formal genetic evaluation are summarised in Table 2 (based on Reaume et al. 2013).

Table 2 Characteristics of hereditary renal cell cancer syndromes and criteria for referral for formal genetic evaluation (based on Reaume et al. 2013)

Patient characteristics	
Renal cell cancer characteristics	Age at diagnosis ≤45 years Bilateral and/or multifocal RCC Non-clear cell histology
Additional syndromic characteristics	Skin abnormalities: fibrofolliculomas, leiomyomas, angiofibromas Pneumothorax Phaeochromocytoma/paraganglioma
Family characteristics	
Renal cell cancer	Any form of RCC in a first- or second-degree relative, especially with age at diagnosis ≤45 years, bilateral and/or multifocal tumours, non-clear cell histology
Additional characteristics	Syndromic features: skin abnormalities: fibrofolliculomas, leiomyomas, angiofibromas Pneumothorax Phaeochromocytoma/paraganglioma

Recently, next-generation sequencing has been introduced in which panels of genes can be analysed in parallel. An example is RenalNext® developed by Ambry Genetics, in which the following 18 genes have been incorporated: *VHL*, *FLCN*, *FH*, *MET*, *SDHA*, *SDHB*, *SDHC*, *SDHD*, *PTEN*, *TSC1*, *TSC2*, *MLH1*, *MSH2*, *EPCAM*, *MSH6*, *PMS2*, *TP53* and *MITF*.

The possible advantages of these panels are obvious. However, these panels also have several disadvantages. First, different panels have been developed, and in some of these panels, genes have been incorporated which have a questionable association with renal cell cancer, for example, the DNA mismatch repair (MMR) genes, associated with Lynch syndrome. Germline mutations in MMR genes may lead to cancer of the pelvis and ureter, but any association with renal cell cancer is questionable.

Second, some of the tested genes may be involved in renal cell cancer but only as medium- or low-penetrance genes, for example *MITF*. Identification of this type of mutation may not fully explain the clinical phenotype. Third, DNA testing of a series of genes will often lead to the identification of variants of unknown clinical significance. Finally, the penetrance of the gene defects found by screening patients without classical features may not necessarily be the same as the penetrance of mutations found in the "classical" patients and families.

We would suggest to incorporate the following genes in a diagnostic panel for renal cell cancer with features suggesting hereditary disease (early-onset and/or bilateral/multifocal disease and/or non-clear cell histology and/or familial occurrence) and without evident syndromic features: *VHL*, *FLCN*, *FH*, *MET*, *SDHB*, *SDHC*, *SDHD* and karyotyping. Further testing for *BAP1* and *TMEM127* mutations might be considered in selected cases, but the more limited experience with these genes means that variant interpretation may be more difficult. The introduction of next-generation sequencing should be the subject of monitoring and evaluation (Domchek et al. 2013).

4 Management

Secondary prevention, i.e. early diagnosis and treatment, is a main goal of diagnosing a hereditary RCC tumour syndrome. For some disorders, such as VHL, renal screening is well established (in addition to screening for other manifestations (see Maher et al. 2011) and annual magnetic resonance imaging (MRI) scanning (MRI is more sensitive than renal ultrasonography and avoids the radiation associated with computerised tomography (CT) scanning) is performed from age 16 years. Small renal tumours are followed by MRI scans until they reach a diameter of 3 cm and then removed by a nephron-sparing approach. For BHD syndrome, a similar approach can be adopted (though from age 20 years). For HLRCC, a consensus statement suggested that annual MRI scans should be considered from age of 8–10 years (though the risk of RCC before 20 years is very low), and because of the aggressive nature of the tumours in this condition, small tumours are removed without delay (i.e. the "3-cm rule" used in VHL disease, and BHD syndrome is not applied). Also, though enucleation of tumours may be suitable for small RCC in VHL disease, BHD syndrome and HPRCC wide excision has been recommended for tumours due to HLRCC and *SDH* mutations (Barrisford et al. 2011; Stamatakis et al. 2013; Metwalli and Linehan 2014). Comprehensive screening protocols have been described for patients with Cowden's syndrome/germline *PTEN* mutations and suggest that renal imaging should be performed every 2 years from age 40 years (Ngeow and Eng 2015). There are standard surveillance schemes for SDH subunit mutation carriers, and renal surveillance can be incorporated into the abdominal imaging protocol employed for detecting phaeochromocytoma/paraganglioma. For SDH subunit mutation carriers and other rare forms of inherited RCC, there is a pressing need for outcome data from surveillance programmes in order to best inform the most appropriate surveillance strategy. For familial non-syndromic RCC without a detectable germline RCC gene mutation, a practical approach might be to offer annual renal ultrasound scans from age 35 years (or 10 years before the earliest age at onset of RCC in the family if there is early-onset RCC).

5 Summary

Hereditary RCC syndromes are clinically indicated by patient and family characteristics, notably young age at diagnosis (≤45 years of age), bilateral or multifocal disease, typical histology, a positive family history for RCC and, in addition, manifestations of specific syndromes.

For DNA-based diagnosis, next-generation sequencing has recently been introduced into clinical practice. Since hereditary renal cell cancer is the umbrella term for about a dozen different syndromes, the simultaneous analysis of a panel of genes has obvious advantages. However, introduction of these techniques also has potential disadvantages and therefore should be subjected to monitoring and evaluation.

Insight into the molecular pathogenesis of renal cell cancer was based on the meticulous study of rare hereditary tumour syndromes. The clarification of signalling pathways has led to targeted therapies for systemic treatment of sporadic RCC. For hereditary tumour syndromes, specific recommendations for local and systemic treatments apply.

6 Ongoing Research and Future Directions

Treatment of metastatic renal cell cancer is a fascinating subject, since new insights in molecular pathogenesis have allowed the development of targeted therapies. Most studies have been performed in sporadic ccRCC, and most targeted therapies have been developed for the treatment of ccRCCs.

Main players in this field are the von Hippel–Lindau tumour suppressor/hypoxia-inducible factor (HIF) pathway, in which HIF stimulates VEGF vascular endothelial growth factor, PDGF platelet-derived growth factor and EGF epidermal growth factor, and the mTOR pathway. Targeted therapies aimed at these signalling pathways include bevacizumab, pazopanib, axitinib, sunitinib, sorafenib, temsirolimus and everolimus (Linehan et al. 2010a, b; Hu et al. 2012; Ljungberg et al. 2013). The VHL/HIF signalling pathway in ccRCC and targeted therapies based on molecular pathogenesis are shown in Fig. 8.

Fewer studies have been performed in non-clear cell RCC. Insight into the HGF (hepatocyte growth factor)/MET pathway has led to targeted therapy of papillary renal cell cancer, for example, with foretinib, aimed at MET and VEGF (Albiges et al. 2014; Fay et al. 2014).

In cancer cells, glucose is preferably metabolised into lactate despite the presence of oxygen. This aerobic glycolysis in cancer cells is referred to as the "Warburg effect" (Otto Warburg 1883–1970). Recently, investigators have concentrated on the metabolic derangements in renal cell cancers, and forms of therapy have been developed which are based on the abnormal cellular metabolic processes, in particular glycolysis and the mitochondrial tricarboxylic acid or Krebs cycle (Linehan et al. 2010a, b; Linehan 2012).

Targeted therapies for the hereditary tumour syndromes have also been developed. For example, sunitinib has been investigated for the treatment of RCC and other syndromic lesions in VHL (Jonasch et al. 2011; Roma et al. 2015).

In hereditary leiomyomatosis and RCC due to germline *FH* (fumarate hydratase) mutations, the accumulation of fumarate may lead to the activation of HIF, increased angiogenesis and increased glycolysis (Bratslavsky et al. 2007; Sudarshan

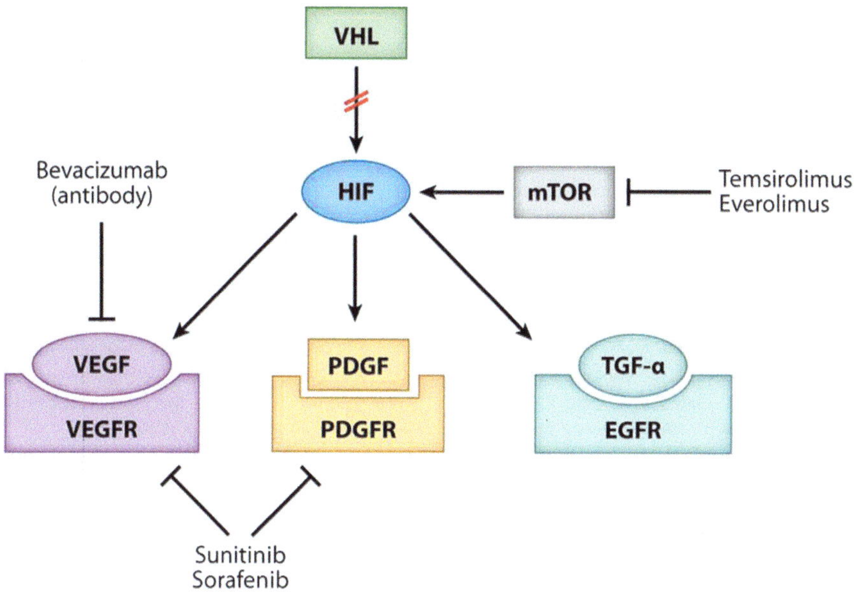

Fig. 8 The VHL/HIF signalling pathway in ccRCC and targeted therapies based on molecular pathogenesis.VEGF (vascular endothelial growth factor), PDGF (platelet-derived growth factor) and EGF (epidermal growth factor) (Linehan et al. 2010b)

et al. 2013). The folliculin defect in Birt–Hogg–Dubé syndrome has been associated with the disruption of multiple signalling pathways including the mTOR pathway, suggesting that mTOR inhibitors might be appropriate for the treatment of the rare cases of BHD syndrome with disseminated RCC (though topical rapamycin did not improve facial fibrofolliculomas). The *TSC1* or *TSC2* gene encodes hamartin and tuberin, respectively, and together these proteins also play a central role in the mTOR pathway. Rapamycin and analogues which inhibit mTOR are of proven benefit in reducing TSC-associated lesions including renal cell carcinoma (Pressey et al. 2010).

The PTEN protein is part of the PTEN-PI3K-AKT-mTOR signalling pathway, and in many sporadic tumours, *PTEN* is inactivated. Insight into the molecular pathogenesis of PHTS has led to the development of targeted treatment in PHTS.

There is hope that as the molecular basis of the various causes of inherited RCC is elucidated, precision therapies will be developed. Nevertheless, the optimal strategy would be early detection of tumours by cost-effective targeted screening. Due to the rarity of the syndromes described above, much emphasis should be put on multicenter and international studies for the collection of clinical, pathological and molecular data from carefully defined clinical cohorts.

References

Alam NA, Barclay E, Rowan AJ et al (2005) Clinical features of multiple cutaneous and uterine leiomyomatosis. An underdiagnosed tumor syndrome. Arch Dermatol 141:199–206

Albiges L, Guegan J, Le Formal A et al (2014) MET is a potential target across all papillary renal cell carcinomas: result from a large molecular study of pRCC with CGH array and matching gene expression array. Clin Cancer Res 20:3411–3421

Bardella C, El-Bahrawy M, Frizzell N et al (2011) Aberrant succination of proteins in fumarate hydratase-deficient mice and HLRCC patients is a robust biomarker of mutation status. J Pathol 225:4–11

Barrisford GW, Singer EA, Rosner IL et al (2011) Familial renal cancer: molecular genetics and surgical management. Int J Surg Oncol ID 658767

Bausch B, Jilg C, Gläsker S et al (2013) Renal cancer in von Hippel-Lindau disease and related syndromes. Nat Rev Nephrol 9:529–538

Benusiglio PR, Gad S, Massard C et al (2014) Case report: Expanding the tumour spectrum associated with the Birt-Hogg-Dubé cancer susceptibility syndrome. F1000Res 3:159

Birt AR, Hogg GR, Dubé WJ (1977) Hereditary multiple fibrofolliculomas with trichodiscomas and acrochordons. Arch Dermatol 113:1674–1677

Bratslavsky G, Sudarshan S, Neckers L et al (2007) Pseudohypoxic pathways in renal cell carcinoma. Clin Cancer Res 13:4667–4671

Bricaire L, Odou M-F, Cardot-Bauters C et al (2013) Frequent large germline *HRPT2* deletions in a French national cohort of patients with primary hyperparathyroidism. J Clin Endocrinol Metab 98:E403–E408

Bubien V, Bonnet F, Brouste V et al (2013) High cumulative risks of cancer in patients with *PTEN* hamartoma tumour syndrome. J Med Genet 50:255–263

Carpten JD, Robbins CM, Villablanca A et al (2002) *HRPT2*, encoding parafibromin, is mutated in hyperparathyroidism-jaw tumor syndrome. Nat Genet 32:676–680

Castro-Vega LJ, Buffet A, De Cubas AA et al (2014) Germline mutations in *FH* confer predisposition to malignant pheochromocytomas and paragangliomas. Hum Mol Genet 23:2440–2446

Chow W-H, Dong LM, Devesa SS (2010) Epidemiology and risk factors for kidney cancer. Nat Rev Urol 7:245–257

Clague J, Lin J, Cassidy A et al (2009) Family history and risk of renal cell carcinoma: results from a case-control study and systematic meta-analysis. Cancer Epidemiol Biomarkers Prev 18:801–807

Clark GR, Sciacovelli M, Gaude E et al (2014) Germline *FH* mutations presenting with pheochromocytoma. J Clin Endocrinol Metab 99:E2046–E2050

Cohen AJ, Li FP, Berg S et al (1979) Hereditary renal-cell carcinoma associated with a chromosomal translocation. N Engl J Med 301:592–595

Crino PB, Nathanson KL, Henske EP (2006) The tuberous sclerosis complex. N Engl J Med 355:1345–1356

Curatolo P, Bombardieri R, Jozwiak S (2008) Tuberous sclerosis. Lancet 372:657–668

Daniels MS, Rich T, Weissman S et al (2012) Lifetime cancer risks of *PTEN* mutation carriers. Clin Cancer Res 18:4213

Delahunt B, Eble N (1997) Papillary renal cell carcinoma: a clinicopathologic and immunohistochemical study of 105 tumors. Mod Pathol 10:537–544

Domchek SM, Bradbury A, Garber JE et al (2013) Multiplex genetic testing for cancer susceptibility: out on the high wire without a net? J Clin Oncol 31:1267–1270

Eble JN, Sauter G, Epstein JI et al (2004) Pathology and Genetics. Tumours of the Urinary System and Male Genital Organs. World Health Organization Classification of Tumours, IARC Press, Lyon

Evenepoel L, Papathomas TG, Krol N et al (2015) Toward an improved definition of the genetic and tumor spectrum associated with *SDH* germ-line mutations. Genet Med 17:610–620

Farley MN, Schmidt LS, Mester JL et al (2013) A novel germline mutation in *BAP1* predisposes to familial clear-cell renal cell carcinoma. Mol Cancer Res 11:1061–1071

Fay AP, Signoretti S, Choueiri TK (2014) MET as a target in papillary renal cell carcinoma. Clin Cancer Res 20:3361–3363

Frank I, Blute ML, Cheville JC et al (2003) Solid renal tumors: an analysis of pathological features related to tumor size. J Urol 170:2217–2220

Gardie B, Remenieras A, Kattygnarath D et al (2011) Novel *FH* mutations in families with hereditary leiomyomatosis and renal cell cancer (HLRCC) and patients with isolated type 2 papillary renal cell carcinoma. J Med Genet 48:226–234

Gill IS, Aron M, Gervais DA et al (2010) Small renal mass. N Engl J Med 362:624–634

Gill AJ, Pachter NS, Clarkson A et al (2011) Renal tumors and hereditary phaeochromocytoma-paraganglioma syndrome type 4. N Engl J Med 364:885–886

Gill AJ, Hes O, Papathomas T et al (2014) Succinate dehydrogenase (SDH)-deficient renal carcinoma: a morphologically distinct entity. A clinicopathologic series of 36 tumors from 27 patients. Am J Surg Pathol 38:1588–1602

Gossage L, Eisen T, Maher ER (2015) VHL, the story of a tumour suppressor gene. Nat Rev Cancer 15:55–64

Haven CJ, Wong FK, van Dam EW et al (2000) A genotypic and histopathological study of a large Dutch kindred with hyperparathyroidism-jaw tumor syndrome. J Clin Endocrinol Metab 85:1449–1454

Hemminki K, Li X (2004) Familial renal cell cancer appears to have a recessive component. J Med Genet 41:e58

Henderson A, Douglas F, Perros P et al (2009) SDHB-associated renal oncocytoma suggests a broadening of the renal phenotype in hereditary paragangliomatosis. Fam Cancer 8:257–260

Houweling AC, Gijezen LM, Jonker MA et al (2011) Renal cancer and pneumothorax risk in Birt-Hogg-Dubé syndrome; an analysis of 115 *FLCN* mutation carriers from 35 BHD families. Br J Cancer 105:1912–1919

Hu B, Lara PN Jr, Evans CP (2012) Defining an individualized treatment strategy for metastatic renal cancer. Urol Clin N Am 39:233–249

Jackson CE, Norum RA, Boyd SB et al (1990) Hereditary hyperparathyroidism and multiple ossifying jaw fibromas: a clinically and genetically distinct syndrome. Surgery 108:1006–1013

Jafri M, Wake NC, Ascher DB et al (2015) Germline mutations in the *CDKN2B* tumor suppressor gene predispose to renal cell carcinoma. Cancer Discov 5:723–729

Jonasch E, McCutcheon IE, Waguespack SG et al (2011) Pilot trial of sunitinib therapy in patients with von Hippel-Lindau disease. Ann Oncol 22:2661–2666

Krueger DA, Northrup H (2013) Tuberous sclerosis complex surveillance and management: recommendations of the 2012 International Tuberous Sclerosis Complex Consensus Conference. Pediatr Neurol 49:255–265

Lachlan KL, Lucassen AM, Bunyan D et al (2007) Cowden syndrome and Bannayan-Riley-Ruvalcaba syndrome represent one condition with variable expression and age-related penetrance: results of a clinical study of *PTEN* mutation carriers. J Med Genet 44:579–585

Latif F, Tory K, Gnarra J et al (1993) Identification of the von Hippel-Lindau tumor suppressor gene. Science 260:1317–1320

Lehtonen HJ (2011) Hereditary leiomyomatosis and renal cell cancer: update on clinical and molecular characteristics. Fam Cancer 10:397–411

Leter EM, Koopmans AK, Gille JJP et al (2008) Birt-Hogg-Dubé syndrome: clinical and genetic studies of 20 families. J Invest Dermatol 128:45–49

Li FP, Decker H-J, Zbar B et al (1993) Clinical and genetic studies of renal cell carcinomas in a family with a constitutional chromosome 3;8 translocation. Genetics of familial renal carcinoma. Ann Intern Med 118:106–111

Lindau A (1926) Studien über Kleinhirncysten. Bau, Pathogenese und Beziehungen zur Angiomatosis retinae. Acta Pathol Microbiol Scand S1:1–128

Linehan WM (2012) Genetic basis of kidney cancer: role of genomics for the development of disease-based therapeutics. Genome Res 22:2089–2100

Linehan WM, Walther MM, Zbar B (2003) The genetic basis of cancer of the kidney. J Urol 170:2163–2172

Linehan WM, Srinivasan R, Schmidt LS (2010a) The genetic basis of kidney cancer: a metabolic disease. Nat Rev Urol 7:277–285

Linehan WM, Bratslavsky G, Pinto PA et al (2010b) Molecular diagnosis and therapy of kidney cancer. Annu Rev Med 61:329–343

Ljungberg B, Bensalah K, Bex A et al (2013) Guidelines: Renal cell carcinoma, European Association of Urology. www.uroweb.org

Lloyd KM II, Dennis M (1963) Cowden's disease. A possible new symptom complex with multiple system involvement. Ann Intern Med 58:136–142

Lonser RR, Glenn GM, Walther M et al (2003) Von Hippel-Lindau disease. Lancet 361:2059–2067

Maffé A, Toschi B, Circo G et al (2011) Constitutional *FLCN* mutations in patients with suspected Birt-Hogg-Dubé syndrome ascertained for non-cutaneous manifestations. Clin Genet 79:345–354

Maher ER (2011) Genetics of familial renal cancers. Nephron Exp Nephrol 118:e21–e26

Maher ER, Yates JRW, Harries R et al (1990) Clinical features and natural history of von Hippel-Lindau disease. Q J Med 77:1151–1163

Maher ER, Neumann HPH, Richard S (2011) Von Hippel-Lindau disease: a clinical and scientific review. Eur J Hum Genet 19:617–623

Malchoff CD, Sarfarazi M, Tendler B et al (2000) Papillary thyroid carcinoma associated with papillary renal neoplasia: genetic linkage analysis of a distinct heritable tumor syndrome. J Clin Endocrinol Metab 85:1758–1764

McKay L, Frydenberg M, Lipton L et al (2011) Case report: renal cell carcinoma segregating with a t(2;3)(q37.3;q13.2) chromosomal translocation in an Ashkenazi Jewish family. Fam Cancer 10:349–353

Menko FH, van Steensel MAM, Giraud S et al (2009) Birt-Hogg-Dubé syndrome: diagnosis and management. Lancet Oncol 10:1199–1206

Menko FH, Johannesma PC, van Moorselaar RJ et al (2013) A de novo *FLCN* mutation in a patient with spontaneous pneumothorax and renal cancer; a clinical and molecular evaluation. Fam Cancer 12:373–379

Menko FH, Maher ER, Schmidt LS et al (2014) Hereditary leiomyomatosis and renal cell cancer (HLRCC): renal cancer risk, surveillance and treatment. Fam Cancer 13:637–644

Mester J, Eng C (2015) Cowden syndrome: recognizing and managing a not-so-rare hereditary cancer syndrome. J Surg Oncol 111:125–130

Mester JL, Zhou M, Prescott N et al (2012) Papillary renal cell carcinoma is associated with *PTEN* hamartoma tumor syndrome. Urology 79:1187.e1–1187.e7

Metwalli AR, Linehan WM (2014) Nephron-sparing surgery for multifocal and hereditary tumors. Curr Opin Urol 24:466–473

Nahorski MS, Lim DHK, Martin L et al (2010) Investigation of the Birt-Hogg-Dubé tumour suppressor gene (*FLCN*) in familial and sporadic colorectal cancer. J Med Genet 47:385–390

Ngeow J, Eng C (2015) PTEN hamartoma tumor syndrome: clinical risk assessment and management protocol. Methods 77–78:11–19

Nickerson ML, Warren MB, Toro JR et al (2002) Mutations in a novel gene lead to kidney tumors, lung wall defects, and benign tumors of the hair follicle in patients with the Birt-Hogg-Dubé syndrome. Cancer Cell 2:157–164

Nieuwenhuis MH, Kets CM, Murphy-Ryan M et al (2014) Cancer risk and genotype-phenotype correlations in *PTEN* hamartoma tumor syndrome. Fam Cancer 13:57–63

Northrup H, Krueger DA (2013) Tuberous sclerosis complex diagnostic criteria update: recommendations of the 2012 International Tuberous Sclerosis Complex Consensus Conference. Pediatr Neurol 49:243–254

Olivero M, Valente G, Bardelli A et al (1999) Novel mutation in the ATP-binding site of the MET oncogene tyrosine kinase in a HPRCC family. Int J Cancer 82:640–643

Papathomas TG, Gaal J, Corssmit EPM et al (2014) Non-pheochromocytoma (PCC)/paraganglioma (PGL) tumors in patients with succinate dehydrogenase-related PCC-PGL syndromes: a clinicopathological and molecular analysis. Eur J Endocrinol 170:1–12

Pavlovich CP, Walther MM, Eyler RA et al (2002) Renal tumors in the Birt-Hogg-Dubé syndrome. Am J Surg Pathol 26:1542–1552

Popova T, Hebert L, Jacquemin V et al (2013) Germline *BAP1* mutations predispose to renal cell carcinomas. Am J Hum Genet 92:974–980

Pressey JG, Wright JM, Geller JI et al (2010) Sirolimus therapy for fibromatosis and multifocal renal cell carcinoma in a child with tuberous sclerosis complex. Pediatr Blood Cancer 54:1035–1037

Qin Y, Deng Y, Ricketts CJ et al (2014) The tumor susceptibility gene *TMEM127* is mutated in renal cell carcinomas and modulates endolysosomal function. Hum Mol Genet 23:2428–2439

Reaume MN, Graham GE, Tomiak E et al (2013) Canadian guideline on genetic screening for hereditary renal cell cancers. Can Urol Assoc J 7:319–323

Reed WB, Walker R, Horowitz R (1973) Cutaneous leiomyomata with uterine leiomyomata. Acta Derm Venereol 53:409–416

Richard S, Gardie B, Couvé S et al (2013) Von Hippel-Lindau: how a rare disease illuminates cancer biology. Semin Cancer Biol 23:26–37

Ricketts C, Woodward ER, Killick P et al (2008) Germline *SDHB* mutations and familial renal cell carcinoma. J Natl Cancer Inst 100:1260–1262

Ricketts CJ, Forman JR, Rattenberry E et al (2010) Tumor risks and genotype-phenotype-proteotype analysis in 358 patients with germline mutations in *SDHB* and *SDHD*. Hum Mutat 31:41–51

Ricketts CJ, Shuch B, Vocke CD et al (2012) Succinate dehydrogenase kidney cancer: an aggressive example of the Warburg effect in cancer. J Urol 188:2063–2071

Roma A, Maruzzo M, Basso U et al (2015) First-line sunitinib in patients with renal cell carcinoma (RCC) in von Hippel-Lindau (VHL) disease: clinical outcome and patterns of radiological response. Fam Cancer 14:309–316

Salvi A, Marchina E, Benetti A et al (2008) Germline and somatic c-met mutations in multifocal/bilateral and sporadic papillary renal carcinomas of selected patients. Int J Oncol 33:271–276

Schmidt LS (2013) Birt-Hogg-Dubé syndrome: from gene discovery to molecularly targeted therapies. Fam Cancer 12:357–364

Schmidt LS, Linehan WM (2014) Hereditary leiomyomatosis and renal cell carcinoma. Int J Nephrol Renovasc Dis 7:253–260

Schmidt L, Duh F-M, Chen F et al (1997) Germline and somatic mutations in the thyrosine kinase domain of the *MET* proto-oncogene in papillary renal carcinomas. Nat Genet 16:68–73

Schmidt LS, Nickerson ML, Angeloni D et al (2004) Early onset hereditary papillary renal carcinoma: germline missense mutations in the tyrosine kinase domain of the *MET* proto-oncogene. J Urol 172:1256–1261

Shuch B, Ricketts CJ, Vocke CD et al (2013a) Adrenal nodular hyperplasia in hereditary leiomyomatosis and renal cell cancer. J Urol 189:430–435

Shuch B, Ricketts CJ, Vocke CD et al (2013b) Germline PTEN mutation Cowden syndrome: an underappreciated form of hereditary kidney cancer. J Urol 190:1990–1998

Shuch B, Vourganti S, Ricketts CJ et al (2014) Defining early-onset kidney cancer: implications for germline and somatic mutation testing and clinical management. J Clin Oncol 32:431–437

Shuch B, Amin A, Armstrong AJ et al (2015) Understanding pathologic variants of renal cell carcinoma: distilling therapeutic opportunities from biologic complexity. Eur Urol 67:85–97

Smit DL, Mensenkamp AR, Badeloe S et al (2011) Hereditary leiomyomatosis and renal cell cancer in families referred for fumarate hydratase germline mutation analysis. Clin Genet 79:49–59

Srigley JR, Delahunt B, Eble JN et al (2013) The International Society of Urological Pathology (ISUP) Vancouver classification of renal neoplasia. Am J Surg Pathol 37:1469–1489

Stamatakis L, Metwalli AR, Middelton LA et al (2013) Diagnosis and management of BHD-associated kidney cancer. Fam Cancer 12:397–402

Sudarshan S, Karam JA, Brugarolas J et al (2013) Metabolism of kidney cancer: from the lab to clinical practice. Eur Urol 63:244–251

Tan M-H, Mester JL, Ngeow J et al (2012) Lifetime cancer risks in individuals with germline *PTEN* mutations. Clin Cancer Res 18:400–407

Teh BT, Farnebo F, Kristoffersson U et al (1996) Autosomal dominant primary hyperparathyroidism and jaw tumor syndrome associated with renal hamartomas and cystic kidney disease: linkage to 1q21-q32 and loss of the wild type allele in renal hamartomas. J Clin Endocrinol Metab 81:4204–4211

Tollefson MK, Boorjian SA, Lohse CM et al (2010) The impact of family history on pathological and clinical outcomes in non-syndromic clear cell renal cell carcinoma. BJU Int 106:1638–1642

Tomlinson IPM, Alam NA, Rowan AJ et al (2002) The Multiple Leiomyoma Consortium. Germline mutations in *FH* predispose to dominantly inherited uterine fibroids, skin leiomyomata and papillary renal cell cancer. Nat Genet 30:406–410

Valle L, Cascón A, Melchor L et al (2005) About the origin and development of hereditary conventional renal cell carcinoma in a four-generation t(3;8) (p14.1;q24.23) family. Eur J Hum Genet 13:570–578

Van Nederveen FH, Gaal J, Favier J et al (2009) An immunohistochemical procedure to detect patients with paraganglioma and phaeochromocytoma with germline *SDHB*, *SDHC*, or *SDHD* gene mutations: a retrospective and prospective analysis. Lancet Oncol 10:764–771

Von Hippel E (1904) Ueber eine sehr seltene Erkrankung der Netzhaut. A von Graefe's Arch Ophthalmol 59:83–106

Wadt KAW, Gerdes A-M, Hansen TV et al (2012) Novel germline *c-MET* mutation in a family with hereditary papillary renal carcinoma. Fam Cancer 11:535–537

Wake NC, Ricketts CJ, Morris MR et al (2013) UBE2QL1 is disrupted by a constitutional translocation associated with renal tumor predisposition and is a novel candidate renal tumor suppressor gene. Hum Mutat 34:1650–1661

Woodward ER, Ricketts C, Killick P et al (2008) Familial non-VHL clear cell (conventional) renal cell carcinoma: clinical features, segregation analysis, and mutation analysis of *FLCN*. Clin Cancer Res 14:5925–5930

Woodward ER, Skytte AB, Cruger DG et al (2010) Population-based survey of cancer risks in chromosome 3 translocation carriers. Genes Chromosomes Cancer 49:52–58

Yang P, Cornejo KM, Sadow PM et al (2014) Renal cell carcinoma in tuberous sclerosis complex. Am J Surg Pathol 38:895–909

Zbar B, Tory K, Merino M et al (1994) Hereditary papillary renal cell carcinoma. J Urol 151:561–566

Zbar B, Glenn G, Lubensky I et al (1995) Hereditary papillary renal cell carcinoma: clinical studies in 10 families. J Urol 153:907–912

Diagnosis and Management of Hereditary Phaeochromocytoma and Paraganglioma

Fiona Lalloo

Abstract

About 30 % of phaeochromocytomas or paragangliomas are genetic. Whilst some individuals will have clinical features or a family history of inherited cancer syndrome such as neurofibromatosis type 1 (NF1) or multiple endocrine neoplasia 2 (MEN2), the majority will present as an isolated case. To date, 14 genes have been described in which pathogenic mutations have been demonstrated to cause paraganglioma or phaeochromocytoma. Many cases with a pathogenic mutation may be at risk of developing further tumours. Therefore, identification of genetic cases is important in the long-term management of these individuals, ensuring that they are entered into a surveillance programme. Mutation testing also facilitates cascade testing within the family, allowing identification of other at-risk individuals. Many algorithms have been described to facilitate cost-effective genetic testing sequentially of these genes, with phenotypically driven pathways. New genetic technologies including next-generation sequencing and whole-exome sequencing will allow much quicker, cheaper and extensive testing of individuals in whom a genetic aetiology is suspected.

Keywords

Paraganglioma · Phaeochromocytoma

F. Lalloo (✉)
Manchester Centre for Genomic Medicine, St Mary's Hospital,
Central Manchester University Hospitals NHS Foundation Trust,
Manchester Academic Health Science Centre, Manchester, UK
e-mail: fiona.lalloo@cmft.nhs.uk

G. Pichert and C. Jacobs (eds.), *Rare Hereditary Cancers*,
Recent Results in Cancer Research 205, DOI 10.1007/978-3-319-29998-3_7

Contents

1 Introduction

A paraganglioma (PG) is a rare neuroendocrine tumour that arises within paraganglia. These can be classified as adrenal or extra-adrenal. Within the adrenal gland, they are referred to as phaeochromocytomas. The extra-adrenal type can be subclassified into sympathetic and parasympathetic tumours. In general, the sympathetic ganglia are found in the trunk and mediastinum along the prevertebral and paravertebral chains. The parasympathetic paraganglia are usually located in the head and neck, along the branches of the glossopharyngeal and vagus nerves.

Clinical symptoms of catecholamine excess are usually associated with the lesions in the sympathetic chains, although some parasympathetic lesions can produce catecholamines. The parasympathetic paraganglia are less likely to be malignant than those on the sympathetic chain. Tumours in paraganglia should be termed either functional or non-functional (Lack et al. 2003). There are over 20 different anatomical sites for paraganglia, but the most common head and neck lesions are carotid body tumours and glomus jugulare tumours (see Fig. 1).

In the general population, the incidence of phaeochromocytomas and paragangliomas is about 0.8 per 100,000 person-years. However, this is influenced by altitude with a higher incidence of head and neck paragangliomas in communities living at altitude. Historically, around 10 % of phaeochromocytomas/paragangliomas have been considered to be genetic.

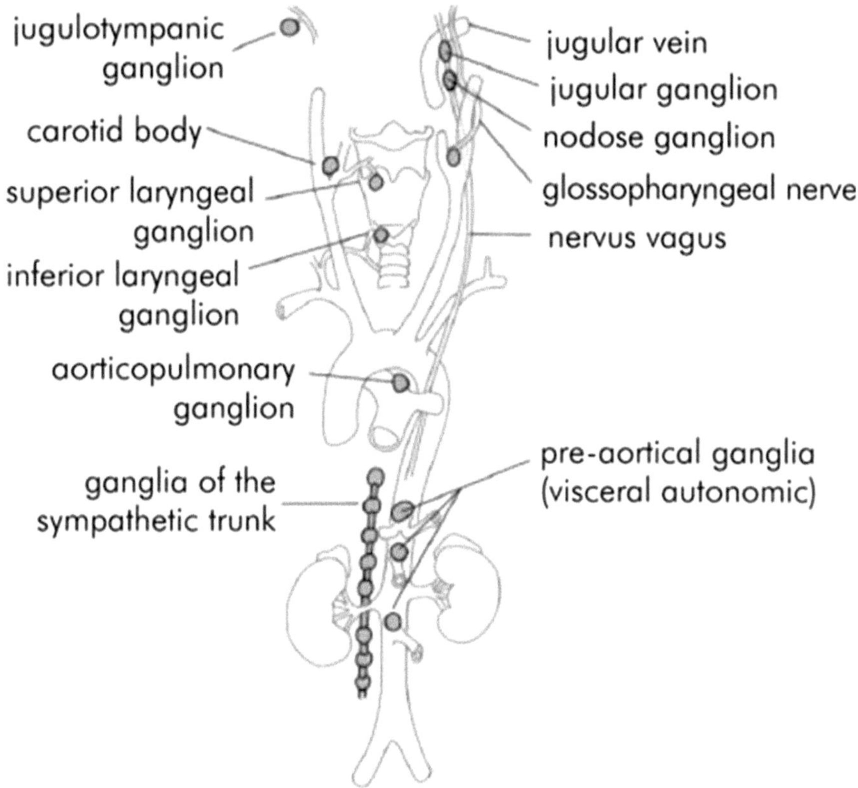

Fig. 1 Anatomical position of paraganglioma *Source* Lips et al. (2006)

In 2002, Neumann et al. studied 271 individuals with non-syndromic phaeochromocytoma. Patients with clinical evidence of neurofibromatosis type 1 (NF1) or a family history of Von Hippel–Lindau syndrome (VHL) and MEN type 2 were excluded. Within this cohort, they demonstrated that 25 % individuals had a genetic aetiology (pathogenic mutations in *RET*, *VHL*, *SDHB* or *SDHD* genes) with a very clear inverse correlation of age at time of diagnosis and probability of identifying a mutation.

Since 2002, a number of other genes have been implicated in hereditary phaeochromocytoma and paraganglioma (see Table 1).

Table 1 Genes in which mutations cause paragangliomas or phaeochromocytomas

Gene	Inheritance	Phenotype	Frequency
NF1	AD	Café au lait spots, axillary freckling, Lisch nodules, peripheral nervous system neurofibromas	1 % patients with NF1 develop phaeochromocytomas 1 % patients with phaoechromocytomas
RET	AD	Multiple endocrine neoplasia type 2—medullary thyroid carcinoma, phaeochromocytomas and hyper parathyroidism	50 % of patients develop phaeochromocytomas 5 % patients with phaeochromocytomas
VHL	AD	Cerebellar and spinal haemangioblastomas, *RET*inal angioma, phaeochromocytomas, renal cell carcinoma	Penetrance varies with mutation, up to about 20 % individuals with VHL 5–10 % patients with paragangliomas or phaeochromocytomas
SDHB	AD	Phaeochromocytomas and paragangliomas. High rate of malignancy. Have been associated with renal tumours	Penetrance about 50 % 10–15 % patients with paragangliomas or phaeochromocytomas
SDHD	AD parent of origin effect	Phaeochromocytomas and paragangliomas. Higher rate of head and neck lesions. Usually non-malignant, frequently multiple. Only develop tumours if inherit from father	Penetrance up to 75 % 5–10 % patients with phaeochromocytomas paragangliomas
SDHC	AD	Phaeochromocytomas and paragangliomas. Mainly head and neck lesions	Rare
SDHA	AD	Phaeochromocytomas and paragangliomas. All locations describe	Penetrance difficult to assess Accounts for less than 1 % inherited paraganglioma
SDHAF2	AD parent of origin effect	Head and neck paragangliomas	Penetrance unclear Rare
MAX	AD parent of origin effect	Phaeochromocytomas and paragangliomas. Malignant cases have been described. Only develop tumours if inherit from father	Penetrance unknown <1 % patients with phaeochromocytomas
TMEM127	AD	Phaeochromocytomas often bilateral and multicentric. Malignancy rare. Paragangliomas have been described	Penetrance unclear 1–2 % patients with phaeochromocytomas
FH	AD	Usually associated with leiomyomatosis and renal carcinoma. Recent association with phaeochromocytomas described	Penetrance is unknown Very rarely found

(continued)

Table 1 (continued)

Gene	Inheritance	Phenotype	Frequency
KIF1Bβ	Ad	Phenotype unclear	Penetrance unknown
			Very rare
ELGN1	AD	Paragangliomas and erythrocytosis	Insufficient data available
EPAS1	AD	Congenital polycythaemia and paragangliomas	Insufficient data available
MDH2	AD	Phaeochromocytomas	Single family described

2 Genes involved with hereditary paragangliomas and phaeochromoctyomas

2.1 *NF1* (17q11)

Neurofibromatosis type 1 (NF1) is an autosomal dominant disorder characterised by café au lait spots, Lisch nodules, axillary freckling, short stature, varying degree of learning disability and peripheral neurofibromatosis (McGaughran et al. 1999). The diagnosis is usually made by clinical examination, although mutation testing is now used routinely for clinical suspicion of mosaicism or to guide reproductive decision making (Rauen et al. 2015). Phaeochromocytomas are a recognised association of NF1 occurring in about 1 % of patients (Riccardi 1981). They usually occur in the 4th decade, around the same time as in the general population and are usually benign, although younger-onset and malignant diseases have been described (Bausch et al. 2006; Giovannoni et al. 2014) *NF1* mutations account for 1 % of patients with phaeochromocytomas.

2.2 *VHL* (3p25)

Von Hippel–Lindau (VHL) disease is an autosomal dominant condition predisposing to cerebellar and spinal haemangioblastomas, retinal angiomas, clear cell renal carcinoma, non-secretory pancreatic neuroendocrine tumours and phaeochromocytomas. The risk of phaeochromocytoma depends on the type of mutation with a higher risk of phaeochromocytoma associated with missense mutations (Ong et al. 2007; Hes et al. 2000). Up to 50 % of phaeochromocytoma may be bilateral or multiple with an average age of diagnosis of 30 years. Head and neck paraganglioma have been described in VHL (Hes et al. 2003; Maher et al. 1996; Gaal et al. 2009; Boedeker et al. 2009). *VHL* mutations are found in 5–10 % of patients with phaeochromocytoma or paragangliomas.

2.3 *RET* (10q11)

Mutations in *RET* cause multiple endocrine neoplasia (MEN) type 2. MEN2 is rare, occurring in about 1 in 200,000 live births. MEN2a accounts for around 70–80 % of cases of MEN2, with MEN2b for about 5 %. Familial medullary thyroid cancer is also caused by mutations in *RET*, but does not cause phaeochromocytoma and will not be discussed further here (Moline and Eng 2011). Medullary thyroid carcinoma (MTC) is the main feature of MEN2a with the majority of patients having biochemical evidence of the disease by 35 years (Ponder et al. 1988). Prophylactic thyroidectomy is advocated in all patients with MEN2a. Whilst MTC is the usual presenting complaint in MEN2a, in around 13–27 % of patients, the phaeochromocytoma will be the presenting complaint (Rodriguez et al. 2008; Frank-Raue et al. 2011). Phaeochromocytoma occurs in about 50 % of patients with MEN2a. Hyperparathyroidism is also a feature of MEN2a, usually caused by a parathyroid adenoma or hyperplasia, and usually occurs after MTC.

MEN2b occurs in about 5 % of cases with MEN2 and is characterised with a very aggressive form of MTC. The untreated natural history of the disease results in death from MTC with an average age of 21 years. As a result, prophylactic thyroidectomy is recommended before the age of 1 year (Shepet et al. 2013). Individuals with MEN2b frequently have a Marfanoid habitus, often with kyphoscoliosis or lordosis. Patients also have mucosal neuromas on the tongue, palate or pharynx. They also have a typical facial appearance with thickened "blubbery lips" appearing over time.

Phaeochromocytoma occurs in 50 % of individuals with MEN2b and is frequently bilateral. The risk of malignant phaeochromocytoma is greater in MEN2b than in MEN2a (Pacak et al. 2009).

MEN2 is caused by mutations in the *RET* proto-oncogene. This codes for a transmembrane receptor tyrosine kinase. The protein has 3 functional domains including an extracellular ligand binding domain, a transmembrane domain and a cytoplasmic tyrosine kinase domain. *RET* is involved with cell signalling pathways for cell survival, proliferation and differentiation of both enteric, neural and renal cells (Krampitz and Norton 2014). There is a very clear genotype–phenotype correlation in *RET*, with the level of risk of MTC being stratified according to the specific mutation (Chen et al. 2010). This then guides management, in particular the age at which preventative thyroidectomy is offered. There does not appear to be any relationship between phenotype and phaeochromocytoma risk. Extra-adrenal lesions are very rare but have been described in MEN2 (Boedeker et al. 2009). About 5 % of sporadic phaeochromocytomas have germline *RET* mutations.

2.4 SDH Mutations

In 2000, mutations were identified in *SDHD* in affected individuals with paraganglia (Baysal et al. 2000). *SDHD* is one of 4 subunits of a heterotetrameric enzyme that is attached to the inner wall of the mitochondria. Succinate dehydrogenase (SDH) has a role in the Krebs cycle and is the complex II component of the electron transport chain. As mutations associated with hereditary paraganglioma were identified in *SDHD*, the other subunits of the enzyme were investigated and mutations identified in *SDHC*, *SDHB* and *SDHA* (Niemann and Müller 2000; Astuti et al. 2001; Burnichon et al. 2010). *SDHAF2* (succinate dehydrogenase assembly factor 2) codes for a protein that ensures flavination of SDHA and therefore correct assembly of the SDH complex (Hao et al. 2009).

2.4.1 *SDHB* (1p36)

SDHB mutations account for up to 40 % of hereditary paraganglioma families (Buffet et al. 2012). Mutations in *SDHB* occur more commonly than mutations in other genes and are more likely to cause phaeochromocytomas and functioning paragangliomas than head and neck paragangliomas (Benn et al. 2006). They are also more likely to be malignant. Van Hulsteijn et al. undertook a meta-analysis of *SDHB* mutation carriers. Those studies including only manifesting mutation carriers demonstrated a pooled incidence of malignant disease of 23 % (van Hulsteijn et al. 2012). Studies including both asymptomatic and manifesting mutation carriers demonstrated an incidence of malignant disease of 17 %. Up to 50 % of individuals presenting with a malignant phaeochromocytomas/paragangliomas may have a germline *SDHB* mutation (Gimenez-Roqueplo et al. 2003; Ricketts et al. 2010; Jafri and Maher 2012).

The average age of tumour development is younger than in the general population with a mean age of about 30 years (Karasek et al. 2013) but with a very wide range from 6 to 77 years. There is a high probability of multiple tumours although less likely than with *SDHD* mutations. The penetrance of *SDHB* is lower than originally thought, with recent studies suggesting that it may be less than 50 % for phaeochromocytomas and less than 30 % for head and neck tumours at the age of 60 years (Ricketts et al. 2010).

There is huge variability in the phenotype with individuals in the same family with the same mutation showing variability in the development, location and severity of the associated lesions (Timmers et al. 2007; Brouwers et al. 2006).

SDHB mutations have also been associated with other tumours, most noticeably renal cell carcinoma (Ricketts et al. 2008). These renal tumours appear to have a specific morphology and may have frank sarcomatous changes (Gill et al. 2014). Mutations have also been described with gastrointestinal stromal tumours (GIST) (Carney and Stratakis 2002; Pasini et al. 2008) and thyroid tumours.

SDHB mutations are inherited in an autosomal dominant fashion. Pathogenic mutations include deletions, splice-site mutations, nonsense–missense and frameshift mutations (Jafri and Maher 2012).

2.4.2 *SDHD* (11q23)

SDHD mutations cause about 30 % mutations in hereditary paraganglioma (Buffet et al. 2012) Mutations in *SDHD* account for the majority of head and neck paragangliomas. These are frequently multifocal and bilateral and are usually non-functional (Benn et al. 2006). Tumours associated with *SDHD* mutations are rarely malignant—in prevalence studies with mutation carriers with manifest disease, the malignancy rate was 3 % (van Hulsteijn et al. 2012). However, head and neck tumours may result in severe morbidity because of their proximity to important vascular and neurological structures (Papaspyrou et al. 2009). The penetrance of mutations in *SDHD* is higher than that of *SDHB* mutations, with an estimated penetrance of head and neck tumours of 71 % and phaeochromocytomas of 29 % (Ricketts et al. 2010).

SDHD mutations are less commonly associated with other tumour types, although mutations have been reported with renal tumours. Whilst an increase in morbidity is recognised, mortality in patients with *SDHD* mutations is not significantly increased (van Hulsteijn et al. 2015).

SDHD mutations are inherited in an autosomal dominant fashion. However, the phenotype demonstrates "parent of origin" with the development of tumours only if the germline mutation is inherited via the paternal line. This was considered to be due to maternal imprinting although subsequently biallelic expression has been demonstrated in a variety of tissues (Baysal et al. 2000). Cases of tumours following maternal transmission, although rare, have been reported and offer insights into the mechanisms underlying the "parent of origin" effect (Bayley et al. 2014).

Pathogenic mutations in *SDHD* include deletions, frameshifts, nonsense, missense and splice-site mutations (Jafri and Maher 2012). There are 2 founder mutations in *SDHD* in the Dutch population and both of these result in a typical phenotype of benign head and neck tumours (van Hulsteijn et al. 2013).

2.4.3 *SDHC* (1q23)

SDHC mutations account for between 4 and 8 % of hereditary paragangliomas (Buffet et al. 2012). *SDHC* mutations are most often associated with head and neck tumours which are usually benign and rarely multifocal (Schiavi et al. 2005). The majority of tumours are head and neck tumours although sympathetic extra-adrenal paragangliomas and phaeochromocytomas have been described with *SDHC* mutations (Burnichon et al. 2012a, b). As mutations are rare, there is little clinical information about the phenotype of *SDHC* mutations. However, the age range at presentation may be very wide.

SDHC mutations are inherited in an autosomal dominant fashion and a wide variety of mutations described encompassing the whole genes.

2.4.4 *SDHA* (5p15)

Biallelic mutations in *SDHA* cause Leigh syndrome, a recessive neurodegenerative condition. Due to the function of the protein within the complex II of the mitochondrion, *SDHA* was studied in patients with paragangliomas and phaeochromocytomas. In 2010, Burnichon et al. (2010) identified mutations in *SDHA* in a patient with and extra-adrenal paraganglioma. Few individuals with mutations have been described to date, but have presented with a range of phenotypes including abdominal and thoracic sympathetic tumours and head and neck tumours (Dwight et al. 2013; Korpershoek et al. 2011).

SDHA mutations only account for 0.5–3 % of familial paragangliomas and are inherited in an autosomal dominant fashion.

2.4.5 *SDHAF2* (11q12)

SDHAF2 was originally mapped in 2009 (originally called *SDH5*) with mutations shown to cause head and neck paragangliomas (Hao et al. 2009). Mutations in this gene have not been associated with phaeochromocytomas, but are known to cause multiple head and neck tumours. Mutations in *SDHAF2* have a high penetrance with a young age at onset and are frequently multifocal. As with *SDHD*, mutations in *SDHAF2* demonstrate a "parent of origin" effect with tumours developing only following paternal transmission of the mutation (Bayley et al. 2010; Kunst et al. 2011). On radiological investigation of a large family with a mutation, a number of individuals were diagnosed with asymptomatic lesions. To date, malignancies have not been reported in families with *SDHAF2* mutations.

Mutations in this gene are rare and account for a very small proportion of families with inherited paragangliomas.

2.4.6 *MAX* (14q23)

Myc-associated factor—*MAX*—is a component of the MYC–MAX–MXD1 network of transcription factors that regulate cell proliferation, differentiation and apoptosis. Mutations in *MAX* were identified as a cause of phaeochromocytomas following exome sequencing of 3 individuals with phaeochromocytomas. Further studies suggested that mutations frequently cause bilateral and malignant disease (Comino-Méndez et al. 2011). A more recent study suggested that 1.12 % of phaeochromocytomas may harbour a mutation in *MAX*. The familial cases present earlier that sporadic cases and that a parent of origin effect (paternal transmission results in tumours) is likely (Burnichon et al. 2012a, b). Cases of paragangliomas were also described, of which a proportion was malignant at presentation. The rate of malignancy associated with *MAX* mutations is much lower than that associated with *SDHB* mutations. These cases presented as a second tumour following an initial phaeochromocytoma.

2.4.7 *TMEM127* (2q11)

Mutations in *TMEM127* (transmembrane protein 127) have been described in phaeochromocytoma (Qin et al. 2010; Elston et al. 2013). The phaeochromocytomas appear to be multicentric and frequently bilateral. Malignancy is rare and the penetrance is considered to be high (Yao et al. 2010; Toledo et al. 2015). Whilst the majority of patients will have adrenal disease, cases of paragangliomas have been described (Neumann et al. 2011). Other rare associations have been noted including with renal cell carcinoma (Hernandez et al. 2015). *TMEM127* mutations account for between 1 and 2 % of phaeochromocytomas.

2.4.8 *FH* (1q43)

The *FH* gene encodes for fumerate hydratase, an enzyme within the Krebs (TCA) cycle. Homozygote mutations cause fumarase deficiency, a mitochondrial encephalopathy that usually results in death in infancy. Heterozygote mutations have been described in hereditary leiomyomatosis and renal cell carcinoma syndrome (Alam et al. 2003)

Recently mutations have been identified in patients with phaeochromocytomas and/or paragangliomas in the absence of renal cell carcinoma (Clark et al. 2014; Castro-Vega et al. 2014). Small numbers of families have been described, but the phenotype appears to include malignant disease. *FH* mutations account for less than 1 % of phaeochromocytomas

2.5 Other Rare Genes

VHL, NF1 and *RET* act in a developmental c-Jun-dependent apoptotic pathway. During normal embryonic development, neuronal progenitor cells compete for growth factors including nerve growth factor (NGF). Mutations in these genes result in enhanced signalling and neuronal survival. Lee et al. demonstrated that *EglN3* (PHD3) mediates this pathway and that SDH gene products were also affected. Members of the EglN family are known to hydroxylate HIF-α in vitro (Lee et al. 2005). It has been demonstrated that KIF1Bβ acts downstream from ElgN3 and missense mutations in *KIF1Bβ* (1p36) have been described in phaeochromocytoma (Schlisio et al. 2008).

ELGN1 (1q42) (previously termed PHD2) encodes for a protein involved in HIF pathway. A mutation has been described in a patient with congenital erythrocytosis and paraganglioma (Ladroue et al. 2008). A handful of cases with polycythaemia and phaeochromocytoma have been described with mutations in this gene (Yang et al. 2015). However, mutations are unlikely to be a common cause of familial paraganglioma syndrome (Astuti et al. 2011).

Both germline and somatic mutations in *EPAS1* (2p21)—previously known as HIF2α—have been described in patients with congenital polycythemia and phaeochromocytomas and paragangliomas (Taïeb et al. 2013; Lorenzo et al. 2013). These are extremely rare.

A recent study undertaking whole-exome screening of individuals with paraganglioma or phaeochromocytoma identified a mutation in *MDH2* (7q11) a gene encoding for an enzyme in the Krebs cycle. This patient had multiple malignant tumours (Cascón et al. 2015).

3 Who to Test

Any patient presenting with phaeochromocytoma or paraganglioma should have a full personal history taken, in particular to assess the probability of features consistent with one of the above inherited syndromes such as VHL, MEN2 or NF1. Appropriate clinical examination should also be undertaken. A third-generation pedigree should be taken on both sides of the family, again checking for other members of the family with phaeochromocytomas, paragangliomas or other associated problems. If there are obvious features of a specific condition, mutation testing should be directed towards the relevant gene.

However, a lack of family history does not exclude an inherited paraganglioma/phaeochromocytoma. For example, the parent of origin effect seen with mutations in *SDHD*, *SDHAF2* and *MAX* means that if the mutations are inherited via mothers, tumours do not occur and the eventual transmission via a father, resulting in a tumour could then look like a sporadic lesion in a family.

As with all cancer genetics, all diagnoses should be confirmed with pathology reports of affected individuals obtained if possible. Other lesions may be assumed to be paragangliomas or phaeochromocytomas on imaging, but on biopsy are shown to be unrelated.

The presence of multiple cases within a family, or multiple tumours, bilateral or multifocal or extra-adrenal disease within an individual increases the probability of a germline mutation. Metastatic disease is also a marker of a germline mutation. Early onset, less than 45 years of age, is suggestive of a mutation. It has been suggested that a diagnosis of a lesion over the age of 50 years is unlikely to be due to a germline mutation (Mannelli et al. 2009). There have been a number of algorithms produced using these clinical features to stratify genetic testing within individuals (Jafri and Maher 2012; Martins and Bugalho 2014; Martucci and Pacak 2014). Traditionally, genes were sequenced sequentially, which is costly. This approach was recommended in a clinical practice guideline from the Endocrine Society (Lenders et al. 2014). A recent UK study suggested that this approach could be cost-effective in the context of clinical practice (Jafri et al. 2013).

The American Society of Clinical Oncology has suggested that all patients with a 10 % chance of identifying a germline genetic mutation should be offered mutation screening (Robson et al. 2010). A recent study by Brito et al. demonstrated a detection rate of mutations of 11–13 % in sporadic phaeochromocytoma and paraganglioma (Brito et al. 2014). This would suggest that all patients with a phaeochromocytoma or paraganglioma should be offered testing.

This is now becoming a possibility with the advent of next-generation sequencing and gene panels. Cheaper massive parallel sequencing of multiple genes (along with the advent of whole-exome and whole-genome sequencing) is resulting in the availability of testing although this then throws up particular challenges. Currently, in the UK, 9–12-gene panels are being offered for a price of £500–800, a substantial saving compared to sequentially sequencing individual genes. Rattenbury (Rattenberry et al. 2013) demonstrated, in a feasibility study of a 9-gene panel, a 98.7 % sensitivity for the genes and demonstrated a high degree of concordance with conventional sequencing. However, there are limitations to this technology and next-generation sequencing (NGS) panels will require considerable work generating new libraries and revalidation to add newly discovered genes to the panels.

Alternatively, whole-exome sequencing and whole-genome sequencing are more comprehensive options with the added advantage of identifying copy number gains or losses. However, the cost at the moment is untenable in most healthcare systems. More importantly, analysis of data generated by these systems and development of analytical pipelines for groups of genes is a major bottleneck for delivery of whole-exome sequencing (WES) and whole-genome sequencing (WGS) in a clinical service (Bamshad et al. 2011). Toledo and Dahia have written an excellent review of NGS in phaeochromocytoma and paraganglioma (Toledo and Dahia 2015).

One of the added complexities of this type of sequencing is the identification of variants of unknown significance—missense mutations—resulting in uninformative results. These become even more difficult to interpret in rare genes about which there is currently little clinical information. All patients should therefore have appropriate counselling about the limitations of genetic testing.

4 Management of Individuals

4.1 Genetic Testing

As with all of clinical genetics, testing can be divided into diagnostic testing of an individual with the disease and predictive or cascade testing within the family. The management of these individuals is very different.

4.1.1 Diagnostic Testing and Management of Affected Individuals

These individuals are offered genetic testing due to the presence of a paraganglioma or phaeochromocytoma. The major management issue for these individuals is the medical management of the initial presenting lesion. Diagnosis often takes a long time due to the variety of non-specific symptoms, although classically phaeochromocytoma presents with triad of headaches, sweating and palpitations (Manger 2009). It is now recommended (Lenders et al. 2014; Därr et al. 2012) that the initial biochemical diagnosis is with urinary fractionated metanephrines or plasma metanephrines and that diagnosis is confirmed using CT as the imaging modality of choice. However, in those patients with potential paragangliomas or metastatic disease, MRI screening should be considered as the efficacy of detection of skull-based lesions is improved (Sahdev et al. 2005). Functional imaging using ^{123}I-MIBG (metaiodobenzylguanidine) is also suggested as secondary imaging and may also indicate multiple lesions or metastatic disease.

Surgical treatment is the treatment of choice if possible although all patients with functioning lesions will require preoperative blockade with α-adrenergic receptor blockers. Phaeochromocytomas may be operated on laparoscopically, although large or multiple tumours may still need an open approach (Martucci and Pacak 2014; Därr et al. 2012). In those patients with genetic disease and therefore an increased probability of bilateral phaeochromocytomas, a small tumour may be treated with cortex-sparing surgery which may negate the need for steroid replacement. Repeated subtotal adrenalectomies may be performed successfully (Grubbs et al. 2013; Fallon et al. 2013). Occasionally, radiofrequency ablation and external beam radiation have been used for inoperable tumours (Martucci and Pacak 2014).

MIBG therapy has been used as a treatment modality, although this is only possible if the MIBG scintigraphy is positive. For those patients with metastatic disease, chemotherapy may be useful in palliation or stabilisation of the tumours. A number of chemotherapeutic agents have been used, but no large randomised studies have been undertaken. Following treatment of the initial lesion, affected individuals should then have life-long follow-up including surveillance for any of the other features of inherited cancer syndromes.

4.1.2 Predictive Testing of Unaffected Family Members

Once a mutation has been identified in an affected patient, predictive testing may be offered to other members of the family. This will identify individuals who may benefit from target screening. The aim of surveillance is to detect any presymptomatic phaeochromocytomas or paragangliomas to facilitate easier treatment. Any individual identified with a mutation in a gene causing one of the classical inherited cancer syndromes should be entered into the recommended screening programmes.

4.2 NF1

Although patients with NF1 have an increased risk of phaeochromocytoma, the likelihood of this is low. However, screening is part of the recommended long-term management of individuals with this condition (Ferner et al. 2007). Children should be assessed on an annual basis and this should include measurement of blood pressure. Assessment of urinary or plasma catecholamines is only recommended if symptoms of phaeochromocytoma are present. Individuals with complex NF1 should be seen in a specialist NF1 clinic with multidisciplinary input.

4.3 MEN2

Predictive testing for MEN2 is particularly important because of the requirement for prophylactic thyroidectomy for individuals with a *RET* mutation. The age at which the thyroid is removed is determined by the mutation, but is usually in childhood if the family are known to genetic services. Following prophylactic thyroidectomy, patients should be followed up on an annual basis and this should include assessment of plasma or urinary catecholamines (Kloos et al. 2009; Waguespack et al. 2011) to assess for the presence of phaeochromocytoma.

4.4 VHL

Asymptomatic patients with VHL mutations should be in an annual surveillance programme. This includes an annual clinical neurological examination, annual abdominal imaging with ultrasound scan (USS) or magnetic resonance imaging (MRI), annual plasma or urinary catecholamines and annual fundoscopy. Some authors would recommend imaging of the cerebellum and spine on an annual basis (Schmid et al. 2014), others on a 3 yearly basis if the patient does not have symptoms (Maher et al. 2011).

Mutations in the remaining genes generally increase the risk of paragangliomas and phaeochromocytomas only, and this has been termed familial paraganglioma syndrome. The screening and surveillance for asymptomatic carriers of this condition is not so clear cut, with differing modalities suggested by different groups. There is broad agreement that screening needs to be lifelong (Bayley et al. 2010; Lenders et al. 2014; Persky et al. 2015) due the potential for multiple tumours and that screening results in detection and early treatment of occult tumours (Heesterman et al. 2012). Periodic screening using whole-body MRI screening has been advocated on a 2–3 yearly basis (Benn et al. 2006; Lenders et al. 2014; Myssiorek et al. 2008) with the addition of functional imaging if a lesion is suspected. Biochemical screening has also been advocated on an annual basis. It is of note that screening is not always advocated if a parent of origin effect has been described—for example, individuals who have inherited an *SDHD* mutation from their mother have a low risk of tumours and therefore should not be enrolled into a surveillance programme.

One of the major differences between familial paraganglioma syndrome and the other inherited cancer syndrome is the potentially low penetrance of some of these genes—in particular *SDHB* mutations (Hes et al. 2010). There is concern that patient anxiety is increased with genetic testing and subsequent screening of individuals with a potential tumour risk of lower than 50 % (Raygada et al. 2014). Only long-term follow-up of these patients in collaborative studies will provide clear guidelines.

5 Conclusion

It is now well recognised that about 30–40 % of phaeochromocytomas and paragangliomas are due to germline mutations in one of (currently) 14 genes. Mutations in these genes are inherited in autosomal dominant fashion although a small number exhibit a parent of origin effect such that tumours only develop if the mutations are inherited via the paternal line. In the last 5 years, advances in genetic technologies have resulted in next-generation gene panels which enable massive parallel sequencing of multiple genes at a reasonable cost. It is therefore now both practicable and cost-effective to offer genetic testing to all cases of young-onset, bilateral, or multiple phaeochromocytomas/paragangliomas. This will result in improved management of these patients in both the short and long terms. It will also facilitate genetic testing to unaffected at-risk relatives. Whilst the utility of screening programmes is not yet proven, long-term follow-up of these individuals in collaborative studies should give further information both about the efficacy of screening and the most appropriate modalities for imaging.

References

Alam NA et al (2003) Genetic and functional analyses of *FH* mutations in multiple cutaneous and uterine leiomyomatosis, hereditary leiomyomatosis and renal cancer, and fumarate hydratase deficiency. Hum Mol Genet 12(11):1241–1252. Available at: http://www.ncbi.nlm.nih.gov/pubmed/12761039

Astuti D et al (2001) Gene mutations in the succinate dehydrogenase subunit *SDHB* cause susceptibility to familial pheochromocytoma and to familial paraganglioma. Am J Hum Genet 69(1):49–54. Available at: http://www.pubmedcentral.nih.gov/articlerender.fcgi?artid=1226047&tool=pmcentrez&rendertype=abstract

Astuti D et al (2011) Mutation analysis of HIF prolyl hydroxylases (PHD/EGLN) in individuals with features of phaeochromocytoma and renal cell carcinoma susceptibility. Endocr Relat Cancer 18(1):73–83. Available at: http://www.pubmedcentral.nih.gov/articlerender.fcgi?artid=3006001&tool=pmcentrez&rendertype=abstract

Bamshad MJ et al (2011) Exome sequencing as a tool for Mendelian disease gene discovery. Nat Rev Genet 12(11):745–755. Available at: http://www.ncbi.nlm.nih.gov/pubmed/21946919

Bausch B, Borozdin W, Neumann HPH (2006) Clinical and genetic characteristics of patients with neurofibromatosis type 1 and pheochromocytoma. N Engl J Med 354(25):2729–2731. Available at: http://www.ncbi.nlm.nih.gov/pubmed/16790714

Bayley J-P et al (2010) *SDHAF2* mutations in familial and sporadic paraganglioma and phaeochromocytoma. Lancet Oncol 11(4):366–372. Available at: http://www.ncbi.nlm.nih.gov/pubmed/20071235

Bayley J-P et al (2014) Paraganglioma and pheochromocytoma upon maternal transmission of *SDHD* mutations. BMC Med Genet 15:111. Available at: http://www.pubmedcentral.nih.gov/articlerender.fcgi?artid=4259087&tool=pmcentrez&rendertype=abstract

Baysal BE et al (2000) Mutations in *SDHD*, a mitochondrial complex II gene, in hereditary paraganglioma. Science 287(5454):848–851. Available at: http://www.ncbi.nlm.nih.gov/pubmed/10657297

Benn DE et al (2006) Clinical presentation and penetrance of pheochromocytoma/paraganglioma syndromes. J Clin Endocrinol Metab 91(3):827–836. Available at: http://www.ncbi.nlm.nih.gov/pubmed/16317055

Boedeker CC et al (2009) Head and neck paragangliomas in von Hippel-Lindau disease and multiple endocrine neoplasia type 2. J Clin Endocrinol Metab 94(6):1938–1944. Available at: http://www.pubmedcentral.nih.gov/articlerender.fcgi?artid=2690424&tool=pmcentrez&rendertype=abstract

Brito JP et al (2014) Testing for germline mutations in sporadic pheochromocytoma/paraganglioma: a systematic review. Clin Endocrinol 1–8

Brouwers FM et al (2006) High frequency of *SDHB* germline mutations in patients with malignant catecholamine-producing paragangliomas: implications for genetic testing. J Clin Endocrinol Metab 91(11):4505–4509. Available at: http://www.ncbi.nlm.nih.gov/pubmed/16912137

Buffet A et al (2012) A decade (2001–2010) of genetic testing for pheochromocytoma and paraganglioma. Hormone and metabolic research = Hormon- und Stoffwechselforschung = Hormones et métabolisme 44(5):359–366. Available at: http://www.ncbi.nlm.nih.gov/pubmed/22517557

Burnichon N et al (2012a) The genetics of paragangliomas. Eur Ann Otorhinolaryngol Head Neck Dis 129(6):315–318. Available at: http://www.sciencedirect.com/science/article/pii/S1879729612000816

Burnichon N et al (2012b) *MAX* mutations cause hereditary and sporadic pheochromocytoma and paraganglioma. Clin Cancer Res (official journal of the American Association for Cancer Research) 18(10):2828–2837. Available at: http://www.ncbi.nlm.nih.gov/pubmed/22452945

Burnichon N et al (2010) *SDHA* is a tumor suppressor gene causing paraganglioma. Hum Mol Genet 19(15):3011–3020. Available at: http://www.pubmedcentral.nih.gov/articlerender.fcgi?artid=2901140&tool=pmcentrez&rendertype=abstract

Carney JA, Stratakis CA (2002) Familial paraganglioma and gastric stromal sarcoma: a new syndrome distinct from the Carney triad. Am J Med Genet 108(2):132–139. Available at: http://www.ncbi.nlm.nih.gov/pubmed/11857563

Cascón A et al (2015) Whole-exome sequencing identifies MDH2 as a new familial paraganglioma gene. J Natl Cancer Inst 107(5). Available at: http://www.ncbi.nlm.nih.gov/pubmed/25766404

Castro-Vega LJ et al (2014) Germline mutations in *FH* confer predisposition to malignant pheochromocytomas and paragangliomas. Hum Mol Genet 23(9):2440–2446. Available at: http://www.ncbi.nlm.nih.gov/pubmed/24334767

Chen H et al (2010) The North American Neuroendocrine Tumor Society consensus guideline for the diagnosis and management of neuroendocrine tumors: pheochromocytoma, paraganglioma, and medullary thyroid cancer. Pancreas 39(6):775–783

Clark GR et al (2014) Germline *FH* mutations presenting with pheochromocytoma. J Clin Endocrinol Metab 99(10):E2046–E2050. Available at: http://www.ncbi.nlm.nih.gov/pubmed/25004247

Comino-Méndez I et al (2011) Exome sequencing identifies *MAX* mutations as a cause of hereditary pheochromocytoma. Nat Genet 43(7):663–667. Available at: http://www.ncbi.nlm.nih.gov/pubmed/21685915

Därr R et al (2012) Pheochromocytoma—update on disease management. Ther Adv Endocrinol Metab 3(1):11–26. Available at: http://www.pubmedcentral.nih.gov/articlerender.fcgi?artid=3474647&tool=pmcentrez&rendertype=abstract

Dwight T et al (2013) Familial *SDHA* mutation associated with pituitary adenoma and pheochromocytoma/paraganglioma. J Clin Endocrinol Metab 98(6):E1103–E1108. Available at: http://www.ncbi.nlm.nih.gov/pubmed/23633203

Elston MS et al (2013) Novel mutation in the *TMEM127* gene associated with phaeochromocytoma. Int Med J 43(4):449–451. Available at: http://www.ncbi.nlm.nih.gov/pubmed/23551308

Fallon SC et al (2013) The utility of cortical-sparing adrenalectomy in pheochromocytomas associated with genetic syndromes. J Pediatr Surg 48(6):1422–1425. Available at: http://www.ncbi.nlm.nih.gov/pubmed/23845641

Ferner RE et al (2007) Guidelines for the diagnosis and management of individuals with neurofibromatosis 1. J Med Genet 44(2):81–88. Available at: http://www.pubmedcentral.nih.gov/articlerender.fcgi?artid=2598063&tool=pmcentrez&rendertype=abstract

Frank-Raue K et al (2011) Risk profiles and penetrance estimations in multiple endocrine neoplasia type 2A caused by germline *RET* mutations located in exon 10. Hum Mutat 32 (1):51–58. Available at: http://ovidsp.ovid.com/ovidweb.cgi?T=JS&PAGE=reference&D=medl&NEWS=N&AN=20979234

Gaal J et al (2009) Parasympathetic paragangliomas are part of the Von Hippel-Lindau syndrome. J Clin Endocrinol Metab 94(11):4367–471. Available at: http://www.ncbi.nlm.nih.gov/pubmed/19808854

Gill AJ et al (2014) Succinate dehydrogenase (SDH)-deficient renal carcinoma: a morphologically distinct entity: a clinicopathologic series of 36 tumors from 27 patients. Am J Surg patholo 38 (12):1588–1602. Available at: http://www.pubmedcentral.nih.gov/articlerender.fcgi?artid=4229399&tool=pmcentrez&rendertype=abstract

Gimenez-Roqueplo A-P et al (2003) Mutations in the *SDHB* gene are associated with extra-adrenal and/or malignant phaeochromocytomas. Cancer Res 63(17):5615–5621. Available at: http://www.ncbi.nlm.nih.gov/pubmed/14500403

Giovannoni I et al (2014) Malignant pheochromocytoma in a 16-year-old patient with neurofibromatosis type 1. Pediatric and developmental pathology (the official journal of the Society for Pediatric Pathology and the Paediatric Pathology) Society 17(2):126–129. Available at: http://www.ncbi.nlm.nih.gov/pubmed/24555864

Grubbs EG et al (2013) Long-term outcomes of surgical treatment for hereditary pheochromocytoma. J Am Coll Surg 216(2):280–289. Available at: http://www.ncbi.nlm.nih.gov/pubmed/23317575

Hao H-X et al (2009) SDH5, a gene required for flavination of succinate dehydrogenase, is mutated in paraganglioma. Science 325(5944):1139–1142. Available at: http://www.pubmedcentral.nih.gov/articlerender.fcgi?artid=3881419&tool=pmcentrez&rendertype=abstract

Heesterman BL et al (2012) High prevalence of occult paragangliomas in asymptomatic carriers of *SDHD* and *SDHB* gene mutations. Euro J Hum Genet 21(4):469–470. Available at: http://dx.doi.org/10.1038/ejhg.2012.203

Hernandez KG et al (2015) Familial pheochromocytoma and renal cell carcinoma syndrome: *TMEM127* as a novel candidate gene for the association. Virchows Arch : Int J Pathol. Available at: http://www.ncbi.nlm.nih.gov/pubmed/25800244

Hes F et al (2000) Genotype-phenotype correlations in families with deletions in the von Hippel-Lindau (VHL) gene. Hum Gene 106(4):425–431. Available at: http://www.ncbi.nlm.nih.gov/pubmed/10830910

Hes FJ, Höppener JWM, Lips CJM (2003) Clinical review 155: Pheochromocytoma in Von Hippel-Lindau disease. J Clin Endocrinol Metab 88(3):969–974. Available at: http://www.ncbi.nlm.nih.gov/pubmed/12629069

Hes FJ et al (2010) Low penetrance of a *SDHB* mutation in a large Dutch paraganglioma family. BMC Med Genet 11(1):92. Available at: http://www.pubmedcentral.nih.gov/articlerender.fcgi?artid=2891715&tool=pmcentrez&rendertype=abstract

Jafri M, Maher ER (2012) The genetics of phaeochromocytoma: using clinical features to guide genetic testing. Euro J Endocrinol Euro Fed Endocr Soc 166(2):151–158. Available at: http://www.ncbi.nlm.nih.gov/pubmed/21896620

Jafri M et al (2013) Evaluation of *SDHB*, *SDHD* and VHL gene susceptibility testing in the assessment of individuals with non-syndromic phaeochromocytoma, paraganglioma and head and neck paraganglioma. Clin Endocrinol 78(6):898–906. Available at: http://www.ncbi.nlm.nih.gov/pubmed/23072324

Karasek D et al (2013) An update on the genetics of pheochromocytoma. J Hum Hypertens 27 (3):141–147. Available at: http://www.pubmedcentral.nih.gov/articlerender.fcgi?artid=4060418&tool=pmcentrez&rendertype=abstract

Kloos R et al (2009) Medullary thyroid cancer: management guidelines of the American Thyroid Association. Thyroid 19(6). Available at: http://online.liebertpub.com/doi/abs/10.1089/thy.2008.0403

Korpershoek E et al (2011) *SDHA* immunohistochemistry detects germline *SDHA* gene mutations in apparently sporadic paragangliomas and pheochromocytomas. J Clin Endocrinol Metab 96(9):E1472–E1476. Available at: http://www.ncbi.nlm.nih.gov/pubmed/21752896

Krampitz GW, Norton JA (2014) *RET* gene mutations (genotype and phenotype) of multiple endocrine neoplasia type 2 and familial medullary thyroid carcinoma. Cancer 120(13):1920–1931. Available at: http://www.ncbi.nlm.nih.gov/pubmed/24699901

Kunst HPM et al (2011) *SDHAF2* (PGL2-SDH5) and hereditary head and neck paraganglioma. Clin Cancer Res (an official journal of the American Association for Cancer Research) 17(2):247–254. Available at: http://www.ncbi.nlm.nih.gov/pubmed/21224366

Lack EE et al (2003) Recommendations for the reporting of extra-adrenal paragangliomas. The Association of Directors of Anatomic and Surgical Pathology. Hum Pathol 34(2):112–113. Available at: http://www.ncbi.nlm.nih.gov/pubmed/12612877

Ladroue C et al (2008) PHD2 mutation and congenital erythrocytosis with paraganglioma. N Engl J Med 359(25):2685–2692. Available at: http://www.ncbi.nlm.nih.gov/pubmed/19092153

Lee S et al (2005) Neuronal apoptosis linked to EglN3 prolyl hydroxylase and familial pheochromocytoma genes: developmental culling and cancer. Cancer Cell 8(2):155–167. Available at: http://www.ncbi.nlm.nih.gov/pubmed/16098468

Lenders JWM et al (2014) Pheochromocytoma and paraganglioma: an endocrine society clinical practice guideline. J Clin Endocrinol Metab 99(6):1915–1942. Available at: http://www.ncbi.nlm.nih.gov/pubmed/24893135

Lips CJM et al (2006). Familial paragangliomas. Hered Cancer Clin Pract, 4(4):169–176. Available at: http://openi.nlm.nih.gov/detailedresult.php?img=2837305_1897-4287-4-4-169-1&req=4

Lorenzo FR et al (2013) A novel EPAS1/HIF2A germline mutation in a congenital polycythemia with paraganglioma. J Mol Med 91(4):507–512. Available at: http://www.pubmedcentral.nih.gov/articlerender.fcgi?artid=3570726&tool=pmcentrez&rendertype=abstract

Maher ER et al (1996) Phenotypic expression in von Hippel-Lindau disease: correlations with germline VHL gene mutations. J Med Genet 33(4):328–332. Available at: http://www.pubmedcentral.nih.gov/articlerender.fcgi?artid=1050584&tool=pmcentrez&rendertype=abstract

Maher ER, Neumann HP, Richard S (2011) von Hippel-Lindau disease: a clinical and scientific review. Euro J Hum Gene: EJHG 19(6):617–623. Available at: http://www.pubmedcentral.nih.gov/articlerender.fcgi?artid=3110036&tool=pmcentrez&rendertype=abstract

Manger WM (2009) The protean manifestations of pheochromocytoma. Hormone and metabolic research = Hormon- und Stoffwechselforschung = Hormones et métabolisme 41(9):658–663. Available at: http://www.ncbi.nlm.nih.gov/pubmed/19242899

Mannelli M et al (2009) Clinically guided genetic screening in a large cohort of Italian patients with pheochromocytomas and/or functional or nonfunctional paragangliomas. J Clin Endocrinol Metab 94(5):1541–1547

Martins R, Bugalho MJ (2014) Paragangliomas/pheochromocytomas: clinically oriented genetic testing. Int J Endocrinol 2014:794187. Available at: http://www.pubmedcentral.nih.gov/articlerender.fcgi?artid=4037125&tool=pmcentrez&rendertype=abstract

Martucci VL, Pacak K (2014) Pheochromocytoma and paraganglioma: diagnosis, genetics, management, and treatment. Curr Prob Cancer 38(1):7–41. Available at: http://dx.doi.org/10.1016/j.currproblcancer.2014.01.001

McGaughran JM et al (1999) A clinical study of type 1 neurofibromatosis in north west England. J Med Genet 36(3):197–203. Available at: http://www.pubmedcentral.nih.gov/articlerender.fcgi?artid=1734324&tool=pmcentrez&rendertype=abstract

Moline J, Eng C (2011) Multiple endocrine neoplasia type 2: an overview. Genet Med (official journal of the American College of Medical Genetics) 13(9):755–764. Available at: http://www.ncbi.nlm.nih.gov/pubmed/21552134

Myssiorek D et al (2008) Screening for familial paragangliomas. Oral Oncol 44(6):532–537. Available at: http://www.ncbi.nlm.nih.gov/pubmed/17936061

Neumann Hartmut PHB (2002) Germ-line mutations in nonsyndromic pheochromocytoma. N Eng J Med 347(11):854–855; author reply 854–855

Neumann HPH et al (2011) Germline mutations of the *TMEM127* gene in patients with paraganglioma of head and neck and extraadrenal abdominal sites. J Clin Endocrinol Metab 96 (8):E1279–E1282. Available at: http://www.ncbi.nlm.nih.gov/pubmed/21613359

Niemann S, Müller U (2000) Mutations in *SDHC* cause autosomal dominant paraganglioma, type 3. Nat Genet 26(3):268–270. Available at: http://www.ncbi.nlm.nih.gov/pubmed/11062460

Ong KR et al (2007) Genotype-phenotype correlations in von Hippel-Lindau disease. Hum Mutat 28(2):143–149. Available at: http://www.ncbi.nlm.nih.gov/pubmed/17024664

Pacak K, Eisenhofer G, Ilias I (2009) Diagnosis of pheochromocytoma with special emphasis on MEN2 syndrome. Hormones 8:111–116

Papaspyrou K, Mann WJ, Amedee RG (2009) Management of head and neck paragangliomas: review of 120 patients. Head Neck 31(3):381–387. Available at: http://www.ncbi.nlm.nih.gov/pubmed/18972432

Pasini B et al (2008) Clinical and molecular genetics of patients with the Carney-Stratakis syndrome and germline mutations of the genes coding for the succinate dehydrogenase subunits *SDHB*, *SDHC*, and *SDHD*. Euro J Hum Genet: EJHG 16(1):79–88. Available at: http://www.ncbi.nlm.nih.gov/pubmed/17667967

Persky MJ et al (2015) The necessity for lifelong follow up of patients with familial paraganglioma syndrome—a case report. Head Neck. Available at: http://www.ncbi.nlm.nih.gov/pubmed/25783443

Ponder BA et al (1988) Risk estimation and screening in families of patients with medullary thyroid carcinoma. Lancet 1(8582):397–401. Available at: http://www.ncbi.nlm.nih.gov/pubmed/2893198

Qin Y et al (2010) Germline mutations in *TMEM127* confer susceptibility to pheochromocytoma. Nat Genet 42(3):229–233. Available at: http://www.pubmedcentral.nih.gov/articlerender.fcgi?artid=2998199&tool=pmcentrez&rendertype=abstract

Rattenberry E et al (2013) A comprehensive next generation sequencing-based genetic testing strategy to improve diagnosis of inherited pheochromocytoma and paraganglioma. J Clin Endocrinol Metab 98(7):E1248–E1256. Available at: http://www.ncbi.nlm.nih.gov/pubmed/23666964

Rauen KA et al (2015) Recent developments in neurofibromatoses and RASopathies: management, diagnosis and current and future therapeutic avenues. Am J Med Genet. Part A 167A (1):1–10. Available at: http://www.ncbi.nlm.nih.gov/pubmed/25393061

Raygada M et al (2014) Counseling patients with succinate dehydrogenase subunit defects: genetics, preventive guidelines, and dealing with uncertainty. J Pediatr Endocrinol Metab: JPEM 27(9–10):837–844. Available at: http://www.ncbi.nlm.nih.gov/pubmed/24854530

Riccardi VM (1981) Von Recklinghausen neurofibromatosis. N Eng J Med 305(27):1617–1627. Available at: http://www.ncbi.nlm.nih.gov/pubmed/6796886

Ricketts C et al (2008) Germline *SDHB* mutations and familial renal cell carcinoma. J Nat Cancer Inst 100(17):1260–1262. Available at: http://www.ncbi.nlm.nih.gov/pubmed/18728283

Ricketts CJ et al (2010) Tumor risks and genotype-phenotype-proteotype analysis in 358 patients with germline mutations in *SDHB* and *SDHD*. Hum Mutat 31(1):41–51. Available at: http://www.ncbi.nlm.nih.gov/pubmed/19802898

Robson ME et al (2010) American society of clinical oncology policy statement update: genetic and genomic testing for cancer susceptibility. J Clin Oncol : official journal of the American Society of Clinical Oncology 28(5):893–901. Available at: http://www.ncbi.nlm.nih.gov/pubmed/20065170

Rodriguez JM et al (2008) Pheochromocytoma in MEN 2A syndrome. Study of 54 patients. World J Surg 32(11):2520–2526. Available at: http://ovidsp.ovid.com/ovidweb.cgi?T=JS&PAGE=reference&D=med5&NEWS=N&AN=18795243

Sahdev A et al (2005) CT and MR imaging of unusual locations of extra-adrenal paragangliomas (pheochromocytomas). Euro Radiol 15(1):85–92. Available at: http://www.ncbi.nlm.nih.gov/pubmed/15290072

Schiavi F et al (2005) Predictors and prevalence of paraganglioma syndrome associated with mutations of the *SDHC* gene. JAMA 294(16):2057–2063. Available at: http://www.ncbi.nlm.nih.gov/pubmed/16249420

Schlisio S et al (2008) The kinesin KIF1Bbeta acts downstream from EglN3 to induce apoptosis and is a potential 1p36 tumor suppressor. Genes Dev 22(7):884–893. Available at: http://www.pubmedcentral.nih.gov/articlerender.fcgi?artid=2279200&tool=pmcentrez&rendertype=abstract

Schmid S et al (2014) Management of von hippel-lindau disease: an interdisciplinary review. Oncol Res Treat 37(12):761–71. Available at: http://www.ncbi.nlm.nih.gov/pubmed/25531723

Shepet K et al (2013) Hereditary medullary thyroid cancer: age-appropriate thyroidectomy improves disease-free survival. Ann Surg Oncol 20(5):1451–1455. Available at: http://ovidsp.ovid.com/ovidweb.cgi?T=JS&PAGE=reference&D=medl&NEWS=N&AN=23188542

Taïeb D et al. (2013) First report of bilateral pheochromocytoma in the clinical spectrum of HIF2A-related polycythemia-paraganglioma syndrome. J Clin Endocrinol Metab 98(5):E908–E913. Available at: http://www.pubmedcentral.nih.gov/articlerender.fcgi?artid=3644612&tool=pmcentrez&rendertype=abstract

Timmers HJLM et al (2007) Clinical presentations, biochemical phenotypes, and genotype-phenotype correlations in patients with succinate dehydrogenase subunit B-associated pheochromocytomas and paragangliomas. J Clin Endocrinol Metab 92(3):779–786. Available at: http://www.ncbi.nlm.nih.gov/pubmed/17200167

Toledo RA, Dahia PLM (2015) Next-generation sequencing for the diagnosis of hereditary pheochromocytoma and paraganglioma syndromes. Curr Opin Endocrinol Diab Obes 22 (3):169–179. Available at: http://www.ncbi.nlm.nih.gov/pubmed/25871962

Toledo SPA et al (2015) Penetrance and clinical features of pheochromocytoma in a six-generation family carrying a germline *TMEM127* mutation. J Clin Endocrinol Metab 100(2):E308–E318. Available at: http://www.ncbi.nlm.nih.gov/pubmed/25389632

Van Hulsteijn LT et al (2012) Risk of malignant paraganglioma in *SDHB*-mutation and *SDHD*-mutation carriers: a systematic review and meta-analysis. J Med Genet 49(12):768–776. Available at: http://www.ncbi.nlm.nih.gov/pubmed/23099648

Van Hulsteijn LT et al (2013) No difference in phenotype of the main Dutch *SDHD* founder mutations. Clin Endocrinol 79(6):824–31. Available at: http://www.ncbi.nlm.nih.gov/pubmed/23586964

Van Hulsteijn LT et al (2015) No evidence for increased mortality in *SDHD* variant carriers compared with the general population. Euro J Hum Genet: EJHG. Available at: http://www.ncbi.nlm.nih.gov/pubmed/25758995

Waguespack SG et al (2011) Management of medullary thyroid carcinoma and MEN2 syndromes in childhood. Nat Rev Endocrinol 7(10):596–607. Available at: http://ovidsp.ovid.com/ovidweb.cgi?T=JS&PAGE=reference&D=medl&NEWS=N&AN=21862994

Yang C et al (2015) Germ-line PHD1 and PHD2 mutations detected in patients with pheochromocytoma/paraganglioma-polycythemia. J Mole Med 93(1):93–104. Available at: http://www.ncbi.nlm.nih.gov/pubmed/25263965

Yao L et al (2010) Spectrum and prevalence of FP/*TMEM127* gene mutations in pheochromocytomas and paragangliomas. JAMA 304(23):2611–2619

Diagnosis and Management of Hereditary Adrenal Cancer

Anna Angelousi, Mihail Zilbermint, Annabel Berthon, Stéphanie Espiard and Constantine A. Stratakis

Abstract

Benign adrenocortical tumours (ACT) are relatively frequent lesions; on the contrary, adrenocortical carcinoma (ACC) is a rare and aggressive malignancy with unfavourable prognosis. Recent advances in the molecular understanding of adrenal cancer offer promise for better therapies in the future. Many of these advances stem from the molecular elucidation of genetic conditions predisposing to the development of ACC. Six main clinical syndromes have been described to be associated with hereditary adrenal cancer. In these conditions, genetic counselling plays an important role for the early detection and follow-up of the patients and the affected family members.

A. Angelousi (✉) · M. Zilbermint · A. Berthon · S. Espiard · C.A. Stratakis (✉)
Section on Endocrinology and Genetics, Program on Developmental Endocrinology and Genetics, Eunice Kennedy Shriver National Institute of Child Health and Human Development, National Institutes of Health, Bethesda, MD, USA
e-mail: a.angelousi@gmail.com

C.A. Stratakis
e-mail: stratakc@mail.nih.gov

M. Zilbermint
e-mail: mihail.zilbermint@nih.gov

A. Berthon
e-mail: annabel.berthon@nih.gov

S. Espiard
e-mail: stephanie.espiard@live.fr

G. Pichert and C. Jacobs (eds.), *Rare Hereditary Cancers*,
Recent Results in Cancer Research 205, DOI 10.1007/978-3-319-29998-3_8

Keywords
Protein Kinase A (PKA) · PRKAR1A gene · Li-Fraumeni syndrome · TP53 gene · Familial polyposis · APC gene

Contents

1 Introduction

Adrenocortical tumours (ACT) represent a group of lesions arising from cells of the adrenal cortex. The incidence of adrenal incidentalomas has been reported to be as high as 8.7 % in autopsy series and 4 % in radiological studies (Arnaldi and Boscaro 2012). However, adrenocortical carcinomas (ACCs) are rare neoplasms with an incidence of 0.5–2 million per year leading to 0.2 % of all cancer deaths in the USA. They are significantly more frequent in females in all ages. ACCs are usually aggressive tumours with poor prognosis and an only 16–44 % 5-year survival rate (Fassnacht and Allolio 2009). The median age of diagnosis is at approximately 46 years; an early peak of the disease between the ages of 5 and 7 years represents a clinically and molecularly different form of ACC. In childhood, ACCs are slightly more frequent compared to adults, representing as many as 1.3 % of the total number of cancers in children (Fassnacht and Allolio 2009; Icard et al. 2001).

The differential diagnosis between a benign ACT and an ACC can be challenging given the frequency of the former and the rarity of the latter. In addition, about 60 % of ACC patients present with some hormone excess, but their detection remains elusive because the steroid hormone secretion is either subclinical or not typical of Cushing's and Conn's syndromes or hyperandrogenism (Arlt et al. 2011).

ACCs exhibit a complex pattern of genetic defects from many chromosomal aberrations to somatic mutations in a number of genes; they can also be caused by inherited mutations in specific cancer development-related genes (Lerario et al. 2014). Aside from genetic predisposition, no other risk factors have been established. High levels of oestrogens have been suggested to increase the incidence of ACC based on the observation of ACC development during pregnancy and the much higher frequency of ACC in females. Indeed, in vitro studies show growth-promoting effects of oestrogen on the ACC (Sirianni et al. 2012).

2 Genetic Syndromes Associated with ACC

The genetic defects and the manifested clinical syndromes associated with ACC are also briefly described and summarized in Table 1.

2.1 Li–Fraumeni Syndrome (LFS)

LFS is a cancer predisposition syndrome first described in 1969; cancer predisposition in this condition is inherited in an autosomal dominant manner. Half of the patients with LFS develop at least one LFS-associated cancer by age 30; 90 % of the patients develop a tumour by 60 years of age (Gonzalez et al. 2009; Sorrell et al. 2013). While many types of tumours can be seen in patients with LFS, the most frequent include breast cancer, sarcoma and brain tumours.

Breast cancer accounts for 25–30 % of all LFS-associated tumours (Sorrell et al. 2013), sarcomas for 25–30 % (Gonzalez et al. 2009; Olivier et al. 2003) and brain tumours for 9–16 % (Gonzalez et al. 2009; Olivier et al. 2003; Palmero et al. 2010). ACC is a less frequent manifestation accounting for 10–14 % of cancers within the context of LFS (Palmero et al. 2010). The next most frequently associated cancers are leukaemia, lung, colorectal, skin, gastric and ovarian cancers (Sorrell et al. 2013; Olivier et al. 2003). As in other cancer predisposition syndromes, all cancers in LFS are diagnosed at much younger ages than their sporadic counterparts.

Table 1 Genetic defects and associated clinical syndromes related to hereditary ACCs

Clinical syndromes	Inheritance	Locus	Gene(s) involved	Mutations	Prevalence of ACC	Genetic tests	Genetic counselling
LFS	AD	17p13	*TP53* (oncosuppressor)	Germline- and somatic missense-inactivating mutations	– 10–14% (adults)–50–80% (children)	– Sanger sequencing – MLPA	*TP53* germline test should be considered in all ACC patients
BWS	AD	11p15.5	– *IGF-2* – *CDKN1C* (oncosuppressor) – *KCNQ10T1* – *H19*	– Loss of methylation of IC2 or gain of methylation of IC1 on the maternal chromosome – Mutation of the maternal *CDKN1C* – UDP of 11p15.5 – Duplication, inversion or translocation of the 11p15.5	<1% (mainly children)	– CGH – MLPA – Sequence analysis of *CDKN1C* – Testing for microdeletions/microduplications of the CDKN1C by other methods	No specific screening recommendation for ACC patients
MEN1	AD	11q13	*Menin* (oncosuppressor)	Germline-inactivating mutation and somatic missense mutation or deletion leading to LOH	1–2% of adults (13% if tumour > 1 cm)	– Testing for partial or whole-gene deletion – Haplotype analysis – MLPA	No regular monitoring for ACC. If pre-existing adrenal lesions, annual or biennial imaging is proposed
FAP	AD	5q12-22	– *APC* (oncosuppressor) – *CTNNB1*	Germline-inactivating mutations: – Nucleotide substitution – Frameshift mutations *APC* promoter methylation	Rare: <1%	– Sanger sequencing – Large rearrangement analysis – MLPA	No recommendation for routine screening in patients with ACC
LS	AD	– 3p22.2 (*MLH1*) –2p21 (*MSH2*) – 2p16.3 (*MSH6*) – 7p22.1 (*PMS2*)	– *MSH2* – *MSH6* – *MLH1* – *PMS2*	Inactivating mutations	3% of adults	– sequencing – Large rearrangement analysis – Immunochemistry – Microsatellite instability analysis – MLPA	Routine screening in ACC tumours by immunochemistry of the 4 genes regardless of the family history

(continued)

Table 1 (continued)

Clinical syndromes	Inheritance	Locus	Gene(s) involved	Mutations	Prevalence of ACC	Genetic tests	Genetic counselling
CNC	AD	– 17q22.24 – 2p16	*PRKAR1A* (oncosuppressor)	– Germline-inactivating mutations: single-nucleotide base substitutions or exonic insertions or deletions (LOH) – c.439A > G (p.S147G)[a]	Rare (only case reports)	– Sanger sequencing – Array-based analysis – MLPA	No routine screening
NF1	AD	– 17q11.2	*NF1* (oncosuppressor)	Loss-of-function mutation or deletion (LOH)	Rare <1%	– dHPLC – FISH – MLPA – CGH – Sanger sequencing	No routine screening

ACC adrenocortical carcinoma, *LFS* Li–Fraumeni syndrome, *WBS* Beckwith–Wiedemann syndrome, *MEN1* multiple endocrine hyperplasia type 1, *FAP* familial adenomatous polyposis, *LS* Lynch syndrome, *CNC* Carney complex syndrome, *NF1* neurofibromatosis type 1, *AD* autosomal dominant, *TP53* tumour protein 53, *MLPA* multiplex ligation-dependent probe amplification analysis, *WGS* whole-genome sequencing, *WES* whole-exome sequencing, *IGF-2* insulin growth factor 2 gene, *CDKNIK1* cyclin-dependent kinase inhibitor 1C, *KCNQ10T1* potassium channel, voltage-gated KQT-like subfamily Q, member 1, *IC1/2* imprinting centre 1/2, *UDP* uniparental disomy, *LOH* loss of heterozygosity, *APC* adenomatous polyposis coli, *CTNNB1* catenin-beta 1, *MLH1* MutL homolog, *MSH1-6* MutS protein homolog 2-6, *PMS2* postmeiotic segregation increased 2, *PRKAR1A* protein kinase regulatory subunit type 1 alpha gene, *dHPLC* denaturing high-performance liquid chromatography, *FISH* fluorescence in situ hybridization, *CGH* array comparative genomic hybridization, *MLPA* Multiple ligation-dependent probe amplification

[a]Mutation associated with ACCs in members of a family with CNC

2.2 LFS: Diagnostic Criteria

The diagnostic criteria of LFS are presented in Table 2. The initial classical criteria of LFS were developed in 1998 (Li et al. 1988) with a low sensitivity of 40 % and a better specificity of 91 % (Gonzalez et al. 2009). Later, new diagnostic efforts led to the adoption of the Birch and Eeles criteria that were developed for the inclusion of families that had genetic defects leading to LFS but did not meet the criteria established in 1998. The term 'Li–Fraumeni-like syndrome' (LFLS) is used for these patients and families; the Birch criteria have a diagnostic sensitivity of 96 % and a specificity of 38 % (Birch et al. 1994; Gonzalez et al. 2009), whereas the Eeles criteria have a sensitivity of 97 % and a specificity of 16 % (Eeles 1995). In 2001, Chompret et al. (2000, 2001) proposed new criteria with a better sensitivity (95 %), but with a lower specificity (52 %) (Gonzalez et al. 2009). The Chompret criteria were most recently updated in 2009 to better identify families with milder phenotypes (Gonzalez et al. 2009; Tinat et al. 2009; Bougeard et al. 2008).

Table 2 Description of the established clinical classification criteria for LFS

Classification scheme	Description of the criteria
Classic LFS (Li et al. 1988)	– Proband diagnosed with sarcoma before 45 years of age, *and* – A first-degree relative with cancer before 45 years of age, *and* – Another first- or second-degree relative with any cancer diagnosed under 45 years of age *or* with sarcoma at any age
Birch (Birch et al. 1994; Gonzalez et al. 2009)	Among families that do not conform to classic LFS: – Proband with any childhood cancer *or* sarcoma, brain tumour *or* adrenocortical carcinoma diagnosed under 45 years of age, *and* – A first- or second-degree relative with a typical LFS-related cancer (sarcoma, breast cancer, brain tumour, leukaemia *or* adrenocortical carcinoma) diagnosed at any age, *and* – A first- or second-degree relative in the same genetic lineage with any cancer diagnosed under the age of 60 years
Eeles Eeles (1995)	Among families that do not conform to classic LFS: – Two different tumours that are part of extended LFS in first- *or* second-degree relatives at any age (sarcoma, breast cancer, brain tumour, leukaemia, adrenocortical tumour, melanoma, prostate cancer and pancreatic cancer)
Chompret Chompret et al. (2000, 2001)	Proband with sarcoma, brain tumour, breast cancer *or* adrenocortical carcinoma before the age of 36 years, *and* – At least one first- or second-degree relative with cancer (other than breast cancer if the proband has breast cancer) under the age of 46 years *or* a relative with multiple primaries at any age, *or* a proband with multiple primary tumours, two of which are sarcoma, brain tumour, breast cancer *and/or* adrenocortical carcinoma, with the initial cancer occurring before the age of 36 years, regardless of the family history, *or* a proband with adrenocortical carcinoma at any age of onset, regardless of the family history

LFS Li–Fraumeni syndrome

2.3 LFS: Genotype–Phenotype Correlations

TP53 germline mutations are the cause of LFS. The *TP53* genotype in LFS is predictive of age of tumour onset and overall tumour risk (Olivier et al. 2006; Palmero et al. 2010). Mutations in the DNA-binding portion of the gene cause highly penetrant disease with early onset cancers; mutations outside the core DNA-binding domain are associated with slower rates of tumour development (Varley et al. 1999). According to clinical studies, *TP53*-mutant ACCs are larger and associated with a more advanced stage of tumour progression and shorter disease-free survival compared to cases without *TP53* mutations; this is similar to non-LFS-associated ACC that carries somatic *TP53* defects (Libe et al. 2007). Furthermore, LFS-associated ACCs and ACCs with somatic *TP53* mutations show greater resistance to chemotherapy and radiation and overall higher rates of relapse (Tabori et al. 2010; Fernandez-Cuesta et al. 2012).

2.4 LFS: Genetic Mutations and Genetic Testing

Germline mutations of the tumour suppressor *TP53* gene are found in 70 % of cases with LFS (Bachinski et al. 2005). The prevalence of germline *TP53* mutations in sporadic ACTs is 3–6 % in the adult population (Herrmann et al. 2012; Raymond et al. 2013a) and significantly higher, approaching 50–80 %, in children (Varley et al. 1999; Libe et al. 2007). *TP53* inactivation in the somatic step is a late step in tumorigenesis (Hollstein et al. 1991), but somatic mutations of the *TP53* gene are frequent in sporadic, non-LFS-associated ACC (Ohgaki et al. 1993).

Most *TP53* mutations are missense alterations that render the gene inactive; however, some reports have shown gain-of-function, oncogenic effects of some *TP53* mutations. A specific germline *TP53* mutation (R337H) of the p53 protein was identified in more than 80 % of children with ACT in Southern Brazil where the incidence of ACT is 15 times higher than that in the rest of the world. The R337H mutation is also seen in 13.5 % of Brazilian adults with ACT (Giacomazzi et al. 2013; Petitjean et al. 2007).

TP53 genotyping is typically performed by DNA Sanger sequence analysis and multiplex ligation-dependent probe assay (MLPA) or other techniques in order to detect large rearrangements of portions of the gene. Molecular genetic testing for *TP53* germline mutations was developed in 1990 by David Malkin and colleagues (Malkin et al. 1990) and was quickly used as a screening tool to identify patients with hereditary forms of cancer. Currently, the growing availability and use of whole-genome sequencing (WGS), whole-exome sequencing (WES), whole-genome arrays and multigene panels increase the likelihood of detecting unintentionally or unexpectedly *TP53* mutation carriers. The National Comprehensive Cancer Network (NCCN) guidelines recommend *TP53* analysis for individuals who meet either the classic LFS criteria, the Chompret criteria, or who were diagnosed with breast cancer under age 30 and are negative for *BRCA1* or *BRCA2* gene mutations.

2.5 LFS: Genetic Counselling

Decisions regarding germline *TP53* testing should be made by healthcare professionals with training in clinical cancer genetics. Most germline *TP53* mutations are inherited from a parent, and only few are de novo. After identifying a mutation, the proband's parent with any pertinent cancer history or family history should be tested first; otherwise, both parents should be tested. Siblings and offspring of the proband should also be tested. If one of the proband's parents carries the *TP53* mutation, each sibling has a 50 % risk of having the mutation. If neither parent carries the mutation, the risk to siblings is low, but they should be tested due to the possibility of germline mosaicism. A family history can appear negative due to a limited family structure or incomplete penetrance of the mutation. The frequency of de novo mutations is not well established; however, based on two studies, the de novo rate has been estimated to be between 7 and 24 % (Chompret et al. 2000; Gonzalez et al. 2009).

LFS: **Key point**: Testing for all at risk for *TP53* mutation should be considered due to emerging evidence showing reduction of morbidity and mortality from *TP53*-related malignancies when an early screening protocol was implemented (Evans et al. 2010).

3 Beckwith–Wiedemann Syndrome (BWS)

BWS is one of the most common paediatric overgrowth disorders with an estimated incidence of 1 in 13,700 neonates, affecting men and women with equal frequency (Shuman et al. 1993). BWS is associated with epigenetic/genetic alterations on chromosome 11p15 and usually occurs sporadically (85 %), although familial transmission can also occur in 15 % of the cases (Weksberg et al. 2010). The overall risk of tumour development in children with BWS has been estimated to 7.5 % (4–21 %) (Rump et al. 2005).

3.1 BWS: Diagnostic Criteria

No consensus diagnostic criteria for BWS have been established; however, the most frequent features are anterior abdominal wall defects (80 %), macroglossia (97 %) and overgrowth. Other features such as external ear cartilage abnormalities (76 %), birth weight or postnatal growth over the 90th centile (88 %), facial naevus flammeus (62 %), neonatal hypoglycaemia, nephromegaly (59 %) and hemihypertrophy (24 %) have been also described (Mazzuco et al. 2012; Elliott et al. 1994), in addition to tumours, including nephro- and hepatoblastoma and adrenal cancer. Thus, the diagnosis of BWS is usually made when there is (i) positive family history (a parent or a sibling with a clinical diagnosis or a history of BWS) and (ii) the following: macroglossia, overgrowth (traditionally defined as height and weight >97th centile), visceromegaly, renal abnormalities (nephrocalcinosis), abdominal wall defect (omphalocele), embryonal tumours (nephroblastoma, hepatoblastoma), foetal adrenocortical cytomegaly, hemihyperplasia, cleft lip/palate and bifid uvula. Conditions that have also been described in association with BWS and may be used in diagnosing the disease, are: prematurity, polyhydramnion, neonatal hypoglycaemia, facial naevi and specific facial features such as prominent eyes, mid-facial hypoplasia, prominent mandible (Weksberg et al. 2010; Shuman et al. 1993).

BWS can be suspected even in utero based on intrauterine findings such as exomphalos, macroglossia, pancreatic hyperplasia, placentomegaly, as well as substantially increased levels of beta-human chorionic gonadotropin (hCG) upon maternal testing (Kagan et al. 2015).

3.2 BWS: Genotype–Phenotype Correlations

Increased insulin growth factor-2 (*IGF2*) signalling is the main molecular cause of the phenotype associated with BWS. IGF2 overexpression has also been linked with the development and progression of sporadic ACCs. In addition, molecular partners of *IGF2*, such as IGF-2 binding protein, have also been correlated with tumour volume in sporadic ACC (Boulle et al. 2001). Somatic hemihyperplasia is associated with mosaicism for paternal disomy of 11p15 or molecular alterations at imprinting centre 2 (IC2) or imprinting centre 1 (IC1) regulating *IGF2* expression (Ohta et al. 2013; Shuman et al. 1993; Enklaar et al. 2006). More recently, mutations in the cyclin-dependent kinase inhibitor 1C (*CDKN1C*) gene or microdeletions at IC1 and rarely microduplication at IC2 were found to explain BWS in cases with germline defects (Hatada et al. 1997; Enklaar et al. 2006; Bliek et al. 2009). Uniparental disomy of 11p15 or gain of methylation at IC1 is associated with the highest risk for Wilms' tumour and hepatoblastoma. Loss of methylation at IC2 is associated with a lower risk for tumour development.

3.3 BWS: Genetic Mutations and Genetic Testing

BWS is associated with abnormal regulation of gene transcription in the imprinted domain on chromosome 11p15.5. Normally, *IGF2* gene is maternally imprinted; therefore, only the paternal allele is expressed. On the other hand, the paternal alleles of *CDKN1C* and *H19* are silenced by imprinting; thus, only the maternal alleles are expressed (Weksberg et al. 2010). It has been shown that the BWS-associated defects on chromosome 11p15.5 result in the expression of the otherwise repressed maternal copy of the *IGF2* gene, and in some cases, this is accompanied by repression and DNA methylation of the maternal (otherwise active) copy of the neighbouring *H19* gene. Thus, in BWS, the more common molecular genetic defects are as follows: (Weksberg et al. 2003, 2005): (1) loss of methylation of the IC2 on the maternal chromosome leading to an increased activity of the *KCNQ1OT1* (opposite strand/antisense transcript 1) gene, (2) gain of methylation of the IC1 on the maternal chromosome, (3) mutation of the maternal *CDKN1C* allele, (4) paternal uniparental disomy of 11p15.5 and (5) duplication, inversion or translocation of the 11p15.5.

The genetic tests that can detect more than 80 % of individuals with BWS are the following: (1) molecular cytogenetic analysis of chromosome 11p and/or (2) methylation studies of IC1 and IC2. Methylation-specific (MS) multiplex ligation-dependent probe amplification (MLPA) is the most recently developed robust testing methodology for these defects. Sequence analysis of *CDKN1C* should be undertaken in familial cases, in individuals with BWS and cleft palate, or in those who meet diagnostic criteria for BWS but have no detectable molecular cytogenetic abnormalities of chromosome 11p, or methylation abnormalities. Chromosome 11p-specific molecular cytogenetic analysis for the detection of microdeletions or duplications may be undertaken in familial cases in which a *CDKN1C* mutation has not been detected and conventional cytogenetics are normal (Niemitz et al. 2004; Prawitt et al. 2005).

3.4 BWS: Genetic Counselling

Prenatal diagnosis for at-risk pregnancies in families with heritable forms of BWS requires prior identification of the disease-causing defect in the family. Most individuals with BWS are reported to have normal chromosome studies or karyotypes. Approximately 85 % of individuals with BWS have no family history of BWS, while about 15 % have a family history consistent with autosomal dominant transmission of BWS (Shuman et al. 1993). Specific prenatal testing is possible by cytogenetic analysis for families with an inherited chromosome abnormality or by molecular genetic testing for families in which the molecular mechanism of BWS has been defined.

Key point: Due to the low incidence of ACC in BWS, no specific screening recommendations for ACC exist (Else et al. 2014). Patients with BWS should be monitored for the development of tumours, including ACC.

4 Multiple Endocrine Neoplasia Type 1 (MEN1)

MEN1 is a tumour syndrome that is caused by defects of the *menin* gene on chromosome 11q13 and in most cases is inherited in an autosomal dominant manner. Parathyroid tumours, resulting in primary hyperparathyroidism, are the most common feature (95 %), followed by pancreatic neuroendocrine tumours (45 %), anterior pituitary tumours (40 %), thymic carcinoids, thyroid adenomas and ACT. Adrenal involvement in MEN1 has been reported in 20–40 % of cases; however, endoscopic ultrasound detected adrenal lesions in up to 73 % of MEN1 patients (Schaefer et al. 2008). ACCs is rare; less than 1 % of patients with MEN1 develop ACC, but the incidence increases to approximately 13 % among patients with MEN1 and adrenal tumours larger than 1 cm (Gatta-Cherifi et al. 2012).

Most patients with MEN1 have bilateral adrenocortical hyperplasia (40 %) that is usually non-functional and benign. Less than 10 % of patients with enlarged adrenal glands have hormonal hypersecretion, and among these, primary aldosteronism and ACTH-independent Cushing's syndrome are the most commonly encountered conditions; hyperandrogenemia has been associated with MEN1-associated ACCs (Gatta-Cherifi et al. 2012).

4.1 MEN1: Diagnostic Criteria

The diagnosis of the MEN1 syndrome is based on the presence of one of the three following criteria:

i. A patient with 2 or more MEN1-associated endocrine tumours;
ii. A patient with MEN1-associated tumours and a first-degree relative with MEN1;
iii. An individual who has a *MEN1* mutation without clinical or biochemical manifestations of MEN1 (Newey and Thakker 2011).

4.2 MEN1: Genotype–Phenotype Correlations

No correlation between the MEN1 genotype and phenotype has yet been clearly identified. A study suggested that adrenal lesions usually develop in patients with mutations in the exons 2 and 10 (Newey and Thakker 2011). Various clinical manifestations may be caused by tissue-dependent factors such as epigenetics, as it is found in parathyroid tumours associated with tissue-specific methylation.

4.3 MEN1: Genetic Mutations and Genetic Testing

MEN1 is caused by (typically) germline mutations of menin (*MEN1* gene), a tumour suppressor gene that predisposes to the development of endocrine and non-endocrine tumours with variable penetrance. Menin is the major regulator of transcription interacting with many molecules and signalling pathways (Wu and Hua 2008; Marini et al. 2009). More than 1133 germline and 203 somatic mutations of the MEN1 have been reported (Lemos and Thakker 2008). A number of *MEN1* polymorphisms have been identified and should be differentiated from pathogenic mutations during genetic analysis (Lemos and Thakker 2008). Loss of heterozygosity (LOH) involving the *MEN1* locus on chromosome 11q13 has also been observed in 5–50 % of sporadic endocrine tumours (Thakker et al. 2012), but somatic MEN1 mutations are relatively rare in tumours compared to other tumour suppressor genes. If *MEN1* coding region mutations are not identified, then testing for partial or whole-gene deletion or haplotype analysis of the *MEN1* locus should be considered.

More than 10 % of *MEN1* germline mutations are found de novo and may be transmitted to subsequent generations. Five to Twenty five percentage of patients with *MEN1* may not harbour germline mutations and these individuals may have partial or whole-gene deletions, or mutations in the promoter or untranslated regions (Newey and Thakker 2011; Thakker et al. 2012). In these cases, MLPA for the detection of exonic deletions is recommended (Tham et al. 2007).

A few patients with *MEN1* may have mutations in others genes, mostly p27 (CDK1NB); however, it is not known if these patients are at risk for ACC.

4.4 MEN1: Genetic Counselling

Relatives of a patient with a known *MEN1* mutation should be offered *MEN1* germline mutational analysis before any biochemical or radiological screening tests for the detection of MEN1 tumours (Thakker et al. 2012).

Briefly, *MEN1* mutational analysis should be undertaken in (i) patients with two or more *MEN1*-associated endocrine tumours (Newey and Thakker 2011). Such mutational analysis may be undertaken in (i) children within the first decade of life; (ii) asymptomatic first-degree relative of a known *MEN1* mutation carrier; and (iii) patients with suspicious or atypical *MEN1*, which includes individuals with parathyroid adenomas occurring before the age of 30 years; or multigland parathyroid disease, gastrinoma and multiple pancreatic neuroendocrine tumour (NET) at any age; or individuals who have two or more *MEN1*-associated tumours that are not part of the classical triad of parathyroid, pancreatic islet and anterior pituitary tumours.

Individuals with *MEN1* mutations undergo biochemical screening at least once per year and also have baseline pituitary and abdominal imaging. Screening begins in early childhood because the disease has developed in some individuals by the age of 5 years, and it should be repeated throughout life, since in some individuals tumour may not develop until they are elderly (Thakker et al. 2012).

Key point: No regular monitoring for ACC is recommended in patients with MEN1. However, because of the increased risk of malignant transformation of pre-existing adrenal lesions, MEN1 patients should be monitored for possible ACC as other patients with radiologically detectable ACTs.

5 Familial Adenomatous Polyposis (FAP) and Lynch Syndrome (LS)

FAP is a disorder inherited in an autosomal dominant manner and is primarily associated with the early development of multiple colonic adenomatous polyps and an increased risk of colorectal cancer; the prevalence of adrenal tumours in patients with FAP varies from 7.4 to 13 %. LS is a disorder inherited in an autosomal dominant manner that is also associated with an increased risk for colorectal cancer as well as other malignancies such as carcinomas of endometrium, ovary, small bowel, hepatobiliary system, central nervous system, lung adenocarcinoma, sarcoma, melanoma and ACCs (Raymond et al. 2013b). Patients with FAP carry a germline-inactivating mutation in the adenomatous polyposis coli (*APC*) gene, whereas patients with LS carry germline mutations of genes important for DNA mismatch repair. Recent studies showed that the prevalence of LS in patients with ACC was 3 % comparable to their prevalence of colorectal and endometrial cancer estimated at 2–5 % (Raymond et al. 2013b; Liu et al. 2014).

5.1 FAP and LS: Diagnostic Criteria

Diagnosis of LS is based on Amsterdam I and II criteria as well the most recently revised Bethesda criteria which include also histological findings (Liu et al., 2014). The revised Bethesda criteria include the following:

i. Colorectal cancer diagnosed in a patient who is less than 50 years of age;
ii. Presence of synchronous or metachronous colorectal or LS associated tumours;
iii. Colorectal cancer with the microsatellite instability-high histology diagnosed in a patient who is less than 60 years of age;
iv. Colorectal cancer or LS-associated tumour diagnosed under the age of 50 years in at least one first-degree relative;
v. Colorectal cancer or LS-associated tumour diagnosed at any age in two first- or second-degree relatives.

5.2 FAP and LS: Genetic Mutations and Genetic Testing

APC-inactivating mutations result in constitutive activation of β-catenin and elevated levels of β-catenin/TCF (T cell factor) target genes. Activation of this pathway may play an important role in adrenocortical tumourigenesis through activating mutations of the β-catenin gene (*CTNNB1*) in ACC. APC is a downstream regulator of the Drosophila melanogaster wingless (*Wnt*) molecular signalling pathway. Abnormal, constitutive Wnt activation is thought to be oncogenic (Karim et al. 2004). The majority of *APC* mutations are nucleotide substitutions and frameshift mutations that result in inactive APC and consequently overactive Wnt signalling. *APC* promoter methylation may also result in suppressed APC activity (Raymond et al. 2013b). Patients with LS have mutations of genes involved in DNA mismatch repair such as *MLH1*, *MSH2*, *MSH6* and *PMS2* (Karamurzin et al. 2012). ACC patients with a family history suggestive of LS should be considered for genetic risk assessment. Immunohistochemical screening in all ACCs may be an effective strategy for identifying these patients (Raymond et al. 2013b). This includes immunochemistry for the 4 gene products as well as microsatellite instability analysis. Full germline genetic testing for LS should include DNA sequencing and large rearrangement analysis. Patients with multiple colorectal adenomas (>10) should be considered for germline genetic testing of *APC*. Similarly, full germline genetic testing for FAP should include DNA sequencing and large rearrangement analysis (Stoffel et al. 2015).

5.3 FAP and LS: Genetic Counselling

Genetic counselling in patients with FAP or LS is necessary for follow-up and therapeutic decisions. For example, in families with classic FAP, sigmoidoscopy or colonoscopy should be carried out every 1–2 years starting at the age of 10–11 years and continued lifelong in mutation carriers. Surgery is indicated if there are large numbers of adenomas or adenomas with high degree of dysplasia. Generally, screening for extracolonic tumours should be considered when colorectal polyposis is diagnosed before the age of 25–30 years.

Key point: Routine screening for LS in ACC tumours by immunochemistry for the protein products of the four responsible genes (*MLH1*, *MSH2*, *MSH6* and *PMS2*) is recommended regardless of the family history (Birch et al. 1994; Else et al. 2014).

6 Carney Complex (CNC)

Carney complex is multiple tumour syndrome inherited in an autosomal dominant disorder. The main endocrine manifestation of CNC is primary pigmented nodular adrenocortical hyperplasia (PPNAD), a rare form of bilateral adrenocortical hyperplasia featuring small to normal-sized adrenal glands that contain multiple small and pigmented, cortical nodules with internodular atrophy (Stratakis et al. 2001). ACCs are extremely rare in this syndrome, and only two cases of ACC in CNC have been reported.

6.1 CNC: Diagnostic Criteria

The diagnosis of CNC is based on the presence of two or more major diagnostic criteria or on the presence of just one major if the patient is a carrier of a known inactivating mutation of the protein kinase regulatory subunit type 1 alpha gene (*PRKAR1A*) (Bossis et al. 2004). The major diagnostic criteria for CNC include the following:

i. Spotty skin pigmentation with typical distribution (lips, conjunctiva and inner or outer canthi, vaginal and penile mucosal (Fig. 1));
ii. Cutaneous myxoma;
iii. Cardiac myxoma;
iv. Breast myxomatosis;
v. PPNAD or paradoxical positive response of urinary glucocorticosteroid excretion to dexamethasone administration during Liddle's test;
vi. Acromegaly due to GH-producing adenoma;
vii. Large cell calcifying Sertoli cell tumours (LCCSCT) or characteristic calcifications on testicular ultrasound;
viii. Thyroid carcinoma or multiple, hypoechoic nodules on thyroid ultrasound in a young patient;
ix. Psammomatous melanotic schwannomas;
x. Blue naevus, epithelioid blue naevus;
xi. Breast ductal adenoma;

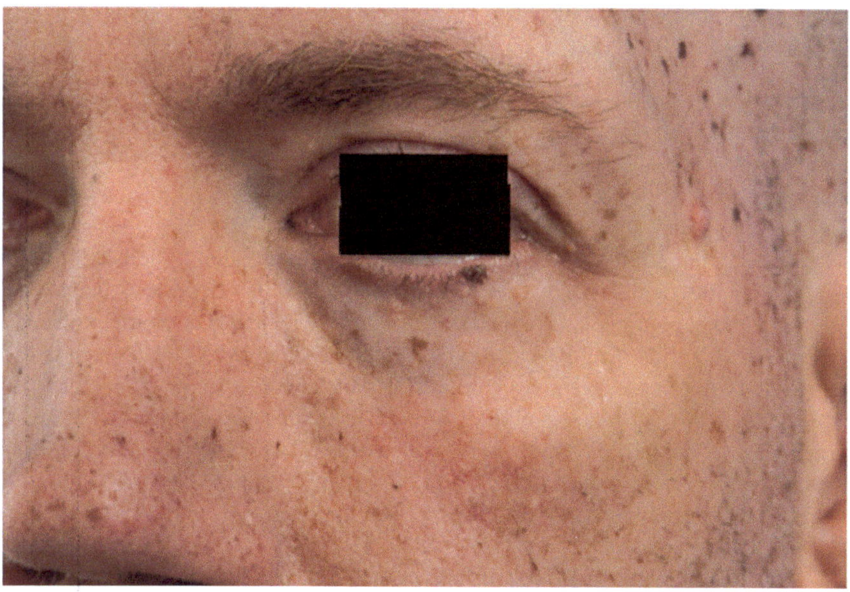

Fig. 1 The classical facies of a patient with CNC and typical distribution

xii. Osteochondromyxomas. Supplementary criteria include (Rodriguez et al. 2012; Boikos and Stratakis 2006): (i) affected first-degree relative and (ii) inactivating mutation of the *PRKAR1A* gene.

6.2 CNC: Genotype–Phenotype Correlations

There seems to be no direct and consistent correlation between *PRKAR1A* mutations described to date and the various CNC phenotypes. Only recently, certain associations between specific mutations and particular sets of CNC manifestations have emerged (Bertherat et al. 2009). Phosphodiesterases type 11A (*PDE11A*) and type 8b (*PDE8B*) mutations have also been found in isolated micronodular adrenocortical disease, a condition that is similar to PPNAD but distinct from CNC. Interestingly, among CNC patients, germline protein-truncating mutations of *PDE11A* predispose to a variety of endocrine tumours. A higher frequency of *PDE11A* variants was found in cases with PPNAD and testicular tumours (LCCSCTs). A base substitution (c.439A > G/p.S147G) in *PRKAR1A* identified to a large family was found to cause a large spectrum of adrenal diseases that ranged from lack of significant manifestations to ACC (Anselmo et al. 2012). Cases with this mutation did not present myxomas, schwannomas or any other tumours associated with CNC.

6.3 CNC: Genetic Mutations and Genetic Testing

Genetic linkage analysis identified two independent loci for CNC, one on chromosome 17p22–24 and the other on chromosome 2p16. Most of the cases of CNC are caused by inactivating mutations in the *PRKAR1A* gene located at 17q22–24 which encodes the most widely expressed of the protein kinase A (PKA) regulatory subunits. Germline heterozygous *PRKAR1A* mutation most often create a premature stop codon, and the resulting RNA is degraded by a mechanism of nonsense-mediated mRNA decay, inactivating fully the mutant allele. More than 125 pathogenic mutations of the *PRKAR1A* gene in CNC patients have been reported to date, but only approximately 70 % of CNC patients are found by Sanger sequencing to carry *PRKAR1A* defects; a significant number (21.6 %) of patients with CNC who are negative by currently available testing may have *PRKAR1A* haploinsufficiency due to genomic defects that are not detected by Sanger sequencing (Salpea et al. 2014). Array-based studies are necessary for diagnostic confirmation of these defects and should be done in patients with unusual and/or severe CNC phenotypes who are *PRKAR1A* mutation negative.

6.4 CNC: Genetic Counselling

CNC–adrenal tumours are typically histologically benign lesions. However, two cases of ACC with CNC have been described (Anselmo et al. 2012; Morin et al. 2012). The rarity of CNC and ACC precludes statistical demonstration of their association.

Key point: ACCs are extremely rare in this syndrome, and therefore, genetic testing for *PRKAR1A* mutation in ACCs should be reserved in cases with other signs of Carney complex.

7 Neurofibromatosis Type 1 (NF1)

NF1 is an autosomal dominant disease with an incidence of one in 3–4000 cases. ACC in patients with NF1 is rare: six case reports are available in the public domain (Menon et al. 2014; Fienman and Yakovac 1970; Sorensen et al. 1986; Wagner et al. 2005; Gutmann et al. 1994; Fraumeni and Miller 1967). Yet, there has not been any clear evidence of a causal association between *NF1* gene mutations and development of adrenocortical tumours.

7.1 NF1: Diagnostic Criteria

Two or more of the following clinical features are sufficient to establish a diagnosis of NF1:

i. Six or more café-au-lait macules (>0.5 cm at largest diameter in a prepubertal child or >1.5 cm in postpubertal individuals);
ii. Axillary freckling or freckling in inguinal regions;
iii. Two or more neurofibromas of any type or one or more plexiform neurofibromas;
iv. Two or more iris hamartomas (Lisch nodules);
v. Osseous lesion (sphenoid wing dysplasia, long-bone dysplasia);
vi. Optic pathway glioma;
vii. A first-degree relative with NF1 diagnosed by the above criteria.

7.2 NF1: Genotype–Phenotype Correlations

Patients with *NF1* microdeletions tend to develop neurofibromas at an earlier age, have a lower mean IQ, manifest abnormal facial features and are at increased risk of developing malignant peripheral nerve sheath tumours (Menon et al. 2014). Patients are susceptible to a variety of malignant tumours, of which the most common are the sarcomas (leiomyosarcoma and neurofibrosarcoma), breast cancer and lung cancers and cancers of the gastrointestinal tract. A novel germline frameshift mutation (c.5452_5453delAT) in exon 37 of the *NF1* gene was recently associated with the ACC development (Menon et al. 2014).

7.3 NF1: Genetic Mutations and Genetic Testing

At present, the diagnosis of NF1 is made using established clinical criteria, reserving NF1 genetic testing for unusual presentations. NF1 results from a loss-of-function mutation or deletion in the *NF1* gene. *NF1* is a tumour suppressor gene encoding neurofibromin. This protein functions as a negative regulator of the Ras proto-oncogene, which is a key signalling molecule in the control of cell growth. About 50 % of individuals with NF1 have no family history of the disease, and the disease is due to de novo mutations. In patients with a heterozygous germline *NF1* mutation, the loss of the other allele will lead to the complete loss of neurofibromin function and the development of tumours, according to the two-hit hypothesis. ACC development is linked to loss of heterozygosity of NF1 gene (Menon et al. 2014). The *NF1* gene mutation is found in approximately 85–95 % of cases using a combination of molecular techniques, including denaturing high-performance liquid chromatography (dHPLC), direct sequencing, fluorescence in situ hybridization (FISH), MLPA and array comparative genomic hybridization (CGH) (Ferner et al. 2007). Prenatal testing is possible by direct mutation testing of foetal DNA extracted from chorionic villous sampling or amniocentesis.

7.4 NF1: Genetic Counselling

Genetic counselling is advised for patients with NF1, as neurofibromas often start to develop in late adolescence. An individual with NF1 has a 50 % risk of passing on the condition to an offspring, but the clinical manifestation cannot be predicted, even within families. It is imperative to examine the parents for cutaneous stigmata or for Lisch nodules. Genetic counselling prior to conception is advised in all NF1 individuals.

Key point: There are no recommendations for NF1 gene mutation screening in patients with ACCs because of the rare cases described up to date in the literature and the lack of a clear evidence of linking NF1 to ACCs (Ferner et al. 2007).

8 Conclusions

Every patient with ACC should receive a basic physical examination aimed at finding clues of hereditary diseases. A detailed family history and a search for malignancies even in second- and third-degree relatives should be obtained. If the clinical history points to a specific disease, corresponding genes should be sequenced. Germline *TP53* mutations have to be considered, since it is the underlying genetic cause in the 50–80 % of all ACC cases in childhood. The possibility of a *TP53* mutation should not be dismissed because of a negative family history as up to 25 % can occur de novo. However, next-generation sequencing now allows sequencing of a panel of genes at the same time. This systematic screening should be performed in the absence of family history. The design of the arrays should include *TP53, IGF-2, CDKN1C, KCNQ1OT1, APC, MSH genes, PRKAR1A, Menin and NF-1*. The use of next-generation sequencing will be especially helpful in permitting guided potential target therapy options.

References

Anselmo J, Medeiros S, Carneiro V, Greene E, Levy I, Nesterova M, Lyssikatos C, Horvath A, Carney JA, Stratakis CA (2012) A large family with Carney complex caused by the S147G PRKAR1A mutation shows a unique spectrum of disease including adrenocortical cancer. J Clin Endocrinol Metab 97:351–359

Arlt W, Biehl M, Taylor AE, Hahner S, Libe R, Hughes BA, Schneider P, Smith DJ, Stiekema H, Krone N, Porfiri E, Opocher G, Bertherat J, Mantero F, Allolio B, Terzolo M, Nightingale P, Shackleton CH, Bertagna X, Fassnacht M, Stewart PM (2011) Urine steroid metabolomics as a biomarker tool for detecting malignancy in adrenal tumors. J Clin Endocrinol Metab 96:3775–3784

Arnaldi G, Boscaro M (2012) Adrenal incidentaloma. Best Pract Res Clin Endocrinol Metab 26:405–419

Bachinski LL, Olufemi SE, Zhou X, Wu CC, Yip L, Shete S, Lozano G, Amos CI, Strong LC, Krahe R (2005) Genetic mapping of a third Li-Fraumeni syndrome predisposition locus to human chromosome 1q23. Cancer Res 65:427–431

Bertherat J, Horvath A, Groussin L, Grabar S, Boikos S, Cazabat L, Libe R, Rene-Corail F, Stergiopoulos S, Bourdeau I, Bei T, Clauser E, Calender A, Kirschner LS, Bertagna X, Carney JA, Stratakis CA (2009) Mutations in regulatory subunit type 1A of cyclic adenosine 5′-monophosphate-dependent protein kinase (PRKAR1A): phenotype analysis in 353 patients and 80 different genotypes. J Clin Endocrinol Metab 94:2085–2091

Birch JM, Hartley AL, Tricker KJ, Prosser J, Condie A, Kelsey AM, Harris M, Jones, PH, Binchy A, Crowther D and et al (1994) Prevalence and diversity of constitutional mutations in the p53 gene among 21 Li-Fraumeni families. Cancer Res 54, 1298–304

Bliek J, Verde G, Callaway J, Maas SM, de Crescenzo A, Sparago A, Cerrato F, Russo S, Ferraiuolo S, Rinaldi MM, Fischetto R, Lalatta F, Giordano L, Ferrari P, Cubellis MV, Larizza L, Temple IK, Mannens MM, Mackay DJ, Riccio A (2009) Hypomethylation at multiple maternally methylated imprinted regions including PLAGL1 and GNAS loci in Beckwith-Wiedemann syndrome. Eur J Hum Genet 17:611–619

Boikos SA, Stratakis CA (2006) Carney complex: pathology and molecular genetics. Neuroendocrinology 83:189–199

Bossis I, Voutetakis A, Bei T, Sandrini F, Griffin KJ, Stratakis CA (2004) Protein kinase A and its role in human neoplasia: the Carney complex paradigm. Endocr Relat Cancer 11:265–280

Bougeard G, Sesboue R, Baert-Desurmont S, Vasseur S, Martin C, Tinat J, Brugieres L, Chompret A, De Paillerets BB, Stoppa-Lyonnet D, Bonaiti-Pellie C, Frebourg T, French LFSWG (2008) Molecular basis of the Li-Fraumeni syndrome: an update from the French LFS families. J Med Genet 45(8), 535–538, England

Boulle N, Baudin E, Gicquel C, Logie A, Bertherat J, Penfornis A, Bertagna X, Luton JP, Schlumberger M, le Bouc Y (2001) Evaluation of plasma insulin-like growth factor binding protein-2 as a marker for adrenocortical tumors. Eur J Endocrinol 144:29–36

Chompret A, Brugieres L, Ronsin M, Gardes M, Dessarps-Freichey F, Abel A, Hua D, Ligot L, Dondon MG, Bressac-de Paillerets B, Frebourg T, Lemerle J, Bonaiti-Pellie C, Feunteun J (2000) P53 germline mutations in childhood cancers and cancer risk for carrier individuals. *Br J Cancer,* 82:1932–1937

Chompret A, Abel A, Stoppa-Lyonnet D, Brugieres L, Pages S, Feunteun J, Bonaiti-Pellie C (2001) Sensitivity and predictive value of criteria for p53 germline mutation screening. J Med Genet 38:43–47

Eeles RA (1995) Germline mutations in the TP53 gene. Cancer Surv 25:101–124

Elliott M, Bayly R, Cole T, Temple IK, Maher ER (1994) Clinical features and natural history of Beckwith-Wiedemann syndrome: presentation of 74 new cases. Clin Genet 46:168–174

Else T, Kim AC, Sabolch A, Raymond VM, Kandathil A, Caoili EM, Jolly S, Miller BS, Giordano TJ, Hammer GD (2014) Adrenocortical carcinoma. Endocr Rev 35:282–326

Enklaar T, Zabel BU, Prawitt D (2006) Beckwith-Wiedemann syndrome: multiple molecular mechanisms. Expert Rev Mol Med 8:1–19

Evans DG, Lunt P, Clancy T, Eeles R (2010) Childhood predictive genetic testing for Li-Fraumeni syndrome. Fam Cancer 9:65–69

Fassnacht M, Allolio B (2009) Clinical management of adrenocortical carcinoma. Best Pract Res Clin Endocrinol Metab 23:273–289

Fernandez-Cuesta L, Oakman C, Falagan-Lotsch P, Smoth KS, Quinaux E, Buyse M, Dolci MS, Azambuja ED, Hainaut P, Dell'Orto P, Larsimont D, Francis PA, Crown J, Piccart-Gebhart M, Viale G, Leo AD, Olivier M (2012) Prognostic and predictive value of TP53 mutations in node-positive breast cancer patients treated with anthracycline- or anthracycline/taxane-based adjuvant therapy: results from the BIG 02-98 phase III trial. Breast Cancer Res 14:R70

Ferner RE, Huson SM, Thomas N, Moss C, Willshaw H, Evans DG, Upadhyaya M, Towers R, Gleeson M, Steiger C, Kirby A (2007) Guidelines for the diagnosis and management of individuals with neurofibromatosis 1. J Med Genet 44:81–88

Fienman NL, Yakovac WC (1970) Neurofibromatosis in childhood. J Pediatr 76:339–346

Fraumeni JF Jr., Miller RW (1967) Adrenocortical neoplasms with hemihypertrophy, brain tumors, and other disorders. J Pediatr 70:129–38

Gatta-Cherifi B, Chabre O, Murat A, Niccoli P, Cardot-Bauters C, Rohmer V, Young J, Delemer B, du Boullay H, Verger MF, Kuhn JM, Sadoul JL, Ruszniewski P, Beckers A, Monsaingeon M, Baudin E, Goudet P, Tabarin A (2012) Adrenal involvement in MEN1. Analysis of 715 cases from the Groupe d'etude des Tumeurs Endocrines database. Eur J Endocrinol 166:269–279

Giacomazzi J, Selistre SG, Rossi C, Alemar B, Santos-Silva P, Pereira FS, Netto CB, Cossio SL, Roth DE, Brunetto AL, Zagonel-Oliveira M, Martel-Planche G, Goldim JR, Hainaut P, Camey SA, Ashton-Prolla P (2013) Li-Fraumeni and Li-Fraumeni-like syndrome among children diagnosed with pediatric cancer in Southern Brazil. Cancer 119:4341–4349

Gonzalez KD, Noltner KA, Buzin CH, Gu D, Wen-Fong CY, Nguyen VQ, Han JH, Lowstuter K, Longmate J, Sommer SS, Weitzel JN (2009) Beyond Li Fraumeni Syndrome: clinical characteristics of families with p53 germline mutations. J Clin Oncol 27:1250–1256

Gutmann DH, Cole JL, Stone WJ, Ponder BA, Collins FS (1994) Loss of neurofibromin in adrenal gland tumors from patients with neurofibromatosis type I. Genes Chromosomes Cancer 10:55–58

Hatada I, Nabetani A, Morisaki H, Xin Z, Ohishi S, Tonoki H, Niikawa N, Inoue M, Komoto Y, Okada A, Steichen E, Ohashi H, Fukushima Y, Nakayama M, Mukai T (1997) New p57KIP2 mutations in Beckwith-Wiedemann syndrome. Hum Genet 100:681–683

Herrmann LJ, Heinze B, Fassnacht M, Willenberg HS, Quinkler M, Reisch N, Zink M, Allolio B, Hahner S (2012) TP53 germline mutations in adult patients with adrenocortical carcinoma. J Clin Endocrinol Metab 97:E476–E485

Hollstein M, Sidransky D, Vogelstein B, Harris CC (1991) p53 mutations in human cancers. Science 253:49–53

Icard P, Goudet P, Charpenay C, Andreassian B, Carnaille B, Chapuis Y, Cougard P, Henry JF, Proye C (2001) Adrenocortical carcinomas: surgical trends and results of a 253-patient series from the French Association of Endocrine Surgeons study group. World J Surg 25:891–897

Kagan KO, Berg C, Dufke A, Geipel A, Hoopmann M, Abele H (2015) Novel fetal and maternal sonographic findings in confirmed cases of Beckwith-Wiedemann syndrome. Prenat Diagn 35 (4):394–399

Karamurzin Y, Zeng Z, Stadler ZK, Zhang L, Ouansafi I, Al-Ahmadie HA, Sempoux C, Saltz LB, Soslow RA, O'Reilly EM, Paty PB, Coit DG, Shia J, Klimstra DS (2012) Unusual DNA mismatch repair-deficient tumors in Lynch syndrome: a report of new cases and review of the literature. Hum Pathol 43:1677–1687

Karim R, Tse G, Putti T, Scolyer R, Lee S (2004) The significance of the Wnt pathway in the pathology of human cancers. Pathology 36:120–128

Lemos MC, Thakker RV (2008) Multiple endocrine neoplasia type 1 (MEN1): analysis of 1336 mutations reported in the first decade following identification of the gene. Hum Mutat 29:22–32

Lerario AM, Moraitis A, Hammer GD (2014) Genetics and epigenetics of adrenocortical tumors. Mol Cell Endocrinol 386:67–84

Li FP, Fraumeni JF Jr, Mulvihill JJ, Blattner WA, Dreyfus MG, Tucker MA, Miller RW (1988) A cancer family syndrome in twenty-four kindreds. Cancer Res 48:5358–5362

Libe R, Groussin L, Tissier F, Elie C, Rene-Corail F, Fratticci A, Jullian E, Beck-Peccoz P, Bertagna X, Gicquel C, Bertherat J (2007) Somatic TP53 mutations are relatively rare among adrenocortical cancers with the frequent 17p13 loss of heterozygosity. Clin Cancer Res 13:844–850

Liu Y, Chew MH, Goh XW, Tan SY, Loi CT, Tan YM, Law HY, Koh PK, Tang CL (2014) Systematic study on genetic and epimutational profile of a cohort of Amsterdam criteria-defined Lynch Syndrome in Singapore. PLoS ONE 9:e94170

Malkin D, LI FP, Strong LC, Fraumeni JF, Jr., Nelson CE, Kim DH, Kassel J, Gryka MA, Bischoff FZ, Tainsky MA, et al (1990) Germ line p53 mutations in a familial syndrome of breast cancer, sarcomas, and other neoplasms. Science 250:1233–1238

Marini F, Falchetti A, Luzi E, Tonelli F, Maria Luisa B (2009) Multiple endocrine neoplasia type 1 (MEN1) Syndrome. In: Riegert-Johnson DL, Boardman LA, Hefferon T, Roberts M (eds) Cancer syndromes. Bethesda (MD), National Center for Biotechnology Information (US)

Mazzuco TL, Durand J, Chapman A, Crespigio J, Bourdeau I (2012) Genetic aspects of adrenocortical tumours and hyperplasias. Clin Endocrinol (Oxf) 77:1–10

Menon RK, Ferrau F, Kurzawinski TR, Rumsby G, Freeman A, Amin Z, Korbonits M, Chung TT (2014) Adrenal cancer in neurofibromatosis type 1: case report and DNA analysis. Endocrinol Diabetes Metab Case Rep 2014:140074

Morin E, Mete O, Wasserman JD, Joshua AM, Asa SL, Ezzat S (2012) Carney complex with adrenal cortical carcinoma. J Clin Endocrinol Metab 97:E202–E206

Newey PJ, Thakker RV (2011) Role of multiple endocrine neoplasia type 1 mutational analysis in clinical practice. Endocr Pract 17(Suppl 3):8–17

Niemitz EL, Debaun MR, Fallon J, Murakami K, Kugoh H, Oshimura M, Feinberg AP (2004) Microdeletion of LIT1 in familial Beckwith-Wiedemann syndrome. Am J Hum Genet 75:844–849

Ohgaki H, Kleihues P, Heitz PU (1993) p53 mutations in sporadic adrenocortical tumors. Int J Cancer 54:408–410

Ohta A, Schumacher FR, Mehellou Y, Johnson C, Knebel A, Macartney TJ, Wood NT, Alessi DR, Kurz T (2013) The CUL3-KLHL3 E3 ligase complex mutated in Gordon's hypertension syndrome interacts with and ubiquitylates WNK isoforms: disease-causing mutations in KLHL3 and WNK4 disrupt interaction. Biochem J 451:111–122

Olivier M, Goldgar DE, Sodha N, Ohgaki H, Kleihues P, Hainaut P, Eeles RA (2003) Li-Fraumeni and related syndromes: correlation between tumor type, family structure, and TP53 genotype. Cancer Res 63:6643–6650

Olivier M, Langerod A, Carrieri P, Bergh J, Klaar S, Eyfjord J, Theillet C, Rodriguez C, Lidereau R, Bieche I, Varley J, Bignon Y, Uhrhammer N, Winqvist R, Jukkola-Vuorinen A, Niederacher D, Kato S, Ishioka C, Hainaut P, Borresen-Dale AL (2006) The clinical value of somatic TP53 gene mutations in 1794 patients with breast cancer. Clin Cancer Res 12:1157–1167

Palmero EI, Achatz MI, Ashton-Prolla P, Olivier M, Hainaut P (2010) Tumor protein 53 mutations and inherited cancer: beyond Li-Fraumeni syndrome. Curr Opin Oncol 22:64–69

Petitjean A, Mathe E, Kato S, Ishioka C, Tavtigian SV, Hainaut P, Olivier M (2007) Impact of mutant p53 functional properties on TP53 mutation patterns and tumor phenotype: lessons from recent developments in the IARC TP53 database. Hum Mutat 28:622–629

Prawitt D, Enklaar T, Gartner-Rupprecht B, Spangenberg C, Lausch E, Reutzel D, Fees S, Korzon M, Brozek I, Limon J, Housman DE, Pelletier J, Zabel B (2005) Microdeletion and IGF2 loss of imprinting in a cascade causing Beckwith-Wiedemann syndrome with Wilms' tumor. Nat Genet, United States

Raymond VM, Else T, Everett JN, Long JM, Gruber SB, Hammer GD (2013a) Prevalence of germline TP53 mutations in a prospective series of unselected patients with adrenocortical carcinoma. J Clin Endocrinol Metab 98:E119–E125

Raymond VM, Everett JN, Furtado LV, Gustafson SL, Jungbluth CR, Gruber SB, Hammer GD, Stoffel EM, Greenson JK, Giordano TJ, Else T (2013b) Adrenocortical carcinoma is a lynch syndrome-associated cancer. J Clin Oncol 31:3012–3018

Rodriguez FJ, Stratakis CA, Evans DG (2012) Genetic predisposition to peripheral nerve neoplasia: diagnostic criteria and pathogenesis of neurofibromatoses, Carney complex, and related syndromes. Acta Neuropathol 123:349–367

Rump P, Zeegers MP, van Essen AJ (2005) Tumor risk in Beckwith-Wiedemann syndrome: a review and meta-analysis. Am J Med Genet A 136:95–104

Salpea P, Horvath A, London E, Faucz FR, Vetro A, Levy I, Gourgari E, Dauber A, Holm IA, Morrison PJ, Keil MF, Lyssikatos C, Smith ED, Sanidad MA, Kelly JC, Dai Z, Mowrey P, Forlino A, Zuffardi O, Stratakis CA (2014) Deletions of the PRKAR1A locus at 17q24.2-q24.3 in Carney complex: genotype-phenotype correlations and implications for genetic testing. J Clin Endocrinol Metab 99:E183–E188

Schaefer S, Shipotko M, Meyer S, Ivan D, Klose KJ, Waldmann J, Langer P, Kann PH (2008) Natural course of small adrenal lesions in multiple endocrine neoplasia type 1: an endoscopic ultrasound imaging study. Eur J Endocrinol 158:699–704

Shuman C, Beckwith JB, Smith AC, Weksberg R (1993) Beckwith-Wiedemann Syndrome. In: Pagon RA, Adam MP, Ardinger HH, Bird TD, Dolan CR, Fong CT, Smith RJH, Stephens K (eds) GeneReviews(R). Seattle (WA), University of Washington, Seattle. All rights reserved

Sirianni R, Zolea F, Chimento A, Ruggiero C, Cerquetti L, Fallo F, Pilon C, Arnaldi G, Carpinelli G, Stigliano A, Pezzi V (2012) Targeting estrogen receptor-alpha reduces adrenocortical cancer (ACC) cell growth in vitro and in vivo: potential therapeutic role of selective estrogen receptor modulators (SERMs) for ACC treatment. J Clin Endocrinol Metab 97:E2238–E2250

Sorensen SA, Mulvihill JJ, Nielsen A (1986) Long-term follow-up of von Recklinghausen neurofibromatosis. Survival and malignant neoplasms. N Engl J Med 314:1010–1015

Sorrell AD, Espenschied CR, Culver JO, Weitzel JN (2013) Tumor protein p53 (TP53) testing and Li-Fraumeni syndrome: current status of clinical applications and future directions. Mol Diagn Ther 17:31–47

Stoffel EM, Mangu PB, Gruber SB, Hamilton SR, Kalady MF, Lau MW, Lu KH, Roach N, Limburg PJ (2015) Hereditary colorectal cancer syndromes: American society of clinical oncology clinical practice guideline endorsement of the familial risk-colorectal cancer: European society for medical oncology clinical practice guidelines. J Clin Oncol 33:209–217

Stratakis CA, Kirschner LS, Carney JA (2001) Clinical and molecular features of the Carney complex: diagnostic criteria and recommendations for patient evaluation. J Clin Endocrinol Metab 86:4041–4046

Tabori U, Baskin B, Shago M, Alon N, Taylor MD, Ray PN, Bouffet E, Malkin D, Hawkins C (2010) Universal poor survival in children with medulloblastoma harboring somatic TP53 mutations. J Clin Oncol 28:1345–1350

Thakker RV, Newey PJ, Walls GV, Bilezikian J, Dralle H, Ebeling PR, Melmed S, Sakurai A, Tonelli F, Brandi ML (2012) Clinical practice guidelines for multiple endocrine neoplasia type 1 (MEN1). J Clin Endocrinol Metab 97:2990–3011

Tham E, Grandell U, Lindgren E, Toss G, Skogseid B, Nordenskjold M (2007) Clinical testing for mutations in the MEN1 gene in Sweden: a report on 200 unrelated cases. J Clin Endocrinol Metab 92:3389–3395

Tinat J, Bougeard G, Baert-Desurmont S, Vasseur S, Martin C, Bouvignies E, Caron O, Bressac-de Paillerets B, Berthet P, Dugast C, Bonaiti-Pellie C, Stoppa-Lyonnet D, Frebourg T (2009) Version of the Chompret criteria for Li Fraumeni syndrome. J Clin Oncol *27*(26):e108–e109, United States

Varley JM, McGown G, Thorncroft M, James LA, Margison GP, Forster G, Evans DG, Harris M, Kelsey AM, Birch JM (1999) Are there low-penetrance TP53 Alleles? evidence from childhood adrenocortical tumors. Am J Hum Genet 65:995–1006

Wagner AS, Fleitz JM, Kleinschmidt-Demasters BK (2005) Pediatric adrenal cortical carcinoma: brain metastases and relationship to NF-1, case reports and review of the literature. J Neurooncol 75:127–133

Weksberg R, Shuman C, Beckwith JB (2010) Beckwith-Wiedemann syndrome. Eur J Hum Genet 18:8–14

Weksberg R, Smith AC, Squire J, Sadowski P (2003) Beckwith-Wiedemann syndrome demonstrates a role for epigenetic control of normal development. Hum Mol Genet 12 Spec No 1:R61–8

Weksberg R, Shuman C, Smith AC (2005) Beckwith-Wiedemann syndrome. Am J Med Genet C Semin Med Genet 137c:12–23

Wu X, Hua X (2008) Menin, histone h3 methyltransferases, and regulation of cell proliferation: current knowledge and perspective. Curr Mol Med 8:805–815

Diagnosis and Management of Hereditary Carcinoids

Sarah Benafif and Rosalind Eeles

Abstract

Carcinoid tumours arise in cells of the diffuse neuroendocrine system and can develop in a number of anatomical sites including the lungs and the gastrointestinal tract. There has been a move away from the use of the term carcinoid tumour to the more appropriate use of neuroendocrine tumour (NET) to highlight the potential for invasion and metastasis associated with some NETs. Although most cases are sporadic, 15–20 % of cases are related to a hereditary syndrome, the most common of these being multiple endocrine neoplasia 1 (MEN1). Other hereditary syndromes include the following: von Hippel–Lindau (VHL), neurofibromatosis 1 and tuberous sclerosis complex (TSC), which are all associated with a germline mutation of the associated tumour suppressor gene and an autosomal dominant inheritance pattern. Familial small intestinal NET (SI NET) is a recently described condition which is also inherited in an autosomal dominant manner. There appears to be more than one causative gene; thus far, only the *IPMK* gene has been identified as a causative germline mutation. This was identified by carrying out whole-exome sequencing of germline and tumour DNA in a family with multiple members diagnosed with SI NET. Identification of NET predisposition genes in other families via these methods will allow the development of dedicated NET gene panels which can be used to screen NET patients and at-risk relatives for hereditary mutations. Close surveillance of at-risk individuals is important to detect NETs early when

S. Benafif · R. Eeles (✉)
The Institute of Cancer Research, Sutton, Surrey, UK
e-mail: Rosalind.Eeles@icr.ac.uk

S. Benafif · R. Eeles
Royal Marsden NHS Foundation Trust, Sutton, Surrey, UK

G. Pichert and C. Jacobs (eds.), *Rare Hereditary Cancers*,
Recent Results in Cancer Research 205, DOI 10.1007/978-3-319-29998-3_9

curative surgery can be offered and the morbidity and mortality of metastatic NETs can be avoided.

Keywords
Neuroendocrine tumour · NET · Carcinoid · Tumour suppressor gene · Genetics

Contents

1 Introduction

Carcinoid tumours arise in cells of the diffuse neuroendocrine system and can develop in a number of anatomical sites including the lungs and the gastrointestinal tract. Historically, the term 'carcinoid' was coined by Siegfried Oberndorfer over 100 years ago to describe tumours of the small bowel which he noted were indolent and slow growing in nature and resembled 'little carcinomas' (Modlin et al. 2004). With the increasing study of carcinoid and neuroendocrine tumours (NETs), we now know that there is a spectrum of disease with some tumours displaying aggressive features such as invasion and metastasis. Carcinoid tumours may be 'functional' and secrete vasoactive peptides such as gastrin, glucagon or serotonin (causing the classic carcinoid syndrome), while others are non-functional and hormonally silent. There has been a call to move away from the term 'carcinoid' (Klimstra et al. 2010; Chetty 2008) due to the connotations of this being associated with a benign condition when in fact all NETs have the propensity for malignant behaviour and metastasis. It is still common for carcinoid and NET to be used synonymously in the literature.

The classification systems for NETs have undergone several changes in recent years as distinct molecular and pathological entities have emerged (Tables 1 and 2). The main distinctions highlighted in these systems are that of well-differentiated versus poorly differentiated tumours as a different management approach is used for each of these categories (Klimstra et al. 2010). Secondly, with the gastroenteropancreatic (GEP-) NETs, the management of pancreatic NETs differs from

Table 1 WHO 2010 classification of gastroenteropancreatic neuroendocrine tumours (GEP-NETs); *hpf* high powered field (Klimstra et al. 2010)

Differentiation	Grade	Proliferative rate	WHO classification
Well differentiated	1 (low grade)	Ki-67 <3 % and <2 mitoses/10 hpf	Neuroendocrine neoplasm
	2 (intermediate grade)	Ki-67 3–20 % or 2–20 mitoses/10 hpf	Neuroendocrine neoplasm
Poorly differentiated	3 (high grade)	Ki-67 >20 % or >20 mitoses/10 hpf	Neuroendocrine carcinoma

Table 2 WHO 2010 classification of lung and thymic NETs; *hpf* high powered field (Klimstra et al. 2010)

Differentiation	Grade	Proliferative rate	WHO classification
Well differentiated	1 (low grade)	No necrosis and <2 mitoses/10 hpf	Typical carcinoid
	2 (intermediate grade)	Focal necrosis or 2–10 mitoses/10 hpf	Atypical carcinoid
Poorly differentiated	3 (high grade)	Extensive necrosis and >10 mitoses/10 hpf	Small cell carcinoma; large cell neuroendocrine carcinoma

non-pancreatic NETs; with the former, targeted agents such as sunitinib and everolimus have been approved for use, whereas with the latter, somatostatin analogues can be considered (Bergsland 2013). These distinctions are also important as they influence eligibility for clinical trials.

The incidence and prevalence of NETs has risen in recent decades (Fig. 1) (Yao et al. 2008). This rise has been ascribed in part to the increased use of diagnostic technology such as computerised tomography, endoscopy, and endoscopic ultrasound, with a proportion of cases being detected incidentally, when patients are investigated for unrelated conditions. The changes in classification of NETs have also contributed to the rise in number of cases as tumours that are low grade and indolent which would previously have been labelled as benign are now termed well-differentiated NET.

Worldwide figures for incidence of NETs are not readily available due to the rarity of the condition as well as the changes in pathological classification described. Instead, population-based data from the USA and various European countries have been published. Based on data analysed from the Surveillance, Epidemiology, and End Results Program (SEER) database in the USA, the incidence of GI NETs is estimated to be 2–5/100,000 with a prevalence of 35/100,000 (Yao et al. 2008). GI NETs are more prevalent than gastric and pancreatic adenocarcinoma, probably due to their indolent progression, and recognition of this has spurred on research in this previously neglected field. Bronchial carcinoid makes up 25 % of NET cases and has an incidence of 1.57/100,000 (Oberg et al. 2012). European incidence rates appear to be similar ranging from 2 to 4/100,000 (Taal and Visser 2004; Hauso et al. 2008). Distribution by gender appears to be equal though the primary site of

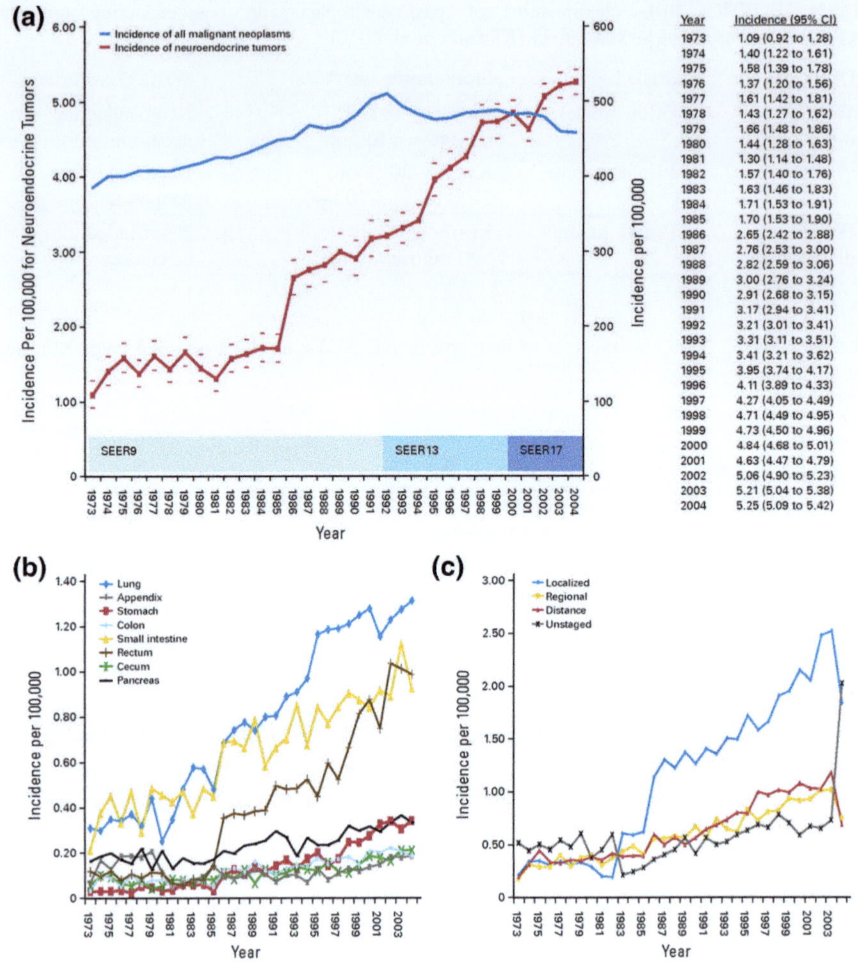

Year	Incidence (95% CI)
1973	1.09 (0.92 to 1.28)
1974	1.40 (1.22 to 1.61)
1975	1.58 (1.39 to 1.78)
1976	1.37 (1.20 to 1.56)
1977	1.61 (1.42 to 1.81)
1978	1.43 (1.27 to 1.62)
1979	1.66 (1.48 to 1.86)
1980	1.44 (1.28 to 1.63)
1981	1.30 (1.14 to 1.48)
1982	1.57 (1.40 to 1.76)
1983	1.63 (1.46 to 1.83)
1984	1.71 (1.53 to 1.91)
1985	1.70 (1.53 to 1.90)
1986	2.65 (2.42 to 2.88)
1987	2.76 (2.53 to 3.00)
1988	2.82 (2.59 to 3.06)
1989	3.00 (2.76 to 3.24)
1990	2.91 (2.68 to 3.15)
1991	3.17 (2.94 to 3.41)
1992	3.21 (3.01 to 3.41)
1993	3.31 (3.11 to 3.51)
1994	3.41 (3.21 to 3.62)
1995	3.95 (3.74 to 4.17)
1996	4.11 (3.89 to 4.33)
1997	4.27 (4.05 to 4.49)
1998	4.71 (4.49 to 4.95)
1999	4.73 (4.50 to 4.96)
2000	4.84 (4.68 to 5.01)
2001	4.63 (4.47 to 4.79)
2002	5.06 (4.90 to 5.23)
2003	5.21 (5.04 to 5.38)
2004	5.25 (5.09 to 5.42)

Fig. 1 Incidence of neuroendocrine tumours (NETs) over time, by site and by disease stage. **a** Annual age-adjusted incidence of NETs by year (1973–2004). The incidence is presented as the number of tumours per 100,000 (with 95 % CIs) age-adjusted for the 2000 US standard population. Cases were selected from the Surveillance, Epidemiology, and End Results database (1973–2004) using International Classification of Diseases for Oncology histology codes 8150–8157, 8240–8246 and 8249. **b** Time-trend analyses of the incidence of NETs by primary tumour site (1973–2004). Statistically significant increases in incidence at all sites are shown ($P < 0.001$). **c** The incidence of NETs by disease stage at diagnosis. Statistically significant increases in incidence at all stages are shown ($P < 0.001$) (Yao et al. 2008). Reprinted with permission.

NET differs depending on gender. According to USA data, females are more likely to have a lung, stomach, appendix or caecum primary NET, whereas the primary site in males is more likely to be thymus, small bowel, pancreas or rectum (Yao et al. 2008). Median age at diagnosis is 63 years though this can vary according to race (median age in black people is 59 and white people is 64) and primary site of NET (appendiceal NET median age 47) (Yao et al. 2008).

There are no known aetiological risk factors for the development of NET, although the rise in gastric NET specifically has been theoretically linked to the increased use of proton pump inhibitors. This has not been directly proven but is proposed to be associated with prolonged achlorhydria secondary to proton pump inhibition leading to gastric G cell hyperplasia and hypergastrinemia (Nikou and Angelopoulos 2012).

Although the majority of NETs are sporadic, 15–20 % of cases are associated with a hereditary syndrome (Kunz 2015) such as multiple endocrine neoplasia 1 (MEN1) which is the most common, neurofibromatosis 1 (NF1) and Von Hippel–Lindau (VHL). In the setting of MEN1, a NET can develop at a much earlier age than that of sporadic NET and earliest reported ages range from 8 to 12 years (Thakker et al. 2012).

Recently, familial small intestinal NET (SI NET) has been described and appears to be inherited in an autosomal dominant pattern. Outside the setting of a hereditary syndrome, there is an increased risk of SI NET development if there is a positive family history in a first-degree relative with a relative risk of 3.6 (Strosberg 2012). The term 'familial ileal endocrine carcinoma' has been coined to describe familial clustering of ileal carcinoid which has been reported by a number of groups. In the largest study of 9 families and a total of 23 cases of ileal carcinoid, an autosomal dominant inheritance pattern is described. Loss of chromosome 18q was found to be an early event in both sporadic and familial ileal NETs, suggesting a shared pathogenetic mechanism, though a specific gene mutation has not yet been identified (Cunningham et al. 2011).

As most cases of hereditary NETs develop within the context of an inherited multisystem disorder, the diagnosis of a hereditary condition may already be known at the time of NET diagnosis. In those without a known hereditary condition, referral of a NET patient for genetic testing may be triggered by a family history of NETs, personal history of conditions related to a particular syndrome associated with NET development or due to a young age at presentation. In this setting, next-generation sequencing (NGS) is now being increasingly used to detect suspected genetic germline mutations. Using NGS, analysis of the coding and non-coding regions as well as regulatory regions of a gene of interest can be carried out simultaneously, thus detecting large intragenic deletions or duplications. It may also reveal unexpected novel causative gene mutations (Marini et al. 2015). In the context of hereditary cancers, hybridisation-based target enrichment can be utilised to analyse large cancer gene panels. Although dedicated gene panels for certain cancers are now offered by some molecular genetics laboratories, there is unlikely to be a dedicated panel targeted to hereditary forms of carcinoid/NET. Instead, genes of interest, e.g. *MEN1*, *NF1* or *VHL*, can be selected from a large cancer gene panel depending on the clinical context or suspected condition.

Summary

- The incidence and prevalence of NETs is rising, possibly due to increased use of diagnostic imaging and due to increased awareness among healthcare professionals.
- Classification of NETs distinguishes between well-differentiated and poorly differentiated tumours and between pancreatic and non-pancreatic tumours as treatment differs for each of these.
- 15–20 % of NETs are associated with a familial syndrome and present at an earlier age than sporadic cases.
- A family history of SI NET confers a relative risk of 3.6 for NET development in first-degree relatives.
- NGS techniques can be utilised to produce cancer gene panels that can be used for mutational analysis in suspected cases of hereditary NET.

2 Hereditary Conditions Associated with NETs

2.1 Multiple Endocrine Neoplasia (MEN1)

MEN1 is a tumour syndrome caused by a germline mutation of the *MEN1* tumour suppressor gene which lies on chromosome 11 at 11q13.1. This mutation can occur sporadically or is inherited in an autosomal dominant manner and has a high penetrance with clinical manifestations developing in 80 % of cases by the age of 50 (Thakker et al. 2012). The three most common tumours in MEN1 are parathyroid adenomas (90–100 %), pituitary adenomas (10–60 %) and pancreatic neuroendocrine tumours (60–70 %). Other tumours have been described as part of MEN1 with over 20 tumour types including cutaneous, adrenal tumours and thymic carcinoids (Toledo et al. 2013). In a Spanish study of 837 GEP-NETs, 5 % of cases were diagnosed with MEN1 (Garcia-Carbonero et al. 2010). Diagnosis of MEN1 is established when one of the following criteria is met (Thakker et al. 2012):

1. Development of ≥2 MEN1-related endocrine tumours (clinical diagnosis)
2. Development of 1 MEN1-related endocrine tumour in the context of a positive family history for MEN1 in a first-degree relative
3. Identification of a germline *MEN1* mutation

The incidence of MEN1 is estimated to be 0.25 %. In those presenting with hyperparathyroidism, the incidence of MEN1 ranges between 1–18 % and in those presenting with gastrinomas 16–38 %. The reported age range for MEN1 patients is wide and lies between 5 and 81 years (Thakker et al. 2012). The pancreatic NETs in MEN1 can be functioning such as gastrinomas, insulinomas and glucagonomas or non-functioning. Non-pancreatic NETs and carcinoid tumours occur in >3 % of patients. Of these, 10 % are gastric, 2 % are bronchial, and 2 % are in the thymus. Thymic carcinoids are more common in male MEN1 patients (male:female 20:1) and are aggressive malignant tumours. This is true for European patients, but in Japanese MEN1 patients with thymic carcinoid, the male:female ratio is 2:1. Median survival from diagnosis of a thymic carcinoid tumour is 9.5 years, and 70 % of patients die of their disease. In contrast, bronchial carcinoids are more frequent in females (male:female ratio 1:4) and are less aggressive tumours (Toledo et al. 2013).

Primary hyperparathyroidism associated with parathyroid adenoma or hyperplasia is commonly a presenting feature of MEN1 and is diagnosed by the ages of 20–35 years in contrast to sporadic hyperparathyroidism which occurs in those over 50 years (Toledo et al. 2013).

The treatment of MEN1-associated tumours is similar to their sporadic counterparts, but unfortunately treatment outcomes are not as good. One of the reasons for this is that tumours tend to be multifocal in MEN1, such as multiple duodenal gastrinomas which are difficult to cure surgically (15 % disease free after surgery compared with 45 % in sporadic gastrinomas). Occult metastatic disease is more common in MEN1 tumours; 50 % of MEN1-associated insulinoma develops metastatic disease compared with 10 % of sporadic insulinoma. Lastly, MEN1 tumours may be larger, more aggressive and more resistant to treatment (Thakker et al. 2012).

2.2 Genetics of MEN1

The *MEN1* gene on chromosome 11q13 is made up of 10 exons encoding the 610-amino acid menin protein. *MEN1* is a tumour suppressor gene, and menin regulates transcription, genome stability and cell division (Thakker et al. 2012). In the first decade after *MEN1* was identified, 1133 germline mutations of the *MEN1* gene were reported, consisting of 459 different mutations (Lemos and Thakker 2008). Seventy-five percent of mutations are inactivating mutations consistent with *MEN1*'s function as a tumour suppressor gene, but there does not appear to be a genotype/phenotype correlation according to the type of mutation seen. Indeed, similar mutations have been observed in MEN1 patients and in familial isolated hyperparathyroidism (FIHP), the latter being a condition that is not associated with the development of other tumours (Lemos and Thakker 2008). Although there is no clear genotype/phenotype correlation, a recently described double substitution in Exon 2 (428T > A; 429C > T, p.Leu143His) of the *MEN1* gene led to a limited penetrance and milder form of MEN1 in affected family members (Ullmann et al. 2013). There was mild hyperparathyroidism, the development of multiple well-differentiated pancreatic NETs and no pituitary adenomas at the time of reporting. This is the only report of a specific genotype/phenotype correlation in MEN1.

Between 5 and 25 % of MEN1 patients may not harbour a mutation in the coding region of the *MEN1* gene. In these cases, a mutation may lie in the gene promoter or in non-coding regions, or there may be whole or partial gene deletions

(Thakker et al. 2012). Published guidelines recommend that in such cases when a *MEN1* mutation is not detected, multiplex ligation-dependent probe amplification (MPLA) analysis to detect exonic deletions should be carried out (Thakker et al. 2012).

Most laboratories use selective PCR-based amplification of *MEN1* exons and splice sites, followed by Sanger sequencing (Marini et al. 2015). If this initial test is negative, only some laboratories carry out MPLA as described above. These approaches can still fail to detect mutations in non-coding and regulatory regions and also would not identify phenocopies. A phenocopy occurs when the clinical manifestations of MEN1 are found to be associated with an alternative aetiology to a *MEN1* mutation; phenocopies have been reported in 5–10 % of MEN1 kindreds (Thakker et al. 2012). Next-generation sequencing (NGS) is now being increasingly used in this setting and would overcome these limitations (Marini et al. 2015).

MEN1 mutation analysis is indicated for the following individuals (Thakker et al. 2012):

1. An index case diagnosed with ≥2 MEN1-related endocrine tumours (parathyroid, pancreatic or pituitary)
2. Asymptomatic first-degree relatives of a known *MEN1* mutation carrier
3. Symptomatic first-degree relative of a *MEN1* mutation carrier (i.e. diagnosed with ≥1 MEN1-related tumour based on radiological or biochemical tests)
4. Suspicion of MEN1 including individuals with parathyroid adenomas under the age of 30 years, or multigland parathyroid disease, multiple gastrinomas or multiple pancreatic NETs at any age
5. An index case with ≥2 MEN1-related tumours not part of the classical triad of MEN1.

Guidelines for MEN1 diagnosis and management published in 2012 recommend that children in MEN1 families undergo *MEN1* mutational analysis in the first decade of life as there have been reports of MEN1-related tumours developing in patients as young as 5 years of age (Thakker et al. 2012).

In a minority of patients with clinical evidence of MEN1 (i.e. 2 or more MEN1-related tumours), mutations in *MEN1* are not found. In 1.5 % of these cases, germline mutation of *CDKN1B* is present which encodes cyclin-dependent kinase inhibitor p27kip1, and in this cohort of patients, the clinical syndrome has been termed MEN4 (Elston et al. 2009; Molatore et al. 2010; Pellegata et al. 2006). *CDKN1B* mutation can be detected as part of a NGS cancer gene panel. Germline mutations in CDK inhibitors p15, p18 and p21 have also been reported as the probable cause of MEN1 in 1, 0.5 and 0.5 % of patients, respectively (Agarwal et al. 2009).

The management approach to NETs in MEN1 patients (as with sporadic NETs) depends on the presence of metastases (to the liver most often) and, if present, whether they are deemed operable to prevent further metastases and improve survival. Over 50 % of GEP-NETs in MEN1 patients are gastrinomas and are most commonly found in the duodenum. In non-MEN1 disease, the risk of hepatic metastases secondary to NETs is related to tumour size with 25–40 % of patients with pancreatic NETs greater than 4 cm developing hepatic metastases. Survival in MEN1 patients with non-metastatic gastrinomas measuring <2.5 cm is 100 % at 15 years, while in those with metastatic disease, survival is 52 % at 15 years. Therefore, surgical excision of pancreatic gastrinomas is recommended in tumours measuring ≥2 cm, whereas with duodenal gastrinomas, management is individualised according to the extent of disease on pre-op and intraoperative imaging, as MEN1 patients may have multiple tumours (unlike sporadic disease where tumours are usually solitary) (Thakker et al. 2012). In patients with metastatic disease, surgery may occasionally be considered. Other treatment options include chemotherapy (streptozocin and 5FU have been used), and somatostatin analogues such as octreotide and hepatic transarterial embolisation (Thakker et al. 2012).

Other functional NETs can also develop in the context of MEN1 such as insulinoma, glucagonoma and VIPomas, and the management approach is similar to that of gastrinoma with surgery being considered when there is limited operable disease.

2.3 Management of Non-functional NETs

Non-functional NETs also occur in the context of MEN1 and may be detected during surveillance imaging. Endoscopic ultrasound detects pancreatic non-functioning NETs in 55 % of MEN1 patients screened (Thomas-Marques et al. 2006). Individuals are likely to be asymptomatic, and these non-functioning NETs can occur in MEN1 carriers under 15 years of age. The management of such asymptomatic tumours is controversial, but their identification is important as malignant pancreatic NET is the most common cause of death in MEN1 individuals (Goudet et al. 2010). Also, non-functioning pancreatic NETs are the most commonly occurring NET in MEN1 patients and carry a worse prognosis than other functioning NETs (Triponez et al. 2006a).

Similar to functional NETs, surgical resection is considered for larger tumours although various guidelines differ in the criteria for resection, ranging from >1 to >2 cm (Thakker et al. 2012; Triponez et al. 2006b). The complications of pancreaticoduodenal surgery such as diabetes mellitus, steatorrhoea and GI symptoms need to be balanced against the prevention of metastatic disease. The rate of growth of a non-functional NET is also a factor that contributes to management decisions, and a doubling in size over 3–6 months is deemed an indication for surgery (Thakker et al. 2012).

Tyrosine kinase inhibitors such as sunitinib are approved for the treatment of metastatic or locally advanced pancreatic NETs (Raymond et al. 2011). Inhibitors of mammalian target of rapamycin (mTOR) such as everolimus are also effective for treatment (Yao et al. 2011). Both targeted treatments showed a doubling of progression-free survival (compared with placebo) in clinical trials treating pancreatic NET patients (Yao et al. 2011; Raymond et al. 2011). Although the majority of these patients were non-MEN1 individuals, it is likely that these results can be extended to MEN1 patients with advanced pancreatic NETs.

2.4 Follow-up and Screening

Regular screening for MEN1 associated tumours is recommended for all known MEN1 individuals so that diagnosis is made at an early stage and appropriate management instituted. The *MEN1* mutation appears to be non-penetrant in those under the age of 5 years and more than 50 % penetrant by the age of 20 years (Thakker et al. 2012). Therefore, screening is advised in those aged 5 years and over. This consists of annual biochemical screening as well as regular imaging of the abdomen and pituitary (Thakker et al. 2012). Biochemical tests include measuring serum calcium and GI hormones such as gastrin, prolactin, fasting glucose, and chromogranin A. The recommended age for the commencement of specific investigations is summarised in Table 3.

Summary

- MEN1 is an autosomal condition with 80 % penetrance by the age of 50.
- MEN1 is associated with the development of parathyroid adenomas (90–100 %), pituitary adenomas (10–60 %) and pancreatic NET (60–70 %). Pancreatic NETs can be functioning or non-functioning.
- Non-pancreatic NETs and carcinoid tumours occur in >3 % of patients.

Table 3 Guidelines for screening MEN1 individuals (Thakker et al. 2012)

Tumour	Age to start screening	Penetrance	Biochemical test (annual)	Imaging test
Anterior pituitary	5	30–40 %	Prolactin IGF-1	MRI 3 yearly
Parathyroid	8	90 %	Calcium PTH	None
Pancreatic NET		30–70 %		
Insulinoma	5	10 %	Fasting glucose, insulin	None
Gastrinoma	20	40 %	Gastrin (±gastric pH)	None
Other pancreatic NET	<10		CgA, pancreatic polypeptide, glucagon, VIP	MRI, CT or EUS annually
Adrenal	<10	Adrenal cortical tumour 40 % Phaeochromocytoma <1 %	None unless symptoms or signs evident, or tumour >1 cm on imaging	MRI or CT annually (alongside pancreatic imaging)
Thymic and bronchial carcinoid	15	2 %	None	CT or MRI every 1–2 years

- MEN1 patients treated for NETs have poorer outcomes compared with sporadic cases as tumours tend to be multifocal and more aggressive, and occult metastatic disease is more common.
- *MEN1* gene mutations can be detected via NGS gene panels which can also include *CDKN1B* which accounts for 1.5 % of MEN cases and is termed MEN4. Children in MEN1 families should be tested for a mutation in the first decade of life.
- Management of MEN1-associated NETs is similar to that of sporadic cases with surgery considered for operable tumours and systemic treatment in metastatic cases or for symptomatic functioning tumours.
- Guidelines recommend commencing screening for MEN1 tumours early from the age of 5 years, and this is continued lifelong.

2.5 Von Hippel–Lindau (VHL)

VHL disease is an autosomal dominant condition caused by mutation of the *VHL* tumour suppressor gene which lies on the short arm of chromosome 3. The incidence is reported to be 1 in 36,000 births, with 20 % of cases arising de novo and a penetrance of up to 95 % by the age of 60 (Maher et al. 2011; Chou et al. 2013). Similar to MEN1, there is marked phenotypic variability although there is an element of genotype–phenotype correlation observed in some VHL families. The three classical clinical features associated with VHL are retinal angiomas, CNS haemangioblastomas and clear cell renal cell carcinomas (ccRCC). The lifetime risk of developing these three features is 70 % although this can vary according to the mutation involved (Woodward and Maher 2006).

Phaeochromocytomas and pancreatic NETs are also observed, and there are reported cases of carcinoid tumours and hyperparathyroidism. VHL families have been subdivided into the following groups according to the clinical manifestations present (Woodward and Maher 2006):

Type 1: retinal and CNS haemangioblastoma and ccRCC; absence of phaeochromocytoma
Type 2: phaeochromocytomas present and further divided into

> **Type 2A**: with retinal and CNS haemangioblastomas, rarely RCC
> **Type 2B**: haemangioblastomas, RCC and phaeochromocytoma
> **Type 2C**: isolated familial phaeochromocytoma

Clinical diagnosis of VHL requires the development of a VHL-associated tumour in an at-risk individual (i.e. a relative of a known VHL patient) or in sporadic cases, the development of two VHL-associated tumours (Maher et al. 2011). Suspected VHL cases should be referred for genetic counselling and VHL mutation analysis, as well as relatives of confirmed *VHL* mutation carriers. In those who test positive for a *VHL* mutation, appropriate screening and surveillance are then commenced.

Pancreatic NETs occur in up to 10 % of VHL patients and are multifocal in 50 % of these. As in the MEN1-associated cases, they occur at an earlier age than sporadic cases with a mean age at diagnosis of 35 years (Maher et al. 2011; Woodward and Maher 2006). Resection of tumours larger than 3 cm in VHL patients has been recommended, while a more conservative approach can be taken for smaller, slowly progressive tumours (Blansfield et al. 2007).

Mutations of the *VHL* gene have been described in more than 900 families (Maher et al. 2011). The majority of these (30–40 %) consist of deletions, removing one or more of the three coding exons. The remainder are made up of missense substitutions and mutations that lead to a truncated protein. Genotype–phenotype correlations have been described for the subgroups of VHL, with Type 1 VHL being most commonly associated with truncating mutations or large deletions. Type 2 VHL individuals are associated with missense mutations that do not have total loss of function. Specific missense mutations are associated with Type 2C isolated phaeochromocytoma (Maher et al. 2011).

There is no specific genotype–phenotype correlation for the development of pancreatic NETs although it appears to be more frequent in VHL individuals developing phaeochromocytomas. In 40 % of VHL patients with a pancreatic NET, adrenal phaeochromocytoma was also confirmed surgically (Marcos et al. 2002).

Regular screening for the complications of VHL as well as associated tumours is commenced at an early age in known VHL individuals. Table 4 summarises the recommended surveillance protocol (Maher et al. 2011).

Summary

- VHL is an autosomal dominant condition due to mutation of the *VHL* gene and arises sporadically in 20 % of cases. Penetrance is 95 % by the age of 60 years.
- The three classical clinical features of VHL are retinal angiomas, CNS haemangioblastomas and ccRCC.
- VHL is divided into type 1 and 2 depending on the absence or presence of phaeochromocytoma, respectively. Type 1 is associated with deletions or truncating mutations, while type 2 is associated with missense mutations.

Table 4 Guidelines for surveillance of VHL individuals (Maher et al. 2011)

Screening test	Age to start screening	Frequency
Ophthalmic examination for retinal angioma	Infancy/early childhood	Annual
MRI scans of head for CNS haemangioblastoma	Adolescence	12–36 months
MRI or USS of abdomen for RCC and pancreatic tumours	16 years	Annual
BP monitoring for phaeochromocytoma[a]	8 years	Annual

[a]If high risk for phaeochromocytoma development, measurement of plasma normetanephrine levels and adrenal imaging should be included. *BP* blood pressure, *USS* ultrasound scan, *MRI* magnetic resonance imaging

- Suspected VHL mutation carriers should be offered genetic testing. Relatives of those who test positive should also be offered genetic testing.
- 10 % of cases develop pancreatic NETs and may be more frequent in VHL individuals with phaeochromocytoma. A conservative approach may be taken to smaller slow-growing tumours.
- Surveillance is commenced in childhood and continues lifelong.

2.6 Neurofibromatosis Type 1

Neurofibromatosis type 1 (NF1) has also been associated with the development of neuroendocrine and carcinoid tumours although these are less common in NF1 than in the previously discussed hereditary conditions. It is an autosomal dominant condition with complete penetrance by the age of 5 years and is caused by a germline mutation of the *NF1* tumour suppressor gene located on chromosome 17 (17q11.2). The condition arises de novo in 50 % of cases, and diagnosis is based on the NIH (National Institutes of Health) criteria which require 2 of 7 clinical features to be present (Box 1). Genetic testing for *NF1* mutations is usually reserved for uncertain cases or in the context of family planning and prenatal diagnosis (Hirbe and Gutmann 2014).

Box 1: NIH Criteria for the diagnosis of NF1 (Hirbe and Gutmann 2014)

NF1 diagnosis requires ≥2 of the following features:

- ≥6 café-au-lait macules (>0.5 cm at largest diameter if prepubertal or >1.5 cm if post-pubertal)
- Freckling in axillae or inguinal regions
- ≥2 neurofibromas of any type or ≥1 plexiform neurofibromas
- ≥2 Lisch nodules (iris hamartomas)
- A distinctive osseous lesion (sphenoid wing dysplasia, long-bone dysplasia)
- An optic pathway glioma
- A first-degree relative with NF1 diagnosed by the above criteria

The worldwide prevalence of NF1 is between 1 in 2500 and 1 in 3000, with no gender or ethnic predisposition. The classical cutaneous features develop in childhood with café-au-lait macules evident by the age of 2 years and axillary and inguinal freckling development between the ages of 5–8 years. Life expectancy for NF1 individuals is reduced compared with the general population (mean age of death 54.5 years versus 70.1 years) (Lin and Gutmann 2013). Death due to malignancy is the predominant cause in those under 30 years and a high proportion of these are due to malignant transformation of peripheral nerve sheath tumours

Table 5 Lifetime risk of malignancy in NF1 (Hirbe and Gutmann 2014)

Malignant condition	Lifetime risk
Optic glioma	15–20 %
Other brain tumour	>5× increase
Malignant PNST	8–13 %
GIST	4–25 %
Breast cancer	5× increase
Leukaemia	7× increase
Phaeochromocytoma	0.1–5.7 %
Duodenal carcinoid tumour	1 %
Rhabdomyosarcoma	1.4–6 %

(MPNST) (Lin and Gutmann 2013). Table 5 shows lifetime risks of various malignancies including NETs in *NF1* patients.

There are a limited amount of data related to genotype–phenotype correlation in NF1, with the most significant finding in the last 20 years consisting of large deletions spanning the whole NF1 gene being associated with a more severe phenotype including intellectual impairment and dysmorphic features (Cnossen et al. 1997). There are no data on genotype correlation with NET development.

Duodenal NETs arise in 1 % of NF1 individuals, often located in the periampullary region, causing jaundice and abdominal pain. They present at an earlier age compared with sporadic cases and are treated with surgery where possible (Hirbe and Gutmann 2014). In advanced disease, systemic treatment can be considered as with sporadic NET. Surveillance for NET development in NF1 individuals is not routinely recommended.

A multidisciplinary approach is taken with the management and follow-up of NF1 individuals, especially in childhood; this includes regular monitoring for spinal and skeletal defects, neurocognitive developmental delay and ophthalmological impairment due to optic glioma. Otherwise, routine screening for other complications of NF1 is not recommended. Monitoring after early adulthood depends on the severity of disease through childhood (Ferner et al. 2007).

Summary

- NF1 is an autosomal dominant condition that demonstrates complete penetrance by the age of 5 years with 50 % of cases arising sporadically.
- The NIH criteria are used to clinically diagnose NF1. Genetic testing is not routinely carried out unless there is uncertainty about the diagnosis. Genetic analysis may be offered in the context of prenatal family planning.
- Duodenal NETs arise in 1 % of NF1 patients and present at an earlier age than sporadic cases.
- Multidisciplinary management is required in children and adolescents, but continued surveillance beyond early adulthood depends on the severity of disease.

2.7 Tuberous Sclerosis Complex (TSC)

TSC is an autosomal dominant disorder characterised by the development of multiple hamartomas in different organs. The incidence is thought to range from 1/6000 to 1/10,000 with a prevalence of 1/20,000 (Northrup et al. 2013). It is caused by a germline mutation in either *TSC1* (9q34) or *TSC2* (16p13.3) genes and has a high frequency of spontaneous development with 80 % of patients not having a familial history of the disease (Dworakowska and Grossman 2009).

There have been multiple case reports of endocrine tumours (e.g. pituitary and parathyroid adenomas) as well as NETs (pancreatic insulinomas and islet cell tumours) in patients with TSC although it is still unclear whether these are truly related to underlying TSC (Dworakowska and Grossman 2009). One of the proposed mechanisms that TSC may lead to NET formation is due to loss of negative regulation of mTOR signalling by the TSC1/TSC2 complex (Dworakowska and Grossman 2009; Larson et al. 2012). The study of sporadic NETs has revealed dysregulation of the mTOR cascade, and this has lead to the use of mTOR inhibitors (e.g. Everolimus) in the treatment of some NETs. Therefore, there is a theoretical rationale for the development of NETs in TSC patients, though there is not sufficient evidence thus far to recommend surveillance for NETs routinely. Despite this, some TSC specialist centres have chosen to incorporate abdominal imaging into their surveillance programs after a small case series of TSC patients showed that the most common pancreatic lesions in these patients were NETs rather than benign angiomyolipomas which are commonly associated with TSC (Larson et al. 2012).

The criteria for diagnosis of TSC were modified in 2013 to include genetic testing results as well as the previously used clinical criteria (Northrup et al. 2013). Surveillance and management of TSC patients should be done in specialist centres within a multidisciplinary team and involves lifelong monitoring from the time of diagnosis (Krueger et al. 2013).

Summary

- TSC is an autosomal dominant condition which occurs sporadically in 80 % of cases and is characterised by the development of multiple hamartomas.
- There are reports of NET development in some TSC patients although a true relationship between the two conditions has not been proven. A proposed mechanism for NET development may be related to loss of regulation of mTOR signalling by the TSC1/2 complex.
- Surveillance guidelines for TSC patients do not include screening for NETs although some centres have chosen to incorporate this into their local programme.

2.8 Hereditary Small Intestinal NET

As mentioned previously, a family history of SI NET confers a relative risk of 3.6 for the development of a SI NET in first-degree relatives. Recent investigation into familial clustering of SI NETs has revealed possible causative germline mutations not previously recognised. As with the hereditary conditions discussed above, SI NETs in these patients tend to be multifocal. In a small prospective American study of 33 families with at least two members diagnosed with SI NET (Sei et al. 2015), screening of asymptomatic relatives resulted in 34 % being diagnosed with a SI NET and were treated with surgery. Linkage analysis and whole-exome sequencing of germline and tumour DNA were carried out on 6 members of one large family. This revealed a germline 4-bp deletion in the inositol polyphosphate multikinase (*IPMK*) gene on chromosome 10. This mutation was subsequently detected in all 11 affected individuals as well as 17 of 35 family members whose carcinoid status was unknown (Sei et al. 2015).

The *IPMK* mutation leads to a truncated protein, and functional studies demonstrate reduced kinase activity and nuclear localisation, which in turn reduces p53 activity and promotes cell survival. The *IPMK* mutation was not found in any of the affected individuals in the other 32 families, but this study did suggest a benefit from screening asymptomatic family members as the detected SI NETs were diagnosed at an earlier stage and were more likely to be operable compared with the individuals who had already had a diagnosis made prior to the study.

Further study of the remaining families using whole-exome sequencing of germline and tumour DNA is needed to identify other susceptibility genes so that at-risk individuals can be identified and appropriate screening offered, as well as being able to offer more refined genetic analysis to SI NET patients where there is the suspicion of a hereditary predisposition (e.g. patients with multifocal tumours).

Summary

- Hereditary SI NET is a recently recognised condition characterised by familial clustering of SI NETs.
- A germline mutation in the *IPMK* gene can lead to familial SI NET and is inherited in an autosomal dominant manner.
- It is likely that a proportion of sporadic NETs that are multifocal and presenting in younger patients are due to a germline mutation.
- In a family with more than one member diagnosed with a SI NET, screening of asymptomatic relatives should be carried out to detect tumours at an early stage when curative treatment can be offered.
- Further study of SI NET families using whole-exome sequencing of germline and tumour DNA is required to identify other NET predisposition genes, so that clinically relevant gene panels can be developed for identifying patients with hereditary SI NETs when there is a high degree of suspicion.

3 Summary

Although the majority of carcinoid and NETs are sporadic, 15–20 % of cases are related to a hereditary syndrome. The most common of these is MEN1 which underlies 5 % of GEP-NET diagnoses. NETs may be diagnosed in patients with familial syndromes during surveillance including regular abdominal imaging or biochemical testing. A hereditary cause for NET development should be suspected in:

Patients with a family history of NET, hyperparathyroidism/parathyroid adenoma or pituitary tumours.

Patients with a personal history of parathyroid adenoma, pituitary tumours or phaeochromocytoma.

Patients without a family history but who present at a young age (e.g. <50–60 years) and/or with multifocal disease.

With the advances in whole-exome sequencing techniques that can be applied to the analysis of germline as well as tumour DNA, it is likely that further NET predisposition genes will be identified in the future and we may find that the proportion of hereditary NETs thus far has been underestimated (e.g. in sporadic patients with younger onset disease). These can then be included in tailored NGS gene panels alongside known genes such as *MEN1*, *VHL*, *NF1* and *TSC1/2* that can be used to identify germline mutations in NET patients where a hereditary cause is suspected or in at-risk relatives of known hereditary NET patients. NET surveillance of at-risk individuals by appropriate imaging or biochemical testing is necessary to diagnose NETs at an early stage when curative surgery can be offered and reduce the risk of development of metastatic disease.

References

Agarwal SK, Mateo CM, Marx SJ (2009) Rare germline mutations in cyclin-dependent kinase inhibitor genes in multiple endocrine neoplasia type 1 and related states. J Clin Endocrinol Metab 94:1826–1834

Bergsland EK (2013) The evolving landscape of neuroendocrine tumors. Semin Oncol 40:4–22

Blansfield JA, Choyke L, Morita SY, Choyke PL, Pingpank JF, Alexander HR, Seidel G, Shutack Y, Yuldasheva N, Eugeni M, Bartlett DL, Glenn GM, Middelton L, Linehan WM, Libutti SK (2007) Clinical, genetic and radiographic analysis of 108 patients with von Hippel-Lindau disease (VHL) manifested by pancreatic neuroendocrine neoplasms (PNETs). Surgery 142:814–818; discussion 818 e1–e2

Chetty R (2008) Requiem for the term 'carcinoid tumour' in the gastrointestinal tract? Can J Gastroenterol 22:357–358

Chou A, Toon C, Pickett J, Gill AJ (2013) von Hippel-Lindau syndrome. Front Horm Res 41:30–49

Cnossen MH, van der Est MN, Breuning MH, van Asperen CJ, Breslau-Siderius EJ, van der Ploeg AT, De Goede-Bolder A, van den Ouweland AM, Halley DJ, Niermeijer MF (1997) Deletions spanning the neurofibromatosis type 1 gene: implications for genotype-phenotype correlations in neurofibromatosis type 1? Hum Mutat 9:458–464

Cunningham JL, Diaz de Stahl T, Sjoblom T, Westin G, Dumanski JP, Janson ET (2011) Common pathogenetic mechanism involving human chromosome 18 in familial and sporadic ileal carcinoid tumors. Genes Chromosomes Cancer 50:82–94

Dworakowska D, Grossman AB (2009) Are neuroendocrine tumours a feature of tuberous sclerosis? A systematic review. Endocr Relat Cancer 16:45–58

Elston MS, McDonald KL, Clifton-Bligh RJ, Robinson BG (2009) Familial pituitary tumor syndromes. Nat Rev Endocrinol 5:453–461

Ferner RE, Huson SM, Thomas N, Moss C, Willshaw H, Evans DG, Upadhyaya M, Towers R, Gleeson M, Steiger C, Kirby A (2007) Guidelines for the diagnosis and management of individuals with neurofibromatosis 1. J Med Genet 44:81–88

Garcia-Carbonero R, Capdevila J, Crespo-Herrero G, Diaz-Perez JA, Martinez Del Prado MP, Alonso Orduna V, Sevilla-Garcia I, Villabona-Artero C, Beguiristain-Gomez A, Llanos-Munoz M, Marazuela M, Alvarez-Escola C, Castellano D, Vilar E, Jimenez-Fonseca P, Teule A, Sastre-Valera J, Benavent-Vinuelas M, Monleon A, Salazar R (2010). Incidence, patterns of care and prognostic factors for outcome of gastroenteropancreatic neuroendocrine tumors (GEP-NETs): results from the National Cancer Registry of Spain (RGETNE). Ann Oncol 21:1794–1803

Goudet P, Murat A, Binquet C, Cardot-Bauters C, Costa A, Ruszniewski P, Niccoli P, Menegaux F, Chabrier G, Borson-Chazot F, Tabarin A, Bouchard P, Delemer B, Beckers A, Bonithon-Kopp C (2010) Risk factors and causes of death in MEN1 disease. A GTE (Groupe d'Etude des Tumeurs Endocrines) cohort study among 758 patients. World J Surg 34:249–255

Hauso O, Gustafsson BI, Kidd M, Waldum HL, Drozdov I, Chan AK, Modlin IM (2008) Neuroendocrine tumor epidemiology: contrasting Norway and North America. Cancer 113:2655–2664

Hirbe AC, Gutmann DH (2014) Neurofibromatosis type 1: a multidisciplinary approach to care. Lancet Neurol 13:834–843

Klimstra DS, Modlin IR, Coppola D, Lloyd RV, Suster S (2010) The pathologic classification of neuroendocrine tumors: a review of nomenclature, grading, and staging systems. Pancreas 39:707–712

Krueger DA, Northrup H, International Tuberous Sclerosis Complex Consensus Group (2013) Tuberous sclerosis complex surveillance and management: recommendations of the 2012 International Tuberous Sclerosis Complex Consensus Conference. Pediatr Neurol 49:255–265

Kunz PL (2015) Carcinoid and neuroendocrine tumors: building on success. J Clin Oncol 33:1855–1863

Larson AM, Hedgire SS, Deshpande V, Stemmer-Rachamimov AO, Harisinghani MG, Ferrone CR, Shah U, Thiele EA (2012) Pancreatic neuroendocrine tumors in patients with tuberous sclerosis complex. Clin Genet 82:558–563

Lemos MC, Thakker RV (2008) Multiple endocrine neoplasia type 1 (MEN1): analysis of 1336 mutations reported in the first decade following identification of the gene. Hum Mutat 29:22–32

Lin AL, Gutmann DH (2013) Advances in the treatment of neurofibromatosis-associated tumours. Nat Rev Clin Oncol 10:616–624

Maher ER, Neumann HP, Richard S (2011) von Hippel-Lindau disease: a clinical and scientific review. Eur J Hum Genet 19:617–623

Marcos HB, Libutti SK, Alexander HR, Lubensky IA, Bartlett DL, Walther MM, Linehan WM, Glenn GM, Choyke PL (2002) Neuroendocrine tumors of the pancreas in von Hippel-Lindau disease: spectrum of appearances at CT and MR imaging with histopathologic comparison. Radiology 225:751–758

Marini F, Giusti F, Brandi ML (2015) Genetic test in multiple endocrine neoplasia type 1 syndrome: an evolving story. World J Exp Med 5:124–129

Modlin IM, Shapiro MD, Kidd M (2004) Siegfried oberndorfer: origins and perspectives of carcinoid tumors. Hum Pathol 35:1440–1451

Molatore S, Marinoni I, Lee M, Pulz E, Ambrosio MR, Degli Uberti EC, Zatelli MC, Pellegata NS (2010) A novel germline CDKN1B mutation causing multiple endocrine tumors: clinical, genetic and functional characterization. Hum Mutat 31:E1825–E1835

Nikou GC, Angelopoulos TP (2012) Current concepts on gastric carcinoid tumors. Gastroenterol Res Pract 2012:287825

Northrup H, Krueger DA, International Tuberous Sclerosis Complex Consensus Group (2013) Tuberous sclerosis complex diagnostic criteria update: recommendations of the 2012 International Tuberous Sclerosis Complex Consensus Conference. Pediatr Neurol 49:243–254

Oberg K, Hellman P, Ferolla P, Papotti M, Group EGW (2012) Neuroendocrine bronchial and thymic tumors: ESMO clinical practice guidelines for diagnosis, treatment and follow-up. Ann Oncol 23(Suppl 7):vii120–vii123

Pellegata NS, Quintanilla-Martinez L, Siggelkow H, Samson E, Bink K, Hofler H, Fend F, Graw J, Atkinson MJ (2006) Germ-line mutations in p27Kip1 cause a multiple endocrine neoplasia syndrome in rats and humans. Proc Natl Acad Sci USA 103:15558–15563

Raymond E, Dahan L, Raoul JL, Bang YJ, Borbath I, Lombard-Bohas C, Valle J, Metrakos P, Smith D, Vinik A, Chen JS, Horsch D, Hammel P, Wiedenmann B, van Cutsem E, Patyna S, Lu DR, Blanckmeister C, Chao R, Ruszniewski P (2011) Sunitinib malate for the treatment of pancreatic neuroendocrine tumors. N Engl J Med 364:501–513

Sei Y, Zhao X, Forbes J, Szymczak S, Li Q, Trivedi A, Voellinger M, Joy G, Feng J, Whatley M, Jones MS, Harper UL, Marx SJ, Venkatesan AM, Chandrasekharappa SC, Raffeld M, Quezado MM, Louie A, Chen CC, Lim RM, Agarwala R, Schaffer AA, Hughes MS, Bailey-Wilson JE, Wank SA (2015) A hereditary form of small intestinal carcinoid associated with a germline mutation in inositol polyphosphate multikinase. Gastroenterology 149:67–78

Strosberg J (2012) Neuroendocrine tumours of the small intestine. Best Pract Res Clin Gastroenterol 26:755–773

Taal BG, Visser O (2004) Epidemiology of neuroendocrine tumours. Neuroendocrinology 80 (Suppl 1):3–7

Thakker RV, Newey PJ, Walls GV, Bilezikian J, Dralle H, Ebeling PR, Melmed S, Sakurai A, Tonelli F, Brandi ML, Endocrine S (2012) Clinical practice guidelines for multiple endocrine neoplasia type 1 (MEN1). J Clin Endocrinol Metab 97:2990–3011

Thomas-Marques L, Murat A, Delemer B, Penfornis A, Cardot-Bauters C, Baudin E, Niccoli-Sire P, Levoir D, Choplin Hdu B, Chabre O, Jovenin N, Cadiot G, Groupe des Tumeurs E (2006) Prospective endoscopic ultrasonographic evaluation of the frequency of nonfunctioning pancreaticoduodenal endocrine tumors in patients with multiple endocrine neoplasia type 1. Am J Gastroenterol 101:266–273

Toledo SP, Lourenço DM Jr, Toledo RA (2013) A differential diagnosis of inherited endocrine tumors and their tumor counterparts. Clinics 68(7):1039–1056

Triponez F, Dosseh D, Goudet P, Cougard P, Bauters C, Murat A, Cadiot G, Niccoli-Sire P, Chayvialle JA, Calender A, Proye CA (2006a) Epidemiology data on 108 MEN 1 patients from the GTE with isolated nonfunctioning tumors of the pancreas. Ann Surg 243:265–272

Triponez F, Goudet P, Dosseh D, Cougard P, Bauters C, Murat A, Cadiot G, Niccoli-Sire P, Calender A, Proye CA, French Endocrine Tumor Study G (2006b) Is surgery beneficial for MEN1 patients with small (< or =2 cm), nonfunctioning pancreaticoduodenal endocrine tumor? An analysis of 65 patients from the GTE. World J Surg 30:654–662; discussion 663–664

Ullmann U, Unuane D, Velkeniers B, Lissens W, Wuyts W, Bonduelle M (2013) A new double substitution mutation in the MEN1 gene: a limited penetrance and a specific phenotype. Eur J Hum Genet 21:695–697

Woodward ER, Maher ER (2006) Von Hippel-Lindau disease and endocrine tumour susceptibility. Endocr Relat Cancer 13:415–425

Yao JC, Hassan M, Phan A, Dagohoy C, Leary C, Mares JE, Abdalla EK, Fleming JB, Vauthey JN, Rashid A, Evans DB (2008) One hundred years after "carcinoid": epidemiology of and prognostic factors for neuroendocrine tumors in 35,825 cases in the United States. J Clin Oncol 26:3063–3072

Yao JC, Shah MH, Ito T, Bohas CL, Wolin EM, van Cutsem E, Hobday TJ, Okusaka T, Capdevila J, de Vries EG, Tomassetti P, Pavel ME, Hoosen S, Haas T, Lincy J, Lebwohl D, Oberg K, RAD001 in advanced neuroendocrine tumors TTSG (2011) Everolimus for advanced pancreatic neuroendocrine tumors. N Engl J Med 364:514–523

Diagnosis and Management of Hereditary Sarcoma

David M. Thomas and Mandy L. Ballinger

Abstract

Sarcomas are rare and heterogeneous diseases that affect a younger population than most epithelial cancers. Epidemiologic studies suggest a strong genetic component to sarcomas, and many familial cancer syndromes have been described, in which sarcomas are a feature. The best known of these are the Li–Fraumeni and retinoblastoma syndromes, study of which has been pivotal to elucidating the molecular basis for the cell response to DNA damage and the cell division. Although much has been learnt about cancer biology from the study of sarcoma families, in general clinical management of increased sarcoma risk has lagged behind other cancer predisposition syndromes. With the advent of genomic tools for genetic testing, it is likely that a substantial fraction of sarcoma patients will be identified as carriers of known risk alleles. The translation of this knowledge into effective risk management programs and cancer treatments will be essential to changes in routine clinical practice.

Keywords

Sarcoma · Genetics · Genomics · TP53

Contents

D.M. Thomas (✉) · M.L. Ballinger
The Kinghorn Cancer Centre & Garvan Institute of Medical Research,
Darlinghurst, NSW, Australia
e-mail: d.thomas@garvan.org.au

G. Pichert and C. Jacobs (eds.), *Rare Hereditary Cancers*,
Recent Results in Cancer Research 205, DOI 10.1007/978-3-319-29998-3_10

1 Introduction

Sarcomas are a diverse set of malignancies of the connective tissues, with an estimated incidence of 50–70 per million of the population (Fletcher et al. 2013). Sarcomas are divided pathologically into those arising in soft tissues and those arising in bone. There are in excess of 50 recognised subtypes of sarcomas, which exacerbates problems of accurate classification and underlines the rarity of these conditions. Sarcomas blur into a much more common group of benign connective tissue tumours, and sarcomas not uncommonly arise in pre-existing benign lesions. The strongest known environmental risk factor for sarcomas in general is ionising radiation, with weaker evidence for arsenicals and herbicides (Thomas and Ballinger 2015). Many of the genes implicated in hereditary sarcomas outlined in this chapter play important roles in the cellular response to DNA damage, which has clinical implications for therapy.

Soft-tissue sarcomas are roughly four times more common than bone tumours. The most common subtypes are undifferentiated pleomorphic sarcomas, followed by liposarcomas, leiomyosarcomas and synovial sarcomas. The most common bone tumours are osteosarcoma, Ewing sarcoma and chondrosarcoma. These categories mask a further degree of genetic, histologic and clinical heterogeneity, further complicating the challenges of accurate diagnosis and clinical management. As an era of increasing targeted therapies emerges, the clinical importance of accurate classification is only increasing.

This complexity is also important from a genetic perspective, because in addition to a broad sarcoma susceptibility for genes, such as *TP53*, mutations in other genes are associated with specific sarcoma subtypes. Because sarcomas often arise at a younger age than most epithelial cancers (Fletcher et al. 2013), they likely carry a significant burden of heritable aetiology. Ethnic variation in sarcoma incidence has not been well mapped, again because of their rarity and difficulties in consistent annotation. For example, Ewing sarcoma appears to be more common in Caucasians (Worch et al. 2010), which suggests ethnic modifier influences for a disease which is not associated with recognised familial clustering. Population-based studies suggest a high frequency of multiple primary and secondary cancers in individuals who develop sarcomas (Fernebro et al. 2006; Hemminki and Li 2001).

Sarcoma-associated syndromes have contributed enormously to our understanding of cancer biology, disproportionate to their incidence. Many of these typically autosomal dominant syndromes are described below, although interestingly many of the sarcomas that arise earlier in life, such as Ewing and synovial sarcoma, are not associated with dominant familial patterns. Despite their contribution to biological knowledge, the clinical management of these syndromes has lagged behind breast cancer and bowel cancer. In part, this may be because of the difficulties in risk modification (for example, by early detection and prevention) of cancers that are not only diverse and rare, but are also not limited to an anatomical organ system. Recent advances in genomics as well as imaging technologies may have a significant impact on our ability to identify and modify sarcoma risk. Generating a comparable evidence base for altering clinical practice may be challenging because of their rarity. We summarise what is currently known about hereditary aspects of sarcomas, consider some of the missing information in our knowledge base and conclude by summarising likely future developments in this fast-moving field of research.

2 Hereditary Conditions Predisposing to Sarcoma

2.1 Li–Fraumeni Syndrome

Li and Fraumeni described several families with a high frequency of bone and soft-tissue sarcoma, breast cancer, brain tumours and leukaemia, suggesting a dominantly inherited predisposition (Li et al. 1988; Li and Fraumeni 1969). Known as Li–Fraumeni syndrome (LFS) (OMIM 151623), this constellation of features was subsequently associated with germline mutations in the *TP53* gene (Srivastava et al. 1990; Malkin et al. 1990). Other genes that may phenocopy LFS include *CHEK2* and perhaps *BRCA2* (Bell et al. 1999; Evans et al. 2008). Clinical criteria for defining LFS and identifying candidates for *TP53* testing have evolved (Table 1) (Li et al. 1988; Bougeard et al. 2008; Chompret et al. 2001; Tinat et al. 2009; Bougeard et al. 2015). A broad range of bone and soft-tissue sarcomas account for approximately 25 % of cancers in LFS families, with osteosarcoma, leiomyosarcoma and rhabdomyosarcoma the most common (Ognjanovic et al. 2012). There are some phenotype–genotype correlations. Missense mutations in the *TP53* DNA-binding domain are associated with the earlier age of tumour onset, while frameshift, splice site and nonsense mutations are associated with leiomyosarcoma in older patients (Ognjanovic et al. 2012). *TP53* mutation carriers have an increased lifetime risk of cancer, with estimates traditionally derived from families meeting classical LFS or Chompret criteria (Table 1). In these families, the cancer risk is almost 100 % for females and 73 % for males over a lifetime (Chompret et al. 2000; Wu et al. 2006), with an early age of onset and increased risk of multiple malig-

Table 1 Modification of LFS classification criteria over time

Classification	Year	Criteria
Classic LFS	1988	Proband with a sarcoma diagnosed <45 years of age AND a first degree relative to any cancer <45 years of age AND a first or second degree relative to any cancer <45 years of age OR a sarcoma at any age
Chompret	2001	Proband with a [a]narrow spectrum LFS cancer <36 years of age AND ≥1 first or second degree relative to a narrow spectrum LFS cancer (except breast cancer if the proband has breast cancer) <46 years of age OR multiple primary cancers **OR** Proband with multiple primary cancers, 2 of which are narrow spectrum LFS cancers and the first occurred <36 years of age, regardless of family history **OR** Proband with adrenocortical carcinoma at any age regardless of family history
	2009	Proband with [b]LFS spectrum cancer <46 years of age AND ≥1 first or second degree relative to a LFS spectrum cancer <56 years of age OR with multiple cancers **OR** Proband with multiple cancers (except multiple breast cancers), 2 of which are LFS spectrum cancers and the first occurred <46 years of age **OR** Proband with adrenocortical carcinoma or choroid plexus tumour regardless of family history
	2015	Proband with [c]LFS spectrum cancer <46 years of age AND ≥1 first or second degree relative to a LFS spectrum cancer (except breast cancer if the proband has breast cancer) <56 years of age OR multiple primary cancers **OR** Proband with multiple primary cancers (except multiple breast cancers), 2 of which are LFS spectrum cancers and the first occurred <46 years of age **OR** Proband with adrenocortical carcinoma, choroid plexus tumour or rhabdomyosarcoma of embryonal anaplastic subtype, regardless of family history **OR** Proband with breast cancer <31 years of age

[a]Narrow spectrum LFS cancers include sarcoma, brain tumour, breast cancer and adrenocortical carcinoma
[b]LFS spectrum cancers include soft-tissue sarcoma, osteosarcoma, brain tumour, premenopausal breast cancer, adrenocortical carcinoma, leukaemia and lung bronchoalveolar cancer
[c]LFS spectrum cancers include soft-tissue sarcoma, osteosarcoma, CNS tumour, premenopausal breast cancer and adrenocortical carcinoma

nancies (Gonzalez et al. 2009; Hisada et al. 1998; Mitchell et al. 2013). A reduced cancer risk may occur in individuals not ascertained on LFS criteria, perhaps reflecting unknown modifier influences that increase the penetrance of alleles in familial settings (Mitchell et al. 2013).

Clinical guidelines for surveillance in *TP53* mutation carriers currently centre on breast and bowel cancer preventative measures (CINSW 2015; NCCN 2014; NICE 2013) with little account for sarcomas and other *TP53*-associated malignancies. Research studies have implemented whole-body surveillance utilising various methods including ^{18}Fluorodeoxyglucose-Positron Emission Tomography/ Computed Tomography (FDG-PET/CT) (Masciari et al. 2008) and whole-body magnetic resonance imaging (MRI; Villani et al. 2011). Although methodologically limited by small sample size and lack of randomisation, screened individuals in the latter study had better clinical outcomes than those who were not screened. A Southern Brazilian study screened neonates for the *TP53* R337H founder mutation and went on to monitor mutation carriers for adrenocortical cancer, one of the commonest malignancies associated with *TP53* seen under 10 years of age (Custodio et al. 2013). Tumours in screened carriers were identified at an earlier stage than those who were not screened. There are several issues to consider in clinical management of TP53 mutation carriers including limiting radiation exposure (Heymann et al. 2010) and the psychological effects and ethical issues associated with potential young age of cancer (Fresneau et al. 2013; Alderfer et al. 2015). Several efforts are underway internationally investigating the many aspects of comprehensive surveillance protocols for *TP53* mutation carriers (Villani et al. 2011; LIFSCREEN 2015; SIGNIFY 2015; ANZCTR 2015; Alderfer et al. 2015; CGP 2015). A surveillance schedule has been proposed to facilitate a consistent international approach while research efforts are ongoing (McBride et al. 2014).

2.2 Gastrointestinal Stromal Tumours (GIST) Predisposition Syndromes

GISTs are a form of soft-tissue sarcoma arising in myenteric cells of Cajal within the gastrointestinal tract, and most commonly affect patients aged 60–65 (Bachet et al. 2013). Most commonly, sporadic may also occur in an autosomally dominant inherited pattern in less than 5 % of cases (Neuhann et al. 2013). The first report of a family displaying characteristics consistent with heritable GIST was made in 1990 (Marshall et al. 1990). In 1998, a gain of function germline mutation in exon 11 of *KIT* was identified in a case of heritable GIST (Nishida et al. 1998). Since then more than 25 kindreds with inherited GIST syndromes (OMIM 606764) have been reported, the majority with *KIT* mutations (Carballo et al. 2005; Robson et al. 2004) reflecting the high frequency (80–85 %) of *KIT* mutations in sporadic GIST (Neuhann et al. 2013). The most common variants are in exon 11 (Nishida et al. 1998; Carballo et al. 2005; Beghini et al. 2001; Maeyama et al. 2001; Adela Avila et al. 2014), but have also been found in exons 8 (Hartmann et al. 2005), 13 (Isozaki et al. 2000; Graham et al. 2007) and 17 (Hirota et al. 1998) of the *KIT* gene. In all reports, an autosomal dominant pattern of inheritance is described with almost 100 % penetrance (Bachet and Emile 2010). GISTs occur most commonly at a young age (40–50 years) often with multiple tumours that are multifocal and arise in the stomach or small intestine (Bachet et al. 2013). In addition to predisposing to GIST, different germline *KIT* mutations are associated with variable phenotypes, including hyperpigmentation, dysphagia and mastocytosis/urticaria pigmentosa (Neuhann et al. 2013), but consistent phenotype–genotype correlations are still to be determined.

Other genes have been linked to familial GIST. GIST families with germline mutations in *PDGFRA* (exons 12 and 14) (de Raedt et al. 2006; Chompret et al. 2004; Pasini et al. 2007) have also been identified, reflecting the incidence (5–10 %) of somatic *PDGFRA* mutations in GIST (Neuhann et al. 2013). GIST clinical manifestations in germline *PDGFRA* mutation carriers are similar to germline *KIT* mutations with the age at GIST onset in these families being 40–50 years. Other clinical observations in these families are variable but include multiple lipomas and polyps in the small intestine (Pasini et al. 2007), intestinal neurofibromas (de Raedt et al. 2006) and large hands (Chompret et al. 2004).

Approximately, 10 % of gastric GISTs have loss of function in the succinate dehydrogenase (SDH) complex and are KIT/PDGFR wild-type (Miettinen et al. 2013). This is indicated by the loss of SDH subunit B (SDHB) staining by immunohistochemistry and tumours are termed SDH-deficient. These SDH-deficient gastric GISTs typically occur in children and young adults, form multiple tumours and often follow an indolent course (Miettinen and Lasota 2014). Carney triad (OMIM 604287) is a non-familial association of pulmonary chondroma, extra-adrenal paraganglioma and SDH-deficient GIST with a strong female predilection (Carney et al. 1977; Zhang et al. 2010). However, the later-described Carney-Stratakis syndrome (CSS) (OMIM 606864) is characterised by SDH-deficient GIST and paragangliomas and is inherited in an autosomal dominant manner with incomplete penetrance (Carney and Stratakis 2002). Germline mutations in the *SDH* genes *SDHB*, *SDHC* and *SDHD* have been identified in these CSS families (Pasini et al. 2008). More recently, *SDHA* germline mutations have been found in SDH-deficient GIST patients (Miettinen et al. 2013; Miettinen and Lasota 2014; Pantaleo et al. 2011).

There are currently no evidence-based guidelines for risk management of hereditary GIST syndromes. Criteria have been outlined for the identification of potential germline *KIT* and *PDGFRA* mutation carriers and surveillance and treatment recommendations made (Bachet et al. 2013). In clinical management of affected individuals, *KIT/PDGFR* mutant tumours respond well to imatinib, while SDH-deficient and wild-type tumours are less likely to respond as well. Patients with advanced wild-type GIST do not respond to imatinib as well as patients with *KIT* exon 11 mutations (Heinrich et al. 2008).

2.3 Neurofibromatosis Type 1 (NF1)

Neurofibromatosis type 1 (OMIM 162200) previously known as von Recklinghausen's disease (Ferner 2007) is a tumour predisposition syndrome characterised by neurofibromas, café au lait pigmentation, Lisch nodules in the eye, optic pathway gliomas and bony dysplasia. Cognitive disabilities in children and cardiovascular problems in adults are also associated with this condition (Ferner 2007). NF1 has an incidence of approximately 1 in 3000 individuals (Evans et al. 2010; Huson et al. 1989; Ratner and Miller 2015). A region on chromosome 17 was identified as being associated with NF1 (Barker et al. 1987) and subsequently the *NF1* gene was cloned and identified as a tumour suppressor (Viskochil et al. 1990; Cawthon et al. 1990; Wallace et al. 1990). Germline *NF1* mutations are inherited in an autosomal dominant manner but phenotypic variability provides little evidence for phenotype–genotype correlations (Ratner and Miller 2015). Type 1 neurofibromatosis is diagnosed on clinical criteria with mutation testing generally limited to the prenatal setting (Ferner 2007). In 1988, the National Institutes of Health Consensus Development Conference on Neurofibromatosis set clinical criteria for NF1 (Agaimy et al. 2012).

Germline *NF1* mutation carriers are at increased risk of several malignancies including malignant peripheral nerve sheath tumour (MPNST) (Evans et al. 2002) and GIST (Miettinen et al. 2006) and more rarely juvenile leukaemias (Stiller et al. 1994), phaeochromocytoma (Walther et al. 1999), glomus tumours (Stewart et al. 2010) and rhabdomyosarcoma (Sung et al. 2004; Crucis et al. 2015). MPNSTs contribute significantly to the mortality associated with NF1 (Evans et al. 2011) and there is an 8–13 % lifetime risk (Evans et al. 2002). Individuals with microdeletions in *NF1* have an increased risk of MPNST compared to other *NF1* mutation carriers (De Raedt et al. 2003). The prevalence of GIST in patients with neurofibromatosis has been reported at 7 % (Zoller et al. 1997), but higher rates have been recorded in autopsy studies (Miettinen et al. 2006). Approximately 10 % of duodenal and jejuno-ileal GISTs were associated with *NF1* mutations in a large study at the Armed Forces Institute of Pathology (Miettinen et al. 2006).

There is no evidence that specific surveillance for MPNST or GIST in *NF1* mutation carriers provides benefit. Risk management guidelines have been formulated by several groups and recommendations relevant to sarcoma include annual physical examination, regular monitoring of central nervous system abnormalities and other studies such as MRI only when clinically indicated (Hersh and American Academy of Pediatrics Committee on 2008; Ferner 2007; Ferner et al. 2007). Diagnosing malignant transformation in the setting of NF1 can be fraught as the emergence of lumps is common, and benign tumours often produce symptoms similar to malignancy (Ferner 2007). There is an increased risk of MPNST following radiotherapy (Sharif et al. 2006), and therefore, the use of radiotherapy should be carefully considered. NF1-associated GIST typically occurs in the small intestine as multiple, small asymptomatic lesions (Miettinen and Lasota 2013) with a low mitotic index; however, clinical malignancy is not uncommon (Agaimy et al. 2012). *KIT* and *PDGFRA* mutations are usually not present in these tumours (Miettinen et al. 2006; Kinoshita et al. 2004) and generally respond incompletely to imatinib (Lee et al. 2006; Mussi et al. 2008).

2.4 Other Sarcoma-Associated Hereditary Syndromes

There is insufficient space to do justice to the many genes associated to date with individual sarcoma subtypes, so a brief survey will suffice (Table 2). Osteosarcomas are cancers of osteoblasts and are associated with germline mutations in some well-known tumour suppressor genes. These include the Retinoblastoma gene (*RB1*) and three helicases: *RECQL4* in Rothmund-Thomson (OMIM 268400) and RAPADILINO (OMIM 266280) syndromes; *RECQL3* (*BLM)* in Bloom syndrome (OMIM 210900); and *RECQL2* (*WRN*) in Werner syndrome (OMIM 277700). These are all extremely rare and in each case are associated with clinical features. Mutations in *RB1* are associated with childhood retinoblastoma (OMIM 180200) (Balmer et al. 2006), while Werner syndrome is an autosomal recessive condition associated with progeric features (Sugimoto 2014). Bloom and Rothmund -Thomson syndromes, also autosomal recessive, are characterised by small stature and growth delay, and skin changes (Veith and Mangerich 2015). It should be noted that other malignancies, including other sarcomas, are also reported in these cancer types. Other syndromes linked to increased bone turnover are associated with osteosarcomas, including Paget's disease of bone (OMIM 602080, *TNFRSF11A, SQSTM1, PDB4*) (Ralston and Albagha 2014) and McCune Albright syndrome (OMIM 174800, *GNAS*) (Turan and Bastepe 2015).

Chondrosarcomas, or tumours of cartilage, are associated with a variety of hereditary and congenital genetic conditions. Unlike osteosarcomas, chondrosarcomas arise at an older age and are not chemo- or radio-sensitive. Early detection and surgery is therefore critical to effective treatment. Frequently, syndromic chondrosarcomas arise in the context of pre-existing benign skeletal lesions, such as multiple osteochondromas due to mutations in *EXT1* or *EXT2* (OMIM 133700, 133701) (Musso et al. 2015; Jones et al. 2014; Ciavarella et al. 2013). Ollier's disease and Maffucci syndrome are the best known congenital (but not hereditary) chondrodysplastic conditions that are associated with an increased risk of chondrosarcomas (Verdegaal et al. 2011). They are associated with early-onset chondroid lesions, and in the case of Maffucci syndrome, associated with vascular anomalies, including a predilection for angiosarcomas (Fletcher et al. 2013). The genetic basis for these diseases includes mutations in *IDH1* and *IDH2* (Amary et al. 2011), and *PTHLH* (Collinson et al. 2010). Perivascular epithelioid cell sarcomas (PEComas) are associated with mutations in *TSC1* and *TSC2* and may respond to mTOR inhibitors (Wagner et al. 2010).

Rhabdomyosarcomas are usually childhood cancers arising from skeletal muscle and are associated with a wide range of syndromes, including LFS, basal cell naevus syndrome (also known as Gorlin syndrome) (OMIM 109400). Gorlin syndrome is due to mutations in *PTCH1* and perhaps other members of the Hedgehog signalling pathway including *PTCH2* and *SUFU* (Pastorino et al. 2009; Fan et al. 2008; Johnson et al. 1996) and clinical manifestations include basal cell carcinomas, medulloblastoma and jaw cysts. Rhabdomyosarcoma is also associated with Beckwith-Wiedemann syndrome (OMIM 130650) a disorder of epigenetic origin

Table 2 Genetic syndromes and conditions predisposing to sarcoma

Genomic class	Sarcoma	Syndrome/condition	Gene
Complex	Osteosarcoma	Li–Fraumeni syndrome	*TP53*
		Retinoblastoma	*RB1*
		Bloom syndrome	*RECQL3 (BLM)*
		Familial Paget disease of bone	*TNFRSF11A*, *SQSTM1*, *PDB4*
		Rothmund-Thomson syndrome	*RECQL4*
		RAPADILINO syndrome	*RECQL4*
		Werner	*RECQL2* (*WRN*)
		McCune Albright syndrome	*GNAS*
	Embryonal rhabdomyosarcoma	Li–Fraumeni syndrome	*TP53*
		Gorlin syndrome	*PTCH1*, *PTCH2*, *SUFU*
		Beckwith-Wiedemann syndrome	*CDKN1C*, *NSD1*, *ICR1*, *H19*, *KCNQ1OT1*
		Neurofibromatosis type 1	*NF1*
		Mosaic variegated aneuploidy	*BUB1B*
		DICER 1 syndrome	*DICER1*
		Costello syndrome	*HRAS*
	Rhabdomyosarcoma (subtype not reported)	Nijmegen Breakage syndrome	*NBS1*
		Li–Fraumeni syndrome	*TP53*
	Leiomyosarcoma/undifferentiated pleomorphic sarcoma	Hereditary leiomyoma and renal cell carcinoma	*FH*
		Neurofibromatosis type 1	*NF1*
	MPNST	Hereditary multiple exostoses	*EXT1*, *EXT2*
	Chondrosarcoma	Retinoblastoma	*RB1*
		Ollier disease[a]	*IDH1*, *IDH2*, *PTHLH*

(continued)

Table 2 (continued)

Genomic class	Sarcoma	Syndrome/condition	Gene
		Maffucci syndrome[a]	*IDH1*, *IDH2*, *PTHLH*
Simple	GIST	Familial GIST	*KIT*, *PDGFRA*
		Carney-Stratakis syndrome	*SDHB*, *SDHC*, *SDHD*
		Neurofibromatosis type 1	*NF1*
	PEComa	Tuberous sclerosis	*TSC1*, *TSC2*
Translocation-associated	Ewing sarcoma	None	
	Myxoid liposarcoma	None	
		None	
	Synovial sarcoma	Retinoblastoma	*RB1*
	Alveolar rhabdomyosarcoma	Costello syndrome	*HRAS*

[a]Not hereditary

involving chromosome 11q15, although the precise genetic basis is not known (Cohen 2005), type-1 neurofibromatosis (Sung et al. 2004; Crucis et al. 2015), Nijmegen breakage syndrome (*NBS*1, a recessive condition associated with short stature and microcephaly and immunodeficiency) (Chrzanowska et al. 2012), mosaic variegated aneuploidy (*BUB1B*, associated with developmental delay and anomalies) (Hanks et al. 2004), DICER1 syndrome (*DICER1*, associated with endocrine phenomena) (Schultz et al. 2014) and Costello syndrome (a congenital myopathy associated with mutations in *HRAS*) (Kratz et al. 2015).

Uterine leiomyosarcomas may be associated with hereditary leiomyomatosis and renal cell carcinoma (HLRCC, OMIM 150800), a cancer predisposition syndrome characterised by cutaneous leiomyomas, multiple benign uterine leiomyomas (fibroids) and early-onset renal tumours with a specific type-II papillary morphology (Schmidt and Linehan 2014; Launonen et al. 2001). Germline mutations in the Fumarate Hydratase (FH) gene are associated with HLRCC (Tomlinson et al. 2002). The estimated lifetime risk of renal cancer is 15 % (Menko et al. 2014). Surveillance recommendations for HLRCC centre around renal cancer risk, but an annual gynaecological review has been suggested as warranted for possible detection of malignancy (Refae et al. 2007). There are reproductive implications for female *FH* mutation carriers to consider also as uterine leiomyomas typically affect young women and may interfere with the ability to bear children.

3 Benign and Intermediate Connective Tissue Tumour Syndromes

It is estimated that there are over 100 benign connective tissue tumours for every sarcoma, and many of these are associated with a hereditary or constitutive genetic basis (Gatta et al. 2011; Myhre-Jensen 1981). In addition to the morbidity due directly to these diseases, the significance of these associations lies in the linkage to both sarcomas and epithelial malignancies. Familial adenomatous polyposis (FAP) should be suspected in individuals presenting with aggressive fibromatosis (AF; also known as desmoid tumour) and is mostly due to germline mutations in the *APC* gene (Fearnhead et al. 2001). This may occur in the absence of a family history, as the de novo rate of APC mutations is estimated at 25 % (Bisgaard et al. 1994). Germline *APC* mutation carriers have a lifetime risk of colorectal cancer nearing 100 % (Burn et al. 1991), and a 12 % risk of AF (Clark and Phillips 1996). Although notionally benign, AF is one of the main causes of death in patients post-colectomy (Sturt and Clark 2006). They are typically non-metastatic but exhibit aggressive local growth patterns, and usually occur in the abdominal wall or mesentery (Lung et al. 2015). Risk management for *APC* mutation carriers focuses primarily on the risk of colorectal cancer but recommendations have included CT or MRI for the detection of AF on an individualised basis (Leoz et al. 2015).

4 Sarcomas not associated with Recognised Syndromes

It is interesting to consider the subset of sarcomas which are not characterised by familial clustering. Many sarcomas are characterised by chromosomal instability (for example, leiomyosarcoma, undifferentiated pleomorphic sarcoma, osteosarcoma), particularly in association with LFS. However, most sarcomas characterised by pathognomonic translocations, such as EWS-FLI1 in Ewing sarcoma (Lessnick and Ladanyi 2012), FUS-CHOP in myxoid liposarcoma (Di Giandomenico et al. 2014) and SYT-SSX in synovial sarcoma (Thway and Fisher 2014), are not associated with known syndromes. This is despite the case that Ewing sarcoma is essentially a paediatric or young adult onset sarcoma, while synovial sarcoma also affects a younger population than most sarcomas. Early age of cancer onset tends to suggest a genetic basis, which makes the absence of reported families a little surprising. Given the historical focus of cancer genetics on dominant cancer families, and single-gene testing based on linkage studies, it is possible that this may be due to non-dominant genetic transmission, or to de novo events that we do not recognise.

5 Future Directions

The traditional focus of cancer genetics on Mendelian dominant families, single-gene testing and breast, bowel and ovarian cancer is going to change over the next decade (Thomas et al. 2015). The driver behind these changes is the impact of genomic tools on mutation identification. The technology ranges from boutique panels comprising a few genes, to whole exome sequencing, and inevitably, whole genome sequencing. A full discussion of this topic is beyond the scope of this chapter. The coming era will see a shift towards ascertainment of risk directly through genetic testing of a broader range of patients than previously. In respect of sarcomas, a recent survey indicated that patients and their families have positive attitudes towards genetic testing for heritable conditions and about genetic research in general (Young et al. 2013).

As these tools are applied to broader populations of cancer patients—and maybe ultimately to the population at large—the architecture of genetic cancer risk will begin to include more quantitative, polygenic elements, as well as the current dominant effects of major cancer genes. It is already clear from studies (predominantly in breast cancer) that common single nucleotide polymorphisms may coincide within individuals with early-onset cancer (Sawyer et al. 2012). However, the effect size attributable to each variant is small, when they overlap their combined effect may be comparable to that seen in individuals carrying known dominant causes of cancer. The key point is that as multiple-gene testing enters the clinic, the ability to discern the effects of multiple variants within an individual will usher in a much more complex era of variant classification. We predict that evidence will accumulate over the next decade of the polygenic contribution to cancer risk at the population level. Of course, we next need to understand how this information is to be used to help carriers.

Population- or clinic-based ascertainment will also identify the hidden burden of de novo mutations in dominant genes in individuals who lack a classic family history. The precise rates of de novo variation are not known for most genes with certainty, and vary quite significantly from apparently negligible in the case of *BRCA1*, to approximately 20 % in the case of *TP53* (Schneider et al. 2013). For sarcomas, it is possible that a combination of unrecognised de novo and polygenic causes may in part account for the group of early-onset, translocation-associated sarcomas.

Genomic studies are already underway in sarcoma populations to begin the journey of mapping genetic risk. The low-hanging fruit from these studies will come from determining the burden of risk attributable to genes already linked to cancer risk in sarcomas, or for cancers in general. Based on current studies in breast and ovarian cancers (Walsh et al. 2011), even the application of limited gene panels will identify about 15–25 % of sarcoma subjects with known oncogenic germline variation. The clinical importance of these early gene panels cannot be overstated, since utility drives change in medical practice. For some of these genes, we have accepted risk management protocols (e.g. for *APC, BRCA1*). Increasingly, germline genetic variation may also be used to select patients for targeted therapies, such as vismodegib for Gorlin's syndrome (Lopez-Lerma et al. 2015) and poly-ADP ribose polymerase inhibitors for carriers of mutations in *BRCA1* or *BRCA2* (Scott et al. 2015). It is also important to recognise that sarcomas are surgically curable if caught at an early stage. The co-development of technologies such as whole-body magnetic resonance imaging will be important to sarcoma-specific risk management and early-detection programs, as is the case for any multiorgan cancer susceptibility syndrome. Finally, it is likely that knowledge of germline variation in DNA repair genes may directly influence decision-making in the treatment of sarcomas. Radiation is the strongest known environmental risk factor for sarcoma development and also forms a key treatment modality for patients with sarcoma—including in the curative management of these diseases. In the future, the decision whether or not to use radiotherapy may be informed by a more detailed knowledge of carriage of variants impairing normal tissue responses to these treatments.

6 Summary

Sarcomas are rare and heterogeneous malignancies that affect the young. Early age of cancer onset is an important guide to genetic risk. While the study of rare families with excess sarcoma has contributed to fundamental insights into cancer biology, including the *TP53* and cell cycle pathways, a genetic basis for the majority of sarcomas remains to be discovered. Clinically, despite long knowledge of syndromes such as those due to mutations in *TP53*, risk management has lagged behind more common hereditary cancer syndromes such as those associated with breast and bowel cancer. This is likely because of the multiorgan nature of most sarcoma susceptibility syndromes and because their rarity impedes the generation of an evidence base for effective risk modification. Future developments in genomics, imaging technologies and molecular therapeutics are likely to present opportunities for both ascertainment of the genetic basis for sarcomas, early detection and treatment of affected patients.

References

Adela Avila S, Penaloza J, Gonzalez F, Abdo I, Rainville I, Root E, Carrero Valenzuela RD, Garber J (2014) Dysphagia, melanosis, gastrointestinal stromal tumors and a germinal mutation of the KIT gene in an Argentine family. Acta Gastroenterol Latinoam 44:9–15

Agaimy A, Vassos N, Croner RS (2012) Gastrointestinal manifestations of neurofibromatosis type 1 (Recklinghausen's disease): clinicopathological spectrum with pathogenetic considerations. Int J Clin Exp Pathol 5:852–862

Alderfer MA, Zelley K, Lindell RB, Novokmet A, Mai PL, Garber JE, Nathan D, Scollon S, Chun NM, Patenaude AF, Ford JM, Plon SE, Schiffman JD, Diller LR, Savage SA, Malkin D, Ford CA, Nichols KE (2015) Parent decision-making around the genetic testing of children for germline TP53 mutations. Cancer 121:286–293

Amary MF, Damato S, Halai D, Eskandarpour M, Berisha F, Bonar F, McCarthy S, Fantin VR, Straley KS, Lobo S, Aston W, Green CL, Gale RE, Tirabosco R, Futreal A, Campbell P, Presneau N, Flanagan AM (2011) Ollier disease and Maffucci syndrome are caused by somatic mosaic mutations of IDH1 and IDH2. Nat Genet 43:1262–1265

ANZCTR (2015) A pilot surveillance study investigating whole body magnetic resonance imaging and other diagnostic procedures in people at high risk of cancer. ACTRN 12613000987763 (Online). Available: https://anzctr.org.au/

Bachet JB, Emile JF (2010) Diagnostic criteria, specific mutations, and genetic predisposition in gastrointestinal stromal tumors. Appl Clin Genet 3:85–101

Bachet JB, Landi B, Laurent-Puig P, Italiano A, le Cesne A, Levy P, Safar V, Duffaud F, Blay JY, Emile JF (2013) Diagnosis, prognosis and treatment of patients with gastrointestinal stromal tumour (GIST) and germline mutation of KIT exon 13. Eur J Cancer 49:2531–2541

Balmer A, Zografos L, Munier F (2006) Diagnosis and current management of retinoblastoma. Oncogene 25:5341–5349

Barker D, Wright E, Nguyen K, Cannon L, Fain P, Goldgar D, Bishop DT, Carey J, Baty B, Kivlin J et al (1987) Gene for von Recklinghausen neurofibromatosis is in the pericentromeric region of chromosome 17. Science 236:1100–1102

Beghini A, Tibiletti MG, Roversi G, Chiaravalli AM, Serio G, Capella C, Larizza L (2001) Germline mutation in the juxtamembrane domain of the kit gene in a family with gastrointestinal stromal tumors and urticaria pigmentosa. Cancer 92:657–662

Bell DW, Varley JM, Szydlo TE, Kang DH, Wahrer DC, Shannon KE, Lubratovich M, Verselis SJ, Isselbacher KJ, Fraumeni JF, Birch JM, Li FP, Garber JE, Haber DA (1999) Heterozygous germ line hCHK2 mutations in Li-Fraumeni syndrome. Science 286:2528–2531

Bisgaard ML, Fenger K, Bulow S, Niebuhr E, Mohr J (1994) Familial adenomatous polyposis (FAP): frequency, penetrance, and mutation rate. Hum Mutat 3:121–125

Bougeard G, Renaux-Petel M, Flaman JM, Charbonnier C, Fermey P, Belotti M, Gauthier-Villars M, Stoppa-Lyonnet D, Consolino E, Brugieres L, Caron O, Benusiglio PR, Bressac-De Paillerets B, Bonadona V, Bonaiti-Pellie C, Tinat J, Baert-Desurmont S, Frebourg T (2015) Revisiting Li-Fraumeni syndrome From TP53 mutation carriers. J Clin Oncol 33:2345–2352

Bougeard G, Sesboue R, Baert-Desurmont S, Vasseur S, Martin C, Tinat J, Brugieres L, Chompret A, de Paillerets BB, Stoppa-Lyonnet D, Bonaiti-Pellie C, Frebourg T,

French LFSWG (2008) Molecular basis of the Li-Fraumeni syndrome: an update from the French LFS families. J Med Genet 45:535–538

Burn J, Chapman P, Delhanty J, Wood C, Lalloo F, Cachon-Gonzalez MB, Tsioupra K, Church W, Rhodes M, Gunn A (1991) The UK Northern region genetic register for familial adenomatous polyposis coli: use of age of onset, congenital hypertrophy of the retinal pigment epithelium, and DNA markers in risk calculations. J Med Genet 28:289–296

Carballo M, Roig I, Aguilar F, Pol MA, Gamundi MJ, Hernan I, Martinez-Gimeno M (2005) Novel c-KIT germline mutation in a family with gastrointestinal stromal tumors and cutaneous hyperpigmentation. Am J Med Genet A 132A:361–364

Carney JA, Stratakis CA (2002) Familial paraganglioma and gastric stromal sarcoma: a new syndrome distinct from the Carney triad. Am J Med Genet 108:132–139

Carney JA, Sheps SG, Go VL, Gordon H (1977) The triad of gastric leiomyosarcoma, functioning extra-adrenal paraganglioma and pulmonary chondroma. N Engl J Med 296:1517–1518

Cawthon RM, Weiss R, Xu GF, Viskochil D, Culver M, Stevens J, Robertson M, Dunn D, Gesteland R, O'connell P et al (1990) A major segment of the neurofibromatosis type 1 gene: cDNA sequence, genomic structure, and point mutations. Cell 62:193–201

Cancer Genetics and Prevention (2015) Li Fraumeni whole body MRI study. http://www.dana-farber.org

Chompret A, Abel A, Stoppa-Lyonnet D, Brugieres L, Pages S, Feunteun J, Bonaiti-Pellie C (2001) Sensitivity and predictive value of criteria for p53 germline mutation screening. J Med Genet 38:43–47

Chompret A, Brugieres L, Ronsin M, Gardes M, Dessarps-Freichey F, Abel A, Hua D, Ligot L, Dondon MG, Bressac-de Paillerets B, Frebourg T, Lemerle J, Bonaiti-Pellie C, Feunteun J (2000) P53 germline mutations in childhood cancers and cancer risk for carrier individuals. Br J Cancer 82:1932–1937

Chompret A, Kannengiesser C, Barrois M, Terrier P, Dahan P, Tursz T, Lenoir GM, Bressac-de Paillerets B (2004) PDGFRA germline mutation in a family with multiple cases of gastrointestinal stromal tumor. Gastroenterology 126:318–321

Chrzanowska KH, Gregorek H, Dembowska-Baginska B, Kalina MA, Digweed M (2012) Nijmegen breakage syndrome (NBS). Orphanet J Rare Dis 7:13

Ciavarella M, Coco M, Baorda F, Stanziale P, Chetta M, Bisceglia L, Palumbo P, Bengala M, Raiteri P, Silengo M, Caldarini C, Facchini R, Lala R, Cavaliere ML, de Brasi D, Pasini B, Zelante L, Guarnieri V, D'Agruma L (2013) 20 novel point mutations and one large deletion in EXT1 and EXT2 genes: report of diagnostic screening in a large Italian cohort of patients affected by hereditary multiple exostosis. Gene 515:339–348

Cancer Institute New South Wales (2015) Risk management for Li Fraumeni syndrome. eviQ Cancer Treatments Online. www.eviq.org.au

Clark SK, Phillips RK (1996) Desmoids in familial adenomatous polyposis. Br J Surg 83:1494–1504

Cohen MM Jr (2005) Beckwith-Wiedemann syndrome: historical, clinicopathological, and etiopathogenetic perspectives. Pediatr Dev Pathol 8:287–304

Collinson M, Leonard SJ, Charlton J, Crolla JA, Silve C, Hall CM, Oglivie C, James MA, Smithson SF (2010) Symmetrical enchondromatosis is associated with duplication of 12p11.23 to 12p11.22 including PTHLH. Am J Med Genet A 152A:3124–3128

Crucis A, Richer W, Brugieres L, Bergeron C, Marie-Cardine A, Stephan JL, Girard P, Corradini N, Munzer M, Lacour B, Minard-Colin V, Sarnacki S, Ranchere-Vince D, Orbach D, Bourdeaut F (2015) Rhabdomyosarcomas in children with neurofibromatosis type I: a national historical cohort. Pediatr Blood Cancer 62(10):1733–1738

Custodio G, Parise GA, Kiesel Filho N, Komechen H, Sabbaga CC, Rosati R, Grisa L, Parise IZ, Pianovski MA, Fiori CM, Ledesma JA, Barbosa JR, Figueiredo FR, Sade ER, Ibanez H, Arram SB, Stinghen ST, Mengarelli LR, Figueiredo MM, Carvalho DC, Avilla SG, Woiski TD, Poncio LC, Lima GF, Pontarolo R, Lalli E, Zhou Y, Zambetti GP, Ribeiro RC,

Figueiredo BC (2013) Impact of neonatal screening and surveillance for the TP53 R337H mutation on early detection of childhood adrenocortical tumors. J Clin Oncol 31:2619–2626

de Raedt T, Brems H, Wolkenstein P, Vidaud D, Pilotti S, Perrone F, Mautner V, Frahm S, Sciot R, Legius E (2003) Elevated risk for MPNST in NF1 microdeletion patients. Am J Hum Genet 72:1288–1292

de Raedt T, Cools J, Debiec-Rychter M, Brems H, Mentens N, Sciot R, Himpens J, de Wever I, Schoffski P, Marynen P, Legius E (2006) Intestinal neurofibromatosis is a subtype of familial GIST and results from a dominant activating mutation in PDGFRA. Gastroenterology 131:1907–1912

di Giandomenico S, Frapolli R, Bello E, Uboldi S, Licandro SA, Marchini S, Beltrame L, Brich S, Mauro V, Tamborini E, Pilotti S, Casali PG, Grosso F, Sanfilippo R, Gronchi A, Mantovani R, Gatta R, Galmarini CM, Sousa-Faro JM, D'Incalci M (2014) Mode of action of trabectedin in myxoid liposarcomas. Oncogene 33:5201–5210

Evans DG, Baser ME, McGaughran J, Sharif S, Howard E, Moran A (2002) Malignant peripheral nerve sheath tumours in neurofibromatosis 1. J Med Genet 39:311–314

Evans DG, Howard E, Giblin C, Clancy T, Spencer H, Huson SM, Lalloo F (2010) Birth incidence and prevalence of tumor-prone syndromes: estimates from a UK family genetic register service. Am J Med Genet A 152A:327–332

Evans DG, O'Hara C, Wilding A, Ingham SL, Howard E, Dawson J, Moran A, Scott-Kitching V, Holt F, Huson SM (2011) Mortality in neurofibromatosis 1: in North West England: an assessment of actuarial survival in a region of the UK since 1989. Eur J Hum Genet 19:1187–1191

Evans DG, Wu CL, Birch JM (2008) BRCA2: a cause of Li-Fraumeni-like syndrome. J Med Genet 45:62–63

Fan Z, Li J, Du J, Zhang H, Shen Y, Wang CY, Wang S (2008) A missense mutation in PTCH2 underlies dominantly inherited NBCCS in a Chinese family. J Med Genet 45:303–308

Fearnhead NS, Britton MP, Bodmer WF (2001) The ABC of APC. Hum Mol Genet 10:721–733

Fernebro J, Bladstrom A, Rydholm A, Gustafson P, Olsson H, Engellau J, Nilbert M (2006) Increased risk of malignancies in a population-based study of 818 soft-tissue sarcoma patients. Br J Cancer 95:986–990

Ferner RE (2007) Neurofibromatosis 1 and neurofibromatosis 2: a twenty first century perspective. Lancet Neurol 6:340–351

Ferner RE, Huson SM, Thomas N, Moss C, Willshaw H, Evans DG, Upadhyaya M, Towers R, Gleeson M, Steiger C, Kirby A (2007) Guidelines for the diagnosis and management of individuals with neurofibromatosis 1. J Med Genet 44:81–88

Fletcher CD, Hogendoorn P, Merterns F, Bridge J (eds) (2013) World Health Organisation classification of tumours of soft tissue and bone. IARC Press, Lyon

Fresneau B, Brugieres L, Caron O, Moutel G (2013) Ethical issues in presymptomatic genetic testing for minors: a dilemma in Li-Fraumeni syndrome. J Genet Couns 22:315–322

Gatta G, Van Der Zwan JM, Casali PG, Siesling S, Dei Tos AP, Kunkler I, Otter R, Licitra L, Mallone S, Tavilla A, Trama A, Capocaccia R, Group RW (2011) Rare cancers are not so rare: the rare cancer burden in Europe. Eur J Cancer 47:2493–2511

Gonzalez KD, Noltner KA, Buzin CH, Gu D, Wen-Fong CY, Nguyen VQ, Han JH, Lowstuter K, Longmate J, Sommer SS, Weitzel JN (2009) Beyond Li Fraumeni syndrome: clinical characteristics of families with p53 germline mutations. J Clin Oncol 27:1250–1256

Graham J, Debiec-Rychter M, Corless CL, Reid R, Davidson R, White JD (2007) Imatinib in the management of multiple gastrointestinal stromal tumors associated with a germline KIT K642E mutation. Arch Pathol Lab Med 131:1393–1396

Hanks S, Coleman K, Reid S, Plaja A, Firth H, Fitzpatrick D, Kidd A, Mehes K, Nash R, Robin N, Shannon N, Tolmie J, Swansbury J, Irrthum A, Douglas J, Rahman N (2004) Constitutional aneuploidy and cancer predisposition caused by biallelic mutations in BUB1B. Nat Genet 36:1159–1161

Hartmann K, Wardelmann E, Ma Y, Merkelbach-Bruse S, Preussner LM, Woolery C, Baldus SE, Heinicke T, Thiele J, Buettner R, Longley BJ (2005) Novel germline mutation of KIT associated with familial gastrointestinal stromal tumors and mastocytosis. Gastroenterology 129:1042–1046

Heinrich MC, Owzar K, Corless CL, Hollis D, Borden EC, Fletcher CD, Ryan CW, von Mehren M, Blanke CD, Rankin C, Benjamin RS, Bramwell VH, Demetri GD, Bertagnolli MM, Fletcher JA (2008) Correlation of kinase genotype and clinical outcome in the North American intergroup phase III trial of imatinib mesylate for treatment of advanced gastrointestinal stromal tumor: CALGB 150105 study by cancer and leukemia group B and Southwest oncology group. J Clin Oncol 26:5360–5367

Hemminki K, Li X (2001) A population-based study of familial soft tissue tumors. J Clin Epidemiol 54:411–416

Hersh JH and American Academy of Pediatrics Committee On Genetics (2008) Health supervision for children with neurofibromatosis. Pediatrics 121:633–642

Heymann S, Delaloge S, Rahal A, Caron O, Frebourg T, Barreau L, Pachet C, Mathieu MC, Marsiglia H, Bourgier C (2010) Radio-induced malignancies after breast cancer postoperative radiotherapy in patients with Li-Fraumeni syndrome. Radiat Oncol 5:104

Hirota S, Isozaki K, Moriyama Y, Hashimoto K, Nishida T, Ishiguro S, Kawano K, Hanada M, Kurata A, Takeda M, Muhammad Tunio G, Matsuzawa Y, Kanakura Y, Shinomura Y, Kitamura Y (1998) Gain-of-function mutations of c-kit in human gastrointestinal stromal tumors. Science 279:577–580

Hisada M, Garber JE, Fung CY, Fraumeni JF Jr, Li FP (1998) Multiple primary cancers in families with Li-Fraumeni syndrome. J Natl Cancer Inst 90:606–611

Huson SM, Compston DA, Clark P, Harper PS (1989) A genetic study of von Recklinghausen neurofibromatosis in south east Wales. I. Prevalence, fitness, mutation rate, and effect of parental transmission on severity. J Med Genet 26:704–711

Isozaki K, Terris B, Belghiti J, Schiffmann S, Hirota S, Vanderwinden JM (2000) Germline-activating mutation in the kinase domain of KIT gene in familial gastrointestinal stromal tumors. Am J Pathol 157:1581–1585

Johnson RL, Rothman AL, Xie J, Goodrich LV, Bare JW, Bonifas JM, Quinn AG, Myers RM, Cox DR, Epstein EH Jr, Scott MP (1996) Human homolog of patched, a candidate gene for the basal cell nevus syndrome. Science 272:1668–1671

Jones KB, Pacifici M, Hilton MJ (2014) Multiple hereditary exostoses (MHE): elucidating the pathogenesis of a rare skeletal disorder through interdisciplinary research. Connect Tissue Res 55:80–88

Kinoshita K, Hirota S, Isozaki K, Ohashi A, Nishida T, Kitamura Y, Shinomura Y, Matsuzawa Y (2004) Absence of c-kit gene mutations in gastrointestinal stromal tumours from neurofibromatosis type 1 patients. J Pathol 202:80–85

Kratz CP, Franke L, Peters H, Kohlschmidt N, Kazmierczak B, Finckh U, Bier A, Eichhorn B, Blank C, Kraus C, Kohlhase J, Pauli S, Wildhardt G, Kutsche K, Auber B, Christmann A, Bachmann N, Mitter D, Cremer FW, Mayer K, Daumer-Haas C, Nevinny-Stickel-hinzpeter C, Oeffner F, Schluter G, Gencik M, Uberlacker B, Lissewski C, Schanze I, Greene MH, Spix C, Zenker M (2015) Cancer spectrum and frequency among children with Noonan, Costello, and cardio-facio-cutaneous syndromes. Br J Cancer 112:1392–1397

Launonen V, Vierimaa O, Kiuru M, Isola J, Roth S, Pukkala E, Sistonen P, Herva R, Aaltonen LA (2001) Inherited susceptibility to uterine leiomyomas and renal cell cancer. Proc Natl Acad Sci USA 98:3387–3392

Lee JL, Kim JY, Ryu MH, Kang HJ, Chang HM, Kim TW, Lee H, Park JH, Kim HC, Kim JS, Kang YK (2006) Response to imatinib in KIT- and PDGFRA-wild type gastrointestinal stromal associated with neurofibromatosis type 1. Dig Dis Sci 51:1043–1046

Leoz ML, Carballal S, Moreira L, Ocana T, Balaguer F (2015) The genetic basis of familial adenomatous polyposis and its implications for clinical practice and risk management. Appl Clin Genet 8:95–107

Lessnick SL, Ladanyi M (2012) Molecular pathogenesis of Ewing sarcoma: new therapeutic and transcriptional targets. Annu Rev Pathol 7:145–159

Li FP, Fraumeni JF Jr (1969) Soft-tissue sarcomas, breast cancer, and other neoplasms. A familial syndrome? Ann Intern Med 71:747–752

Li FP, Fraumeni JF Jr, Mulvihill JJ, Blattner WA, Dreyfus MG, Tucker MA, Miller RW (1988) A cancer family syndrome in twenty-four kindreds. Cancer Res 48:5358–5362

LIFSCREEN (2015) Evaluation of whole body MRI for early detection of cancers in subjects with P53 mutation (Online). Available: https://clinicaltrials.gov/ct2/show/record/NCT01461086

Lopez-Lerma I, Mollet J, Garcia-Patos V (2015) Trichodysplasia spinulosa in gorlin syndrome treated with vismodegib. JAMA Dermatol 151:458–459

Lung MS, Trainer AH, Campbell I, Lipton L (2015) Familial colorectal cancer. Intern Med J 45:482–491

Maeyama H, Hidaka E, Ota H, Minami S, Kajiyama M, Kuraishi A, Mori H, Matsuda Y, Wada S, Sodeyama H, Nakata S, Kawamura N, Hata S, Watanabe M, Iijima Y, Katsuyama T (2001) Familial gastrointestinal stromal tumor with hyperpigmentation: association with a germline mutation of the c-kit gene. Gastroenterology 120:210–215

Malkin D, Li FP, Strong LC, Fraumeni JF Jr, Nelson CE, Kim DH, Kassel J, Gryka MA, Bischoff FZ, Tainsky MA et al (1990) Germ line p53 mutations in a familial syndrome of breast cancer, sarcomas, and other neoplasms. Science 250:1233–1238

Marshall JB, Diaz-Arias AA, Bochna GS, Vogele KA (1990) Achalasia due to diffuse esophageal leiomyomatosis and inherited as an autosomal dominant disorder. Report of a family study. Gastroenterology 98:1358–1365

Masciari S, Van Den Abbeele AD, Diller LR, Rastarhuyeva I, Yap J, Schneider K, Digianni L, Li FP, Fraumeni JF Jr, Syngal S, Garber JE (2008) F18-fluorodeoxyglucose-positron emission tomography/computed tomography screening in Li-Fraumeni syndrome. JAMA 299:1315–1319

McBride KA, Ballinger ML, Killick E, Kirk J, Tattersall MH, Eeles RA, Thomas DM, Mitchell G (2014) Li-Fraumeni syndrome: cancer risk assessment and clinical management. Nat Rev Clin Oncol 11:260–271

Menko FH, Maher ER, Schmidt LS, Middelton LA, Aittomaki K, Tomlinson I, Richard S, Linehan WM (2014) Hereditary leiomyomatosis and renal cell cancer (HLRCC): renal cancer risk, surveillance and treatment. Fam Cancer 13:637–644

Miettinen M, Fetsch JF, Sobin LH, Lasota J (2006) Gastrointestinal stromal tumors in patients with neurofibromatosis 1: a clinicopathologic and molecular genetic study of 45 cases. Am J Surg Pathol 30:90–96

Miettinen M, Killian JK, Wang ZF, Lasota J, Lau C, Jones L, Walker R, Pineda M, Zhu YJ, Kim SY, Helman L, Meltzer P (2013) Immunohistochemical loss of succinate dehydrogenase subunit A (SDHA) in gastrointestinal stromal tumors (GISTs) signals SDHA germline mutation. Am J Surg Pathol 37:234–240

Miettinen M, Lasota J (2013) Gastrointestinal stromal tumors. Gastroenterol Clin North Am 42:399–415

Miettinen M, Lasota J (2014) Succinate dehydrogenase deficient gastrointestinal stromal tumors (GISTs)—a review. Int J Biochem Cell Biol 53:514–519

Mitchell G, Ballinger ML, Wong S, Hewitt C, James P, Young MA, Cipponi A, Pang T, Goode DL, Dobrovic A, Thomas DM, International Sarcoma Kindred Study (2013) High frequency of germline TP53 mutations in a prospective adult-onset sarcoma cohort. PLoS One 8:e69026

Mussi C, Schildhaus HU, Gronchi A, Wardelmann E, Hohenberger P (2008) Therapeutic consequences from molecular biology for gastrointestinal stromal tumor patients affected by neurofibromatosis type 1. Clin Cancer Res 14:4550–4555

Musso N, Caronia FP, Castorina S, Lo Monte AI, Barresi V, Condorelli DF (2015) Somatic loss of an EXT2 gene mutation during malignant progression in a patient with hereditary multiple osteochondromas. Cancer Genet 208:62–67

Myhre-Jensen O (1981) A consecutive 7-year series of 1331 benign soft tissue tumours. Clinicopathologic data. Comparison with sarcomas. Acta Orthop Scand 52:287–293

National Comprehensive Cancer Network (NCCN) (2014) Genetic/familial high risk assessment: breast and ovarian. Li Fraumeni syndrome management. NCCN Clincal Practgice Guidelines in Oncology, USA

Neuhann TM, Mansmann V, Merkelbach-Bruse S, Klink B, Hellinger A, Hoffkes HG, Wardelmann E, Schildhaus HU, Tinschert S (2013) A novel germline KIT mutation (p. L576P) in a family presenting with juvenile onset of multiple gastrointestinal stromal tumors, skin hyperpigmentations, and esophageal stenosis. Am J Surg Pathol 37:898–905

National Institute for Health and Care Excellence (NICE) (2013) Familial breast cancer: classification and care of people at risk of familial breast cancer and management of breast cancer and related risks in people with a family history of breast cancer. NICE clinical guideline 164, UK

Nishida T, Hirota S, Taniguchi M, Hashimoto K, Isozaki K, Nakamura H, Kanakura Y, Tanaka T, Takabayashi A, Matsuda H, Kitamura Y (1998) Familial gastrointestinal stromal tumours with germline mutation of the KIT gene. Nat Genet 19:323–324

Ognjanovic S, Olivier M, Bergemann TL, Hainaut P (2012) Sarcomas in TP53 germline mutation carriers: a review of the IARC TP53 database. Cancer 118:1387–1396

Pantaleo MA, Astolfi A, Indio V, Moore R, Thiessen N, Heinrich MC, Gnocchi C, Santini D, Catena F, Formica S, Martelli PL, Casadio R, Pession A, Biasco G (2011) SDHA loss-of-function mutations in KIT-PDGFRA wild-type gastrointestinal stromal tumors identified by massively parallel sequencing. J Natl Cancer Inst 103:983–987

Pasini B, Matyakhina L, Bei T, Muchow M, Boikos S, Ferrando B, Carney JA, Stratakis CA (2007) Multiple gastrointestinal stromal and other tumors caused by platelet-derived growth factor receptor alpha gene mutations: a case associated with a germline V561D defect. J Clin Endocrinol Metab 92:3728–3732

Pasini B, McWhinney SR, Bei T, Matyakhina L, Stergiopoulos S, Muchow M, Boikos SA, Ferrando B, Pacak K, Assie G, Baudin E, Chompret A, Ellison JW, Briere JJ, Rustin P, Gimenez-Roqueplo AP, Eng C, Carney JA, Stratakis CA (2008) Clinical and molecular genetics of patients with the Carney-Stratakis syndrome and germline mutations of the genes coding for the succinate dehydrogenase subunits SDHB, SDHC, and SDHD. Eur J Hum Genet 16:79–88

Pastorino L, Ghiorzo P, Nasti S, Battistuzzi L, Cusano R, Marzocchi C, Garre ML, Clementi M, Scarra GB (2009) Identification of a SUFU germline mutation in a family with Gorlin syndrome. Am J Med Genet A 149A:1539–1543

Ralston SH, Albagha OM (2014) Genetics of Paget's disease of bone. Curr Osteoporos Rep 12:263–271

Ratner N, Miller SJ (2015) A RASopathy gene commonly mutated in cancer: the neurofibromatosis type 1 tumour suppressor. Nat Rev Cancer 15:290–301

Refae MA, Wong N, Patenaude F, Begin LR, Foulkes WD (2007) Hereditary leiomyomatosis and renal cell cancer: an unusual and aggressive form of hereditary renal carcinoma. Nat Clin Pract Oncol 4:256–261

Robson ME, Glogowski E, Sommer G, Antonescu CR, Nafa K, Maki RG, Ellis N, Besmer P, Brennan M, Offit K (2004) Pleomorphic characteristics of a germ-line KIT mutation in a large kindred with gastrointestinal stromal tumors, hyperpigmentation, and dysphagia. Clin Cancer Res 10:1250–1254

Sawyer S, Mitchell G, McKinley J, Chenevix-Trench G, Beesley J, Chen XQ, Bowtell D, Trainer AH, Harris M, Lindeman GJ, James PA (2012) A role for common genomic variants in the assessment of familial breast cancer. J Clin Oncol 30:4330–4336

Schmidt LS, Linehan WM (2014) Hereditary leiomyomatosis and renal cell carcinoma. Int J Nephrol Renovasc Dis 7:253–260

Schneider K, Zelley K, Nichols K, Garber J (2013) Li Fraumeni syndrome (Online). Available: http://www.ncbi.nlm.nih.gov/books/NBK1311/

Schultz KA, Yang J, Doros L, Williams GM, Harris A, Stewart DR, Messinger Y, Field A, Dehner LP, Hill DA (2014) DICER1-pleuropulmonary blastoma familial tumor predisposition syndrome: a unique constellation of neoplastic conditions. Pathol Case Rev 19:90–100

Scott CL, Swisher EM, Kaufmann SH (2015) Poly (adp-ribose) polymerase inhibitors: recent advances and future development. J Clin Oncol 33:1397–1406

Sharif S, Ferner R, Birch JM, Gillespie JE, Gattamaneni HR, Baser ME, Evans DG (2006) Second primary tumors in neurofibromatosis 1 patients treated for optic glioma: substantial risks after radiotherapy. J Clin Oncol 24:2570–2575

SIGNIFY (2015) Magnetic Resonance Imaging Screening in Li Fraumeni Syndrome (Online). Available: https://clinicaltrials.gov/ct2/show/record/NCT01443468

Srivastava S, Zou ZQ, Pirollo K, Blattner W, Chang EH (1990) Germ-line transmission of a mutated p53 gene in a cancer-prone family with Li-Fraumeni syndrome. Nature 348:747–749

Stewart DR, Sloan JL, Yao L, Mannes AJ, Moshyedi A, Lee CC, Sciot R, de Smet L, Mautner VF, Legius E (2010) Diagnosis, management, and complications of glomus tumours of the digits in neurofibromatosis type 1. J Med Genet 47:525–532

Stiller CA, Chessells JM, Fitchett M (1994) Neurofibromatosis and childhood leukaemia/lymphoma: a population-based UKCCSG study. Br J Cancer 70:969–972

Sturt NJ, Clark SK (2006) Current ideas in desmoid tumours. Fam Cancer 5:275–85; discussion 287–8

Sugimoto M (2014) A cascade leading to premature aging phenotypes including abnormal tumor profiles in Werner syndrome (review). Int J Mol Med 33:247–253

Sung L, Anderson JR, Arndt C, Raney RB, Meyer WH, Pappo AS (2004) Neurofibromatosis in children with Rhabdomyosarcoma: a report from the Intergroup Rhabdomyosarcoma study IV. J Pediatr 144:666–668

Thomas DM, Ballinger ML (2015) Etiologic, environmental and inherited risk factors in sarcomas. J Surg Oncol 111:490–495

Thomas DM, James PA, Ballinger ML (2015) Clinical implications of genomics for cancer risk genetics. Lancet Oncol 16:e303–e308

Thway K, Fisher C (2014) Synovial sarcoma: defining features and diagnostic evolution. Ann Diagn Pathol 18:369–380

Tinat J, Bougeard G, Baert-Desurmont S, Vasseur S, Martin C, Bouvignies E, Caron O, Bressac-de Paillerets B, Berthet P, Dugast C, Bonaiti-Pellie C, Stoppa-Lyonnet D, Frebourg T (2009) 2009 version of the Chompret criteria for Li Fraumeni syndrome. J Clin Oncol 27: e108-e109; author reply e110

Tomlinson IP Alam NA Rowan AJ Barclay E, Jaeger EE, Kelsell D, Leigh I, Gorman P, Lamlum H, Rahman S, Roylance RR, Olpin S, Bevan S, Barker K, Hearle N, Houlston RS, Kiuru M, Lehtonen R, Karhu A, Vilkki S, Laiho P, Eklund C, Vierimaa O, Aittomaki K, Hietala M, Sistonen P, Paetau A, Salovaara R, Herva R, Launonen V, Aaltonen LA, Multiple Leiomyoma C (2002) Germline mutations in FH predispose to dominantly inherited uterine fibroids, skin leiomyomata and papillary renal cell cancer. Nat Genet 30:406–410

Turan S, Bastepe M (2015) GNAS spectrum of disorders. Curr Osteoporos Rep 13:146–158

Veith S, Mangerich A (2015) RecQ helicases and PARP1 team up in maintaining genome integrity. Ageing Res Rev 23:12–28

Verdegaal SH, Bovee JV, Pansuriya TC, Grimer RJ, Ozger H, Jutte PC, San Julian M, Biau DJ, Van der Geest IC, Leithner A, Streitburger A, Klenke FM, Gouin FG, Campanacci DA, Marec-Berard P, Hogendoorn PC, Brand R, Taminiau AH (2011) Incidence, predictive factors, and prognosis of chondrosarcoma in patients with Ollier disease and Maffucci syndrome: an international multicenter study of 161 patients. Oncologist 16:1771–1779

Villani A, Tabori U, Schiffman J, Shlien A, Beyene J, Druker H, Novokmet A, Finlay J, Malkin D (2011) Biochemical and imaging surveillance in germline TP53 mutation carriers with Li-Fraumeni syndrome: a prospective observational study. Lancet Oncol 12:559–567

Viskochil D, Buchberg AM, Xu G, Cawthon RM, Stevens J, Wolff RK, Culver M, Carey JC, Copeland NG, Jenkins NA et al (1990) Deletions and a translocation interrupt a cloned gene at the neurofibromatosis type 1 locus. Cell 62:187–192

Wagner AJ, Malinowska-Kolodziej I, Morgan JA, Qin W, Fletcher CD, Vena N, Ligon AH, Antonescu CR, Ramaiya NH, Demetri GD, Kwiatkowski DJ, Maki RG (2010) Clinical activity of mTOR inhibition with sirolimus in malignant perivascular epithelioid cell tumors: targeting the pathogenic activation of mTORC1 in tumors. J Clin Oncol 28:835–840

Wallace MR, Marchuk DA, Andersen LB, Letcher R, Odeh HM, Saulino AM, Fountain JW, Brereton A, Nicholson J, Mitchell AL et al (1990) Type 1 neurofibromatosis gene: identification of a large transcript disrupted in three NF1 patients. Science 249:181–186

Walsh T, Casadei S, Lee MK, Pennil CC, Nord AS, Thornton AM, Roeb W, Agnew KJ, Stray SM, Wickramanayake A, Norquist B, Pennington KP, Garcia RL, King MC, Swisher EM (2011) Mutations in 12 genes for inherited ovarian, fallopian tube, and peritoneal carcinoma identified by massively parallel sequencing. Proc Natl Acad Sci U S A 108:18032–18037

Walther MM, Herring J, Enquist E, Keiser HR, Linehan WM (1999) von Recklinghausen's disease and pheochromocytomas. J Urol 162:1582–1586

Worch J, Matthay KK, Neuhaus J, Goldsby R, Dubois SG (2010) Ethnic and racial differences in patients with Ewing sarcoma. Cancer 116:983–988

Wu CC, Shete S, Amos CI, Strong LC (2006) Joint effects of germ-line p53 mutation and sex on cancer risk in Li-Fraumeni syndrome. Cancer Res 66:8287–8292

Young MA, Herlihy A, Mitchell G, Thomas DM, Ballinger M, Tucker K, Lewis CR, Neuhaus S, International Sarcoma Kindred S, Halliday J (2013) The attitudes of people with sarcoma and their family towards genomics and incidental information arising from genetic research. Clin Sarcoma Res 3:11

Zhang L, Smyrk TC, Young WF Jr, Stratakis CA, Carney JA (2010) Gastric stromal tumors in Carney triad are different clinically, pathologically, and behaviorally from sporadic gastric gastrointestinal stromal tumors: findings in 104 cases. Am J Surg Pathol 34:53–64

Zoller ME, Rembeck B, Oden A, Samuelsson M, Angervall L (1997) Malignant and benign tumors in patients with neurofibromatosis type 1 in a defined Swedish population. Cancer 79:2125–2131

Diagnosis and Management of Hereditary Basal Cell Skin Cancer

Susan Shanley and Christopher McCormack

Abstract

Basal cell carcinoma (BCC) is the most common cancer in Caucasians worldwide and its incidence is rising. It is generally considered a sporadic tumour, most likely to affect fair-skinned individuals exposed to ultraviolet (UV) radiation. This chapter focusses on the approach to recognising the relatively few individuals in whom a high-risk hereditary susceptibility may be present. Gorlin syndrome is the main consideration and the gene most commonly mutated is *PTCH1*, a key regulator of the Hedgehog developmental pathway. Recently, loss of function of another gene in the same pathway, SUFU, has been found to explain a subset of families. Understanding the pathogenesis of familial BCCs has advanced the understanding of the biology of sporadic tumours and led to targeted therapy trials. The management of familial BCCs remains a challenge due to significant unmet needs for non-surgical treatments and a high burden of disease for the individual. Together with the prospect of advances in gene discovery and translation, these challenges highlight the need for ongoing review of at-risk and affected individuals by a multidisciplinary team.

S. Shanley (✉)
Familial Cancer Clinic, Peter MacCallum Cancer Centre, Melbourne, Australia
e-mail: Sue.Shanley@petermac.org

C. McCormack
Dermatology Unit, Department of Surgical Oncology,
Peter MacCallum Cancer Centre, Melbourne, Australia

G. Pichert and C. Jacobs (eds.), *Rare Hereditary Cancers*,
Recent Results in Cancer Research 205, DOI 10.1007/978-3-319-29998-3_11

Keywords
Basal cell carcinoma • Non-melanoma skin cancer • Gorlin syndrome • Naevoid basal cell carcinoma syndrome • PATCHED (PTCH1) • SUFU • Falcine calcification • Odontogenic keratocysts • Palmar and plantar pits • Medulloblastoma • Bazex-Dupré-Christol syndrome • Rombo syndrome

Contents

1 Introduction

1.1 Basal Cell Carcinoma Biology

Basal cell carcinomas arise from progenitor cells located within the hair follicle and the interfollicular epidermis (Youssef et al. 2012). Morphological subtypes include nodular, micronodular, superficial and morpheaform tumours but a range of variants is described (Wade and Ackerman 1978). Some subtypes, e.g. morpheaform, are associated with increased risk of local infiltration and recurrence (Rubin et al. 2005). Basal cell carcinomas are generally slow-growing and rarely metastasise, a behaviour which is not well understood. It has been suggested that this may be due to a stable genome but recent evidence is against this as sequencing of whole exomes from 12 sporadic BCCs (subtypes not described) supports their having a very high mutation rate (Jayaraman et al. 2014). Other explanations for a low metastatic potential include the possibility that BCCs require specific stromal conditions that are rarely met in metastatic environments (Epstein 2008).

1.2 Basal Cell Carcinoma Epidemiology

The highest incidence rates for BCCs are in Australia, where the last national survey in 2002 reported 884 BCCs per 100,000 (age-standardised incidence) (Staples et al. 2006). In the USA, rates are 166–310 per 100,000 in New Hampshire (Karagas et al. 1999) and in the UK, 60 per 100,000 person years from 1996 to 2003 (Bath-Hextall et al. 2007). Lifetime risk in the 2012 Australian Non-Melanoma Skin Cancer Survey (www.scfa.edu.au) was estimated at 52 % for men by age 70 and 38 % for women. Elsewhere, lifetime risk in Caucasians is about 33–39 % in men and 23–28 % in women (www.americanskin.org and www.pcds.org.uk). Much lower figures are reported for people with dark skin, with lifetime risks about 5 times less than for light-skinned individuals (cited by Herbst M.C., www.cansa.org.za).

1.3 What Proportion of Basal Cell Carcinomas Are Due to Hereditary Syndromes?

High-risk genetic predisposition accounts for very few instances of basal cell carcinoma. The main consideration is Gorlin syndrome, also known as naevoid basal cell carcinoma syndrome. This had an estimated prevalence in 2005 of about 1 in 40,000 in the United Kingdom (Farndon 2005). Other high-risk hereditary conditions (such as Bazex-Dupré-Christol and Rombo syndromes) are extremely rare. Smaller influences on BCC risk are being sought by genome-wide association studies. One such investigation, for example, of over 2000 Icelanders has identified the locus *TGM3*, where a particular risk allele confers an odds ratio (OR) of 1.29 while a protective allele of *RGS22* reduces the OR to 0.77. *TGM3* has a role in epidermal differentiation but the role of *RGS22* is unknown (Stacey et al. 2014).

1.4 Risk Factors for Basal Cell Carcinoma

1.4.1 Ultraviolet Light (UV) and Determinants of Susceptibility to Exposure

The rise in many countries in the incidence of BCCs may be due to increased UV exposure, possibly from ozone depletion, sun exposure, and the use of tanning beds. Molecular studies support a substantial role for UV radiation in BCC development, as 75 % of mutations in a recent sequencing study of tumour exomes were of the C- to T-type known to be UV-induced (Jayaraman et al. 2014).

Susceptibility to UV radiation comes with fair skin, light-coloured eyes, northern European ancestry and childhood freckling (Gallagher et al. 1995). Three variants in the MCR1 (melanocortin receptor 1 gene) increase risk of fair skin and red hair and raise the odds ratio of non-melanoma skin cancer, including BCCs, to 3.15 (95 % CI 1.7–5.82) (Box et al. 2001). Other modifiers of UV response could include variants in the DNA repair gene, *XRCC3*, as homozygotes for rarer alleles have reduced BCC risk (OR 0.61, 95 % CI 0.41–0.92) compared to those with more common homozygous alleles (Surdu et al. 2014). Heightened susceptibility to UV exposure is also part of the clinical picture of the rare high-risk BCC syndromes, discussed later in this chapter.

1.4.2 Ionising Radiation

Ionising radiation increases the risk of cancers in the radiation field after a latency of usually 20 years (Karagas et al. 1996; Lichter et al. 2000). This effect is more marked in specific hereditary conditions such as Gorlin syndrome, where the latency is more likely to be within 5 years.

1.4.3 Immune Suppression

A Dutch series of renal transplant patients studied between 1966 and 1988 showed an increase in BCC risk by a factor of 10 compared to those who did not undergo transplants (Hartevelt et al. 1990). Acute intermittent sunburn further increases BCC risk post-transplant, suggesting that immune suppressive medication interacts with UV radiation (Ramsay et al. 2003).

1.4.4 Arsenic

Chronic ingestion of trivalent inorganic arsenic in sources, such as water or in medications, increases BCC risk (Boonchai et al. 2000), through unclear mechanisms, which could include immune effects (Soto-Pena and Vega 2008).

2 Risk Assessment

The main considerations in looking for a hereditary basal cell carcinoma syndrome are features that could point to a diagnosis of Gorlin syndrome, or the rarer Bazex-Dupré-Christol or Rombo syndromes. Two major features or one major and two minor features are usually required to make a clinical diagnosis of Gorlin syndrome.

2.1 Diagnostic Criteria for Gorlin Syndrome (Jones et al. 2011)

2.1.1 Major Criteria

- Lamellar (sheet-like) calcification of the falx (membrane between the cerebral hemispheres) or clear evidence of calcification in an individual younger than 20 years of age. (Fig. 1)
- Jaw keratocyst (Fig. 2)
- Palmar or plantar pits (two or more) (Fig. 3)

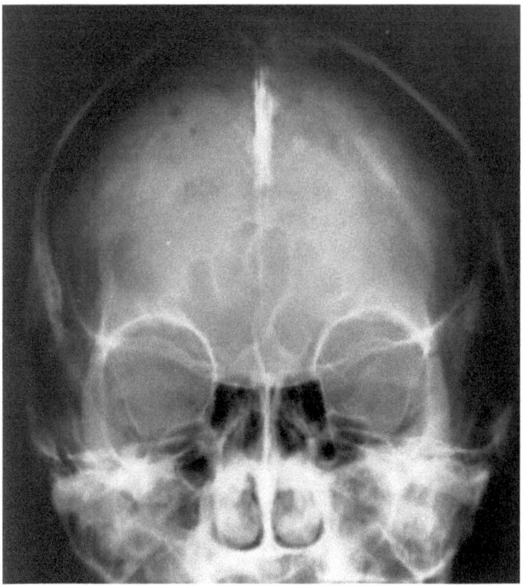

Fig. 1 Calcification of falx membrane between cerebral hemispheres is the vertical opaque line at the *top* of the image (reproduced with permission from Gorlin 2004)

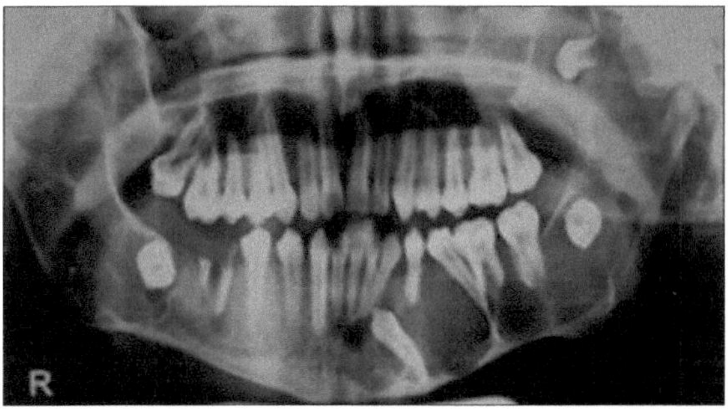

Fig. 2 Jaw cysts appear as lucent areas on X-ray and can displace teeth, reproduced with the permission from Manjima et al. (2015)

- Multiple or early onset BCCs* (Fig. 4). This criterion refers to a single BCC occurring before age 30 or five or more BCCs* [five occurring at any age in low prevalence countries is suggested by (Jones et al. 2011)]. Five BCCs before age 40 in higher prevalence countries is a reasonable modification, as the incidence of multiple BCCs in the general population rises in Australia, for example, after age 40 (Richmond-Sinclair et al. 2009)
- First-degree relative with Gorlin syndrome

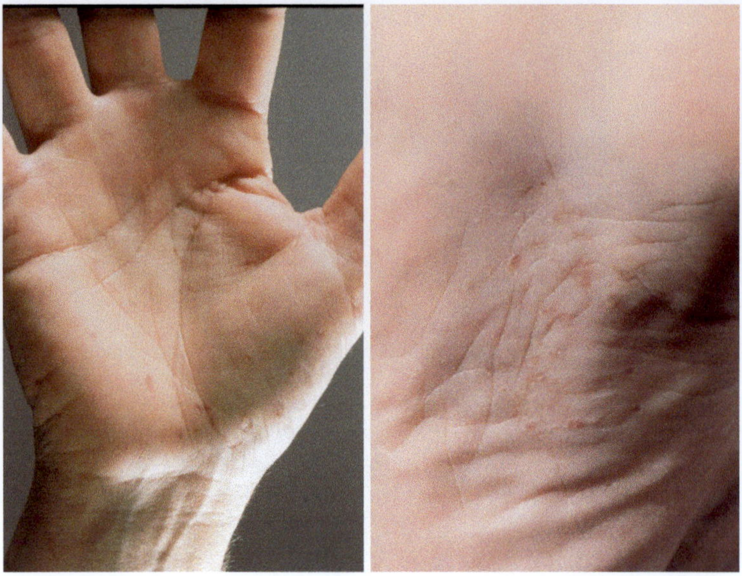

Fig. 3 Palmar pits (*left*) and plantar pits (*right*) present as depressions in the skin which may be *colourless* or *red* and vary from pinpricks to slightly larger defects in the skin (courtesy of Charles Frewen Medical Visuals P/L)

Fig. 4 Basal cell carcinomas in Gorlin syndrome show a range of forms, including nodular, pigmented and superficial forms (courtesy of Charles Frewen Medical Visuals P/L)

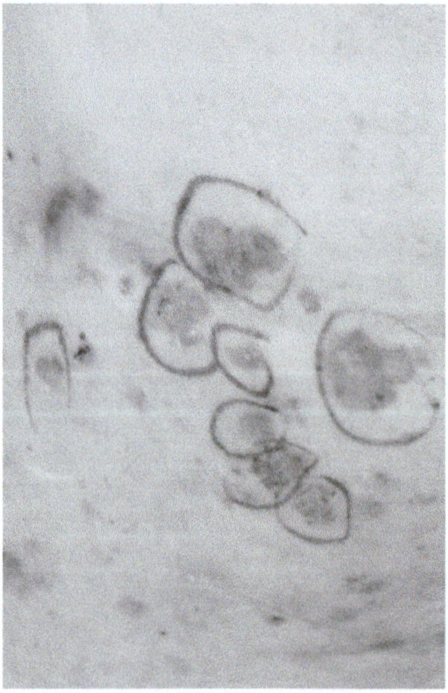

2.1.2 Minor Criteria (Jones et al. 2011)

- Childhood medulloblastoma
- Lympho-mesenteric or pleural cysts
- Macrocephaly (occipitofrontal circumference >97th centile), adjusted for height
- Cleft lip/palate
- Bifid/splayed/extra ribs; bifid vertebrae seen on X-ray
- Preaxial or postaxial polydactyly
- Ovarian/cardiac fibromas
- Ocular anomalies (cataract, developmental defects and pigmentary changes of the retinal epithelium)

Potential triggers to undertake a full clinical evaluation for a basal cell carcinoma syndrome therefore include:

- Early onset BCC before age 30 or 5 or more as described above
- Multiple BCCs in a radiation field, particularly with a latency of 5 years or less
- Any individual with an odontogenic (jaw) keratocyst
- Any child with a medulloblastoma before 3 years of age
- Any child with macrocephaly and other developmental anomalies such as cleft lip/palate; structural eye anomalies, polydactyly or bifid ribs or butterfly vertebrae
- Anyone with a family history of the above features in a close relative

2.2 The Approach to the Assessment

An approach to identifying a BCC predisposition syndrome includes seeking environmental risk factors and genetic features in the history and examination.

1. Enquire about environmental risk factors for BCCs including:
   - sun exposure history and how their skin reacts to sun exposure (Fitzpatrick 1988)
   - the countries a person has the person lived in
   - use of sunbeds
   - use of medications that may have contained arsenic (e.g. Fowler's solution, Bell's asthma mixture and some homeopathic therapies)
   - occupational arsenic exposure, e.g. in tanning animal skins
   - previous radiotherapy treatments
2. Construct a three generational family history noting diagnoses of cancers, with particular attention to 'skin cancers' and other diagnostic criteria in relatives.
3. Enquire about a personal history of childhood problems, such as congenital anomalies (including cleft lip/palate, polydactyly, cardiac fibromas, structural eye anomalies), medulloblastoma, teenage onset problems such as jaw cysts and note the number, type and location of any skin cancers reported, including the ages of diagnoses.

4. Examine the patient for evidence of UV exposure and UV sensitivity. This is ideally done in a multidisciplinary setting where genetic and dermatological expertise is available. Note the skin pigmentation, the degree of freckling and nevi, hair colour, eye colour, other skin cancers or photodamage.
5. Examine for diagnostic features of Gorlin syndrome (as listed by Jones et al. 2011) and for other associated morphological features, namely head circumference (adjusted for height) over 97th percentile, a prominent forehead (frontal bossing) and arched eyebrows (Fig. 5). It is useful to soak the patient's hands in water for a few minutes as this can make the indentations of the palmar pits (Fig. 3) more evident. Look for features that could indicate Bazex-Dupré-Christol or Rombo syndromes—such as sparse hair, milia (small white keratin-containing cysts, usually facial) and atrophoderma (localised areas of skin atrophy). Examining parents and siblings may assist in determining whether pattern on inheritance fits with autosomal (Gorlin or Rombo syndromes) or X-linked (Bazex-Dupré-Christol syndrome).
   Investigations:

   X-ray of the skull: One of the most useful tests in establishing a clinical diagnosis of Gorlin syndrome is the skull X-ray. Arrange for review of old X-rays where possible to avoid unnecessary irradiation or order a skull anteroposterior (AP) X-ray to assess falcine calcification. Dense calcification is seen in 79–92 % of individuals when systematically sought (Ratcliffe et al. 1995; Kimonis et al. 2004). It is either double-layered (bi-lamellar) or a 2–3-mm single layer. If falcine calcification is absent over age 25, then the diagnosis of Gorlin is very unlikely. Conversely, calcification is only seen in around 37 % of patients with Gorlin syndrome aged less than 20 years

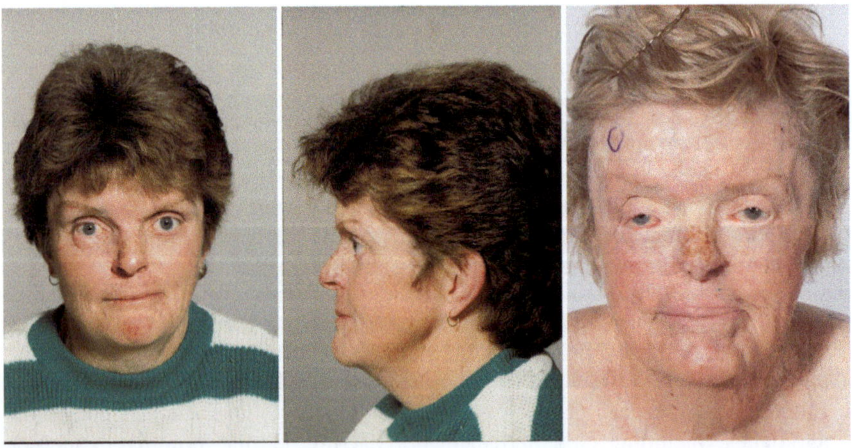

Fig. 5 Facial features of Gorlin syndrome include macrocephaly, prominent forehead, arched eyebrows and wide-set eyes. The photograph on the *right* is 30 years on from those on the *left* and demonstrates surgical scarring and alopecia from medication effects, in addition to the ageing process (courtesy of Charles Frewen, Medical Visuals P/L)

(Kimonis et al. 2004), so the greatest benefit as a diagnostic tool is in adults. Calcification may also be seen on CT but MRI is likely to be less sensitive.
X-ray of the jaw [orthopantomogram (OPG)]: This is indicated to look for jaw keratocysts in an individual aged 8 or above.
X-ray of spine and vertebrae: If the finding or one or two more minor diagnostic criteria would make a clinical diagnosis, then it is useful to review or arrange for X-rays of spine and vertebrae to look for features such as bifid ribs or butterfly vertebrae. This can be of particular help in evaluating a child where other age-dependent features of Gorlin syndrome including falcine calcification may not yet have manifest.

6. Genetic testing: If a patient has sufficient clinical criteria to warrant a clinical diagnosis of Gorlin syndrome, then mutation analysis of their germline DNA is indicated.
   Other situations that make a mutation highly likely include the following:
   - an individual with an odontogenic keratocyst before age 35 (Pastorino et al. 2012)
   - a child with desmoplastic medulloblastoma before age 3 (Garre et al. 2009)

Identifying a mutation may allow predictive testing of other relatives and guide surveillance advice.

2.3 Genes Responsible for Hereditary Basal Cell Carcinoma Syndromes

2.3.1 *PTCH1*

This is the most significant BCC susceptibility gene, found by linkage studies on chromosome 9q22 (Hahn et al. 1996; Johnson et al. 1996) in families with clinical diagnoses of Gorlin syndrome. Mutations are found in up to 67 % of individuals with Gorlin syndrome (Smith et al. 2014) and in a similar proportion of sporadic BCCs. Reifenberger et al. (2005) analysed 42 sporadic tumours, demonstrating *PTCH1* mutations in 28/42 (67 %) tumours, with 42 % demonstrating inactivation of both alleles via mutation and loss of the second allele. Epigenetic inactivation of PTCH1 in the germline has not been documented [although has been seen as somatic event (Pan et al. 2010)].

PTCH1 encodes a transmembrane receptor protein which regulates a key developmental process, the Hedgehog signalling pathway, responsible for determining embryonic patterning. Figure 6 (Epstein 2008) shows how loss of *PTCH1* function upregulates the Hedgehog pathway, driving cellular proliferation. It also impairs radiation-induced cell cycle checkpoints (the *ATR-CHK1* checkpoint), causing genomic instability (Leonard et al. 2008). Loss of *PTCH1* function could also contribute to the development of other tumours, including lung, breast, prostate and pancreas (Jacob and Lum 2007).

PTCH1 gain of function mutations, including duplication, are also described in a separate non-tumour predisposition condition. They confer a variable phenotype

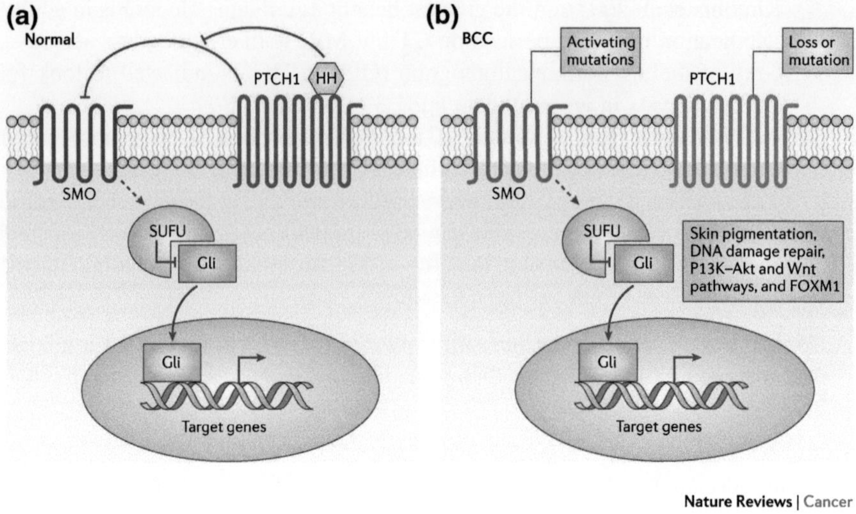

Fig. 6 A basic schematic of the hedgehog (HH) signalling pathway reproduced with permission from Epstein (2008). **a** The family of extracellular HH ligands, of which there are three in mammals [sonic hedgehog (SHH), Indian hedgehog (IHH) and desert hedgehog (DHH)] bind to the patched 1 (PTCH1) receptor. This relieves the inhibition of smoothened (SMO) by PTCH1, and SMO sends signals through a series of interacting proteins, including suppressor of fused (SUFU), resulting in activation of the downstream Gli family of transcription factors: GLI1, GLI2 and GLI3. **b** Loss of *PTCH1* in patients with basal cell naevus syndrome predisposes them to basal cell carcinoma (BCC) development. Sporadic BCCs routinely carry mutations in *PTCH1* and *TP53*, consistent with their having been produced by ultraviolet radiation and, in 10 % of instances, in *SMO*. Other mutations have been implicated in BCC development, including genes that regulate skin colour, DNA damage repair genes, members of the phosphoinositide 3-kinase (PI3K)–Akt and the Wnt pathways and FOXM1

that includes degrees of holoprosencephaly (structural forebrain anomaly) and impairment of intellect and facial formation.

The *PTCH1* gene has 23 exons covering 34 kb, encoding 1447 amino acids (Lo Muzio 2008). More than 224 mutations have been described, over 100 in the germline, with most predicted to truncate the protein (Lindstrom et al. 2006). Inheritance of *PTCH1* mutations is autosomal dominant with apparently complete penetrance but very variable expressivity. Up to 30 % of diagnoses may represent de novo mutations [Evans and Farndon 2002 (updated 2013)] but mosaicism is not well described in the literature. Mutations are clustered within loops within the protein but no correlation has been seen between mutation location and phenotype.

PTCH1 has a homologue, *PTCH2*, located on chromosome 1p32, which has 23 exons and covers 15 kb encoding 1203 amino acids. Very rare mutations in *PTCH2* have been demonstrated in BCCs and medulloblastomas (Smyth et al. 1999). A frameshift *PTCH2* mutation has been found in a 13-year-old Japanese girl with multiple jaw cysts and rib anomalies (Fujii et al. 2013) but without sufficient features yet to meet official criteria for diagnosing Gorlin syndrome. One Chinese family has been described with a possible missense mutation but overall the role of the *PTCH2* gene is not well characterised.

2.3.2 SUFU (Suppressor of Fused)

SUFU is another hedgehog pathway gene (Fig. 6) which acts downstream of *PTCH1* to transmit signals to Gli family transcription factors. Germline mutations were first described in children with medulloblastoma (Brugieres et al. 2012). Pastorino et al. (2012) and Smith et al. (2014) have described the SUFU phenotype in 10 people. The *SUFU* phenotype seems to involve more BCCs and medulloblastomas than jaw cysts. A higher frequency of medulloblastomas than is expected in *PTCH1* carriers needs to be verified. Similarly, ovarian fibromas were frequent, seen in 3/6 *SUFU* mutation carriers in one study, but greater numbers are needed to establish how much phenotype may vary between *PTCH1* and *SUFU* mutation carriers and the mechanisms behind any differences.

2.4 Differential diagnosis (of individuals presenting with a personal or family history of multiple BCC predisposition)

2.4.1 Gorlin Syndrome (naevoid basal cell carcinoma syndrome)

Three large studies from the United Kingdom, Australia and America examined the clinical features of Gorlin syndrome. Basal cell carcinomas were seen in 90–97 % of participants, jaw cysts in 71–90 % and pitting in 71–87 %. There is striking variation in expressivity, however, within and between families, which may be due to the influences such as unknown modifier genes and epigenetic events. Timing of the inactivation of the second *PTCH1* allele in mouse models has been shown to influence the type of BCC that developed (Zibat et al. 2009), so it has been suggested that similarly this could explain some of the variation in humans (Jones et al. 2011).

Basal cell carcinomas in Gorlin Syndrome

BCCs have been reported in children before age 10, but this has been after exposure to carcinogens, namely arsenic in asthma medication and cranial irradiation (Shanley et al. 1994). In the UK, the cumulative incidence of BCCs in Gorlin syndrome patients by age 20 is 12 % (Jones et al. 2011), compared to 47 % in Australia (Shanley et al. 1994). Numbers of BCCs in an individual can range from a few, for example, 5 in countries with little UV exposure, to hundreds to thousands in Australian patients, hence a huge potential cosmetic and health impact (Figs. 4 and 5). In African American individuals with Gorlin syndrome, the proportion of people reported to develop BCCs is less at 28 % (Goldstein et al. 1994) but tumours can still develop at an early age.

Jaw cysts—a single keratocyst is a major feature at any age
Keratocystic odontogenic tumours (KCOTs) usually present as painless jaw swellings in the mid-teenage years, but they may be asymptomatic and found on X-ray (Fig. 2). They may also cause misplaced teeth or abnormal taste due to infection. They have characteristic microscopic features (summarised in Pastorino et al. 2012). The likelihood of an individual with a KCOT having Gorlin syndrome varies between studies from 1.4 to 25.6 %. Features highly suggestive of Gorlin syndrome are onset before age 20 or multiple lesions, especially in the maxilla, as sporadic lesions are more likely to affect only the mandible (Guo et al. 2013). Cyst numbers range from 1 to 18 with 75 % manifesting by age 20 (Kimonis et al. 1997).

Pits
Pits appear as colourless or pink/red pinpricks in the palmar and plantar epithelium (Fig. 3). They may be a difficult sign to interpret as they can be subtle but soaking the hands in water for a few minutes can make the indentations more pronounced. In some families, the observation of pitting has not correlated with the presence of a known family *PTCH1* mutation, so it is wise to be cautious in making a clinical diagnosis if this feature is the tipping point (Wicking et al. 1997).

Other tumours in the Gorlin spectrum
Medulloblastoma is the most common brain malignancy in childhood in the general population and affects up to 5 % of Gorlin syndrome patients. Recent evidence suggests that risk may seem to be more relevant to those with SUFU than with PTCH1-related disease, but confirming this in other studies is needed before modifying advice. Tumours are mainly of the desmoplastic subtype occurring before age 3 (Smith et al. 2014) compared to non-syndromic patients where median onset is by about 5 years (Rudin et al. 2009). Other tumours in the Gorlin spectrum include ovarian fibromas in 14–24 % of study participants, reviewed in (Kimonis et al. 1997) as well as cardiac fibromas in 2.5 % of UK participants in Evans et al. (1993) and occasional individuals with multiple meningiomas after cranial irradiation (Kimonis et al. 1997).

Non-tumour features of Gorlin Syndrome
Ectopic calcification in the falx membrane between the cerebral hemispheres is particularly useful as a diagnostic aid (see section on assessment). Other radiological features are congenital anomalies in the ribs and spine, which can be most useful in evaluating a child. This can be particularly helpful where a parent has a clinical diagnosis of Gorlin syndrome but no mutation is available for predictive testing. These features include bifid ribs, ribs with bony bridging or spina bifida occulta. Rib anomalies were seen on 49 % of X-rays in individuals with a confident clinical diagnosis of Gorlin syndrome based on other features. This frequency is far greater than the 0.5–1 % prevalence in the general population (Ratcliffe et al. 1995).

Other congenital anomalies in Gorlin Syndrome
There are many other congenital features [summarised in Evans and Farndon 2002 (updated 2013)] that are considered part of Gorlin syndrome. Macrocephaly occurs

in at least 50 % of individuals and may affect delivery of an affected child, sometimes requiring a Caesarean. Cleft lip and palate are seen in 3–5 % individuals and severe eye anomalies, such as microphthalmia, occur rarely (Ragge et al. 2005).

2.4.2 Other conditions to consider

1 **Bazex-Dupre-Christol syndrome**: First described in 1964, this X-linked dominant condition has been described in approximately 20 families (Parren and Frank 2011). Earliest features are usually sparseness of hair, with BCCs developing from the first decade, earliest reported as at age 3. Other main features are atrophoderma (localised skin atrophy) and milia (white small keratin-filled facial cysts), while additional features include hyperpigmentation of the face and trichoepitheliomas (benign hair follicle tumours). A candidate region on *Xq25-27*.1 has been located but no gene has been identified to date.

2 **Rombo syndrome**: Rombo syndrome is a condition very similar to Bazex-Christol-Dupré syndrome but with a dominant pattern of inheritance. It is recorded in only a few families. Michaelsson et al. (1981) were first to report patients with atrophoderma of the cheeks, elbows and hands and feet, together with cyanosis of lips and extremities, milia and a BCC predisposition manifesting in the thirties.

3 **Familial clustering of basal cell carcinomas:** Some families ascertained while seeking Gorlin syndrome patients have manifested only BCCs but no other features sufficient to make a clinical diagnosis. Some may represent clustering due to shared UV exposure and UV sensitivity due to skin type or other shared genes that are yet to be identified.

2.4.3 Basal cell cancers may form part of a clinical spectrum in other disorders where they are not the primary feature

1 **Xeroderma pigmentosum (XP)**: This recessive condition is usually diagnosed in infancy with severe skin sun sensitivity or marked development of lentigines (freckling), seen by age 2. This is followed by the development of squamous cell carcinomas (SCCs) as well as BCCs, melanomas and in some forms, neurological abnormalities. The median age for the onset of non-melanoma skin cancers in a study by the National Institute for Health was 9 years of age and 22 years of age for melanoma (Bradford et al. 2011). Clinical features guide the molecular analysis of potential genes which include 8 nucleotide excision repair genes and one polymerase, (reviewed in Kraemer and DiGiovanna 1993). Multigene panel testing is available.

2 **Oculocutaneous albinism(OCA):** Patients, particularly in African populations, with OCA have been described as having an increase in a mixture of skin

cancers, but the predominance of SCCs over BCCs appears more marked than in XP (Luande et al. 1985). The diagnosis is usually clinical, based on the striking reduction in pigment in skin, hair and the iris, but molecular testing of genes such as the TYR tyrosinase gene and the OCA2 gene is available (Lewis 1993).

3. **Epidermolysis bullosa (EB) simplex, Dowling-Meara type:** (Fine et al. 2009): A single record of registry data notes a lifetime risk of 44 % by age 55, but no increase in SCC risk, unlike other EB conditions. This is an autosomal dominant condition due to mutations in the *KRT5* or *KRT14* genes, where the main feature is severe skin blistering from birth.
4. **Uveal melanoma families:** A recent report describes four families in which *BAP1* mutation carriers developed BCCs of which two tumours had lost *BAP1* protein expression but this has yet to be investigated in depth (Wadt et al. 2014).

Other conditions may clinically mimic multiple BCCs, such as cylindromatosis (Brooke–Spiegeler syndrome, turban tumour syndrome). This autosomal dominant condition has strikingly variable expression and manifests as mainly head and neck firm lesions, where the tumours are actually trichoepitheliomas and spiroadenomas (tumours thought to originate from hair or sweat or sebaceous glands) (Poblete Gutierrez et al. 2002).

2.5 Genetic Testing

***PTCH1* testing**: The sensitivity of exon sequencing in Gorlin syndrome patients in one UK study of 171 individuals was 56 % but large rearrangement studies using MLPA, and RNA studies increased this to 67 % (Smith et al. 2014). Intronic splicing mutations have been described in occasional individuals (Bholah et al. 2014). Large chromosomal deletions of 9q22.3 that include *PTCH1* have been described. These would be considered if a patient had marked developmental delay/intellectual disability and other features as described by Muller et al. (2012).

Clinical testing by sequencing and large rearrangement testing is available, both for *PTCH1* alone and as part of panel testing.

***PTCH2* testing**: PTCH2 testing is not routinely available as interpretation of results remains difficult due to limited phenotypic data.

SUFU: Sensitivity of detection is difficult to estimate due to limited numbers of individuals tested but clinical testing is available using sequencing and MLPA.

3 Management of BCC predisposition syndromes

3.1 Surveillance—Childhood

Specialist skin examination by a dermatologist or multidisciplinary unit from infancy is recommended, despite a lack of evidence of the impact, as this may give maximum opportunity for early treatment and may improve morbidity (Jones et al. 2011).

Developmental assessment from infancy for the first few years of life may be offered along with routine plotting of growth during childhood [Evans and Farndon 2002 (updated 2013)]. Imaging for medulloblastoma is not recommended universally (although undertaken with 6-monthly imaging at some centres). It is not widely recommended due to low absolute level of tumour risk, lack of evidence for the benefit of imaging and the need to sedate children for imaging.

Specialist dental review yearly from age 8 is advised for odontogenic keratocysts (Farndon 2005).

3.2 Therapeutic Options

BCCs in patients with Gorlin syndrome have histologies indistinguishable from sporadic tumours, but the challenge is to manage what may be hundreds to thousands of lesions and to tailor the treatment to the patient and each lesion. The most effective treatment for the majority of BCCs in any patient is surgical excision. Superficial lesions may be treated with topical therapies such as the immune modifying agent, imiquimod. Complete clearing of superficial lesions and partial responses in nodular tumours are reported in a couple of very small studies of Gorlin patients (Micali et al. 2002; Stockfleth et al. 2002). Photodynamic therapy is another option. It generally uses a topically applied photosensitising agent such as 5 aminolaevulinic acid and light to target tumours, but the agents can also be delivered systemically. One study of 33 Gorlin patients with 138 tumours showed local control in 56 % of tumours at one year. Responses were similar in tumours <2 mm (treated topically) and thicker lesions treated with systemic agents (Loncaster et al. 2009) but this and other reports have only short follow-up. Consensus guidelines for the use of photodynamic therapy (PDT) in Gorlin syndrome have been developed (Basset-Seguin et al. 2014).

3.3 Targeted Therapies for BCCs

The targeted therapy, vismodegib is the first of its kind, a drug that blocks the Hedgehog pathway by inhibiting the protein smoothened (SMO), to which *PTCH1* binds (see Fig. 6). Following very promising results of Phase 1 studies in a range of solid tumours, including locally advanced and metastatic BCCs (Cowey 2013), 42 individuals with Gorlin syndrome were enrolled in a double-blind placebo-controlled study. In patients treated daily for up to 18 months, there was a significant reduction in new tumours and shrinkage of existing BCCs, but side effects including weight loss, hair loss, altered taste and muscle cramps led 54 % of participants to stop the medication and the rate of tumour formation increased with medication cessation (Tang et al. 2014). Resistance to vismodegib can occur due to acquired mutations in *SMO* (Pricl et al. 2015) and highlights the need for additional targeting, for example with combinations of agents (Gonnissen et al. 2015). Agents acting further along the pathway would also be necessary to manage tumours with *SUFU* mutations where the site of pathway activation is downstream of *SMO*.

Vismodegib is licensed for the treatment of advanced BCCs where surgery is not indicated but it is not indicated for chemoprevention and patient access remains extremely limited outside of trials (see, clinicaltrials.gov).

3.4 Treatment of Keratocysts

Keratocysts (KCOTs) are surgically treated but recurrence is a risk as daughter cysts can form in the tumour wall (Shear 2002). Four of six Gorlin syndrome patients treated with vismodegib had a reduction in size maintained for 9 months while others had stable KCOTs on the medication (Ally et al. 2014). Side effects and access to vismodegib limit its use, as they do for control of BCCs.

3.5 Prevention of BCCs in Gorlin Syndrome

Isotretinoin treatment has produced a decrease in new tumour formation in small numbers of patients with Gorlin syndrome and is considered reasonable by some to trial in individuals (Bettoli et al. 2013). It requires careful follow-up and avoidance of pregnancy during treatment and for one month afterwards due to teratogenicity. Vismodegib has shown effect in reducing new tumour development but is difficult to tolerate and not readily available outside of trial settings. Avoidance of radiation exposure is recommended, where possible, including maximal sun protection.

3.6 Quality of Life

The burden of disease with Gorlin syndrome can be very high, particularly due to the BCC burden and the amount of time away from work in recovering from multiple procedures (Ali et al. 2014). Mathias et al. (2014) are exploring emotional, social and physical functioning, identifying reduced activities and the impact of scarring as important themes in early data. This supports the role of regular review of a patient and a family's overall management, ideally by a multidisciplinary team who can also signpost other supports. Peer support services have been established in a number of countries and have important roles in education and advocacy.

Current research in familial BCC syndromes continues to look for more mutations in the known genes and new candidates. Approaches include more detailed conventional genetic analysis by sequencing and large rearrangement analysis and germline exome sequencing. Unknown modifier genes are thought to influence expression of *PTCH* and *SUFU*. Understanding the landscape of mutations in BCCs from patients with Gorlin syndrome versus sporadic tumours may help find to understand pathways, but is challenging as mutation rates in tumours appear high. Ongoing trials are examining the optimal dosing of *PTCH1*-targeted therapies such as vismodegib (see, www.clinicaltrials.gov) and exploring the impact of other points of hedgehog pathway inhibition.

4 Summary

Rare inherited susceptibility syndromes are important as they may be associated with profuse BCCs, other cancers and specific management implications. Gorlin syndrome is the exemplar, with autosomal dominant inheritance, complete penetrance but highly variable expressivity. It is the result of mutations in the Sonic Hedgehog (SHH) developmental signalling pathway, most commonly in the *PTCH1* tumour suppressor gene and to a lesser extent, the *SUFU* gene. Diagnostic testing is available for these two genes but other rarer BCC syndromes rely on clinical diagnosis. Management is challenging and includes minimising exposure to ionising and UV radiation, careful surveillance to minimise cosmetic issues with repeated excisions, limited use of topical agents and recently the use of targeted therapies in trials. There is much still to learn about the critical events in BCC pathways that may inform understanding of tumour formation in multiple tissues. Given the high disease burden for individuals, there is a marked need for better support, including registries of those with high genetic risk to facilitate access to targeted therapies and clinical trials.

Acknowledgements We would like to thank the patient who so kindly permitted the use of her clinical photographs and medical photographer Mr Charles Frewen (Medical Visuals P/L) for their production.

References

Ali FR, Collier NJ, Evans DG, Costello M, Webster S, Lear JT (2014) National survey of patients with Gorlin syndrome highlights poor awareness, multiple treatments and profound psychosocial impact of disease. J Eur Acad Dermatol Venereol

Ally MS, Tang JY, Joseph T, Thompson B, Lindgren J, Raphael MA, Ulerio G, Chanana AM, Mackay-Wiggan JM, Bickers DR, Epstein EH Jr (2014) The use of vismodegib to shrink keratocystic odontogenic tumors in patients with basal cell nevus syndrome. JAMA Dermatol 150:542–545

Basset-Seguin N, Bissonnette R, Girard C, Haedersdal M, Lear JT, Paul C, Piaserico S (2014) Consensus recommendations for the treatment of basal cell carcinomas in Gorlin syndrome with topical methylaminolaevulinate-photodynamic therapy. J Eur Acad Dermatol Venereol 28:626–632

Bath-Hextall F, Leonardi-Bee J, Smith C, Meal A, Hubbard R (2007) Trends in incidence of skin basal cell carcinoma. Additional evidence from a UK primary care database study. Int J Cancer 121:2105–2108

Bettoli V, Zauli S, Virgili A (2013) Retinoids in the chemoprevention of non-melanoma skin cancers: why, when and how. J Dermatolog Treat 24:235–237

Bholah Z, Smith MJ, Byers HJ, Miles EK, Evans DG, Newman WG (2014) Intronic splicing mutations in PTCH1 cause Gorlin syndrome. Fam Cancer 13:477–480

Boonchai W, Green A, Ng J, Dicker A, Chenevix-Trench G (2000) Basal cell carcinoma in chronic arsenicism occurring in Queensland, Australia, after ingestion of an asthma medication. J Am Acad Dermatol 43:664–669

Box NF, Duffy DL, Irving RE, Russell A, Chen W, Griffyths LR, Parsons PG, Green AC, Sturm RA (2001) Melanocortin-1 receptor genotype is a risk factor for basal and squamous cell carcinoma. J Invest Dermatol 116:224–229

Bradford PT, Goldstein AM, Tamura D, Khan SG, Ueda T, Boyle J, Oh KS, Imoto K, Inui H, Moriwaki S, Emmert S, Pike KM, Raziuddin A, Plona TM, Digiovanna JJ, Tucker MA, Kraemer KH (2011) Cancer and neurologic degeneration in xeroderma pigmentosum: long term follow-up characterises the role of DNA repair. J Med Genet 48:168–176

Brugieres L, Remenieras A, Pierron G, Varlet P, Forget S, Byrde V, Bombled J, Puget S, Caron O, Dufour C, Delattre O, BRESSAC-DE PAILLERETS B, GRILL J (2012) High frequency of germline SUFU mutations in children with desmoplastic/nodular medulloblastoma younger than 3 years of age. J Clin Oncol 30:2087–2093

Cowey CL (2013) Targeted therapy for advanced Basal-cell carcinoma: vismodegib and beyond. Dermatol Ther (Heidelb) 3:17–31

Epstein EH (2008) Basal cell carcinomas: attack of the hedgehog. Nat Rev Cancer 8:743–754

Evans DG, Farndon PA (2002) (updated 2013) Nevoid basal cell carcinoma syndrome. In: Pagon RA, Adam MP, Ardinger HH, Bird TD, Dolan CR, Fong CT, Smith RJH, Stephens K (eds) GeneReviews(R). Seattle (WA)

Evans DG, Ladusans EJ, Rimmer S, Burnell LD, Thakker N, Farndon PA (1993) Complications of the naevoid basal cell carcinoma syndrome: results of a population based study. J Med Genet 30:460–464

Farndon PA (2005) Gorlin syndrome (nevoid basal cell carcinoma syndrome). In: Cassidy SB and Allanson JE (ed) Management of genetic syndromes. Wiley-Liss, Inc., New York

Fine JD, Johnson LB, Weiner M, Li KP, Suchindran C (2009) Epidermolysis bullosa and the risk of life-threatening cancers: the National EB Registry experience, 1986–2006. J Am Acad Dermatol 60:203–211

Fitzpatrick TB (1988) The validity and practicality of sun-reactive skin types I through VI. Arch Dermatol 124:869–871

Fujii K, Ohashi H, Suzuki M, Hatsuse H, Shiohama T, Uchikawa H, Miyashita T (2013) Frameshift mutation in the PTCH2 gene can cause nevoid basal cell carcinoma syndrome. Fam Cancer 12:611–614

Gallagher RP, Hill GB, Bajdik CD, Fincham S, Coldman AJ, McLean DI, Threlfall WJ (1995) Sunlight exposure, pigmentary factors, and risk of nonmelanocytic skin cancer. I. Basal cell carcinoma. Arch Dermatol 131:157–163

Garre ML, Cama A, Bagnasco F, Morana G, Giangaspero F, Brisigotti M, Gambini C, Forni M, Rossi A, Haupt R, Nozza P, Barra S, Piatelli G, Viglizzo G, Capra V, Bruno W, Pastorino L, Massimino M, Tumolo M, Fidani P, Dallorso S, Schumacher RF, Milanaccio C, Pietsch T (2009) Medulloblastoma variants: age-dependent occurrence and relation to Gorlin syndrome—a new clinical perspective. Clin Cancer Res 15:2463–2471

Goldstein AM, Pastakia B, Digiovanna JJ, Poliak S, Santucci S, Kase R, Bale AE, Bale SJ (1994) Clinical findings in two African-American families with the nevoid basal cell carcinoma syndrome (NBCC). Am J Med Genet 50:272–281

Gonnissen A, Isebaert S, Haustermans K (2015) Targeting the Hedgehog signaling pathway in cancer: beyond Smoothened. Oncotarget 6:13899–13913

Gorlin RJ (2004) Nevoid basal cell carcinoma (Gorlin) syndrome. Genet Med 6:530–539

Guo YY, Zhang JY, Li XF, Luo HY, Chen F, Li TJ (2013) PTCH1 gene mutations in Keratocystic odontogenic tumors: a study of 43 Chinese patients and a systematic review. PLoS ONE 8: e77305

Hahn H, Wicking C, Zaphiropoulous PG, Gailani MR, Shanley S, Chidambaram A, Vorechovsky I, Holmberg E, Unden AB, Gillies S, Negus K, Smyth I, Pressman C, Leffell DJ, Gerrard B, Goldstein AM, Dean M, Toftgard R, Chenevix-Trench G, Wainwright B, Bale AE

(1996) Mutations of the human homolog of Drosophila patched in the nevoid basal cell carcinoma syndrome. Cell 85:841–851

Hartevelt MM, Bavinck JN, Kootte AM, Vermeer BJ, Vandenbroucke JP (1990) Incidence of skin cancer after renal transplantation in The Netherlands. Transplantation 49:506–509

Jacob L, Lum L (2007) Deconstructing the hedgehog pathway in development and disease. Science 318:66–68

Jayaraman SS, Rayhan DJ, Hazany S, Kolodney MS (2014) Mutational landscape of basal cell carcinomas by whole-exome sequencing. J Invest Dermatol 134:213–220

Johnson RL, Rothman AL, Xie J, Goodrich LV, Bare JW, Bonifas JM, Quinn AG, Myers RM, Cox DR, Epstein EH Jr, SCOTT M (1996) Human homolog of patched, a candidate gene for the basal cell nevus syndrome. Science 272:1668–1671

Jones EA, Sajid MI, Shenton A, Evans DG (2011) Basal cell carcinomas in gorlin syndrome: a review of 202 patients. J Skin Cancer 2011:217378

Karagas MR, McDonald JA, Greenberg ER, Stukel TA, Weiss JE, Baron JA, Stevens MM (1996) Risk of basal cell and squamous cell skin cancers after ionizing radiation therapy. For The Skin Cancer Prevention Study Group. J Natl Cancer Inst 88:1848–1853

Karagas MR, Greenberg ER, Spencer SK, Stukel TA, Mott LA (1999) Increase in incidence rates of basal cell and squamous cell skin cancer in New Hampshire, USA. New Hampshire Skin Cancer Study Group. Int J Cancer 81:555–559

Kimonis VE, Goldstein AM, Pastakia B, Yang ML, Kase R, Digiovanna JJ, Bale AE, Bale SJ (1997) Clinical manifestations in 105 persons with nevoid basal cell carcinoma syndrome. Am J Med Genet 69:299–308

Kimonis VE, Mehta SG, Digiovanna JJ, Bale SJ, Pastakia B (2004) Radiological features in 82 patients with nevoid basal cell carcinoma (NBCC or Gorlin) syndrome. Genet Med 6:495–502

Kraemer KH, DiGiovanna JJ (1993) Xeroderma pigmentosum. In: Pagon RA, Adam MP, Ardinger HH, Wallace SE, Amemiya A, Bean LJH, Bird TD, Dolan CR, Fong CT, Smith RJH, Stephens K (eds) GeneReviews(R), Seattle (WA)

Leonard JM, Ye H, Wetmore C, Karnitz LM (2008) Sonic Hedgehog signaling impairs ionizing radiation-induced checkpoint activation and induces genomic instability. J Cell Biol 183:385–391

Lewis RA (1993) Oculocutaneous albinism type 2. In: Pagon RA, Adam MP, Ardinger HH, Wallace SE, Amemiya A, Bean LJH, Bird TD, Dolan CR, Fong CT, Smith RJH, Stephens K (eds) GeneReviews(R). Seattle (WA)

Lichter MD, Karagas MR, Mott LA, Spencer SK, Stukel TA, Greenberg ER (2000) Therapeutic ionizing radiation and the incidence of basal cell carcinoma and squamous cell carcinoma. The New Hampshire Skin Cancer Study Group. Arch Dermatol 136:1007–1011

Lindstrom E, Shimokawa T, Toftgard R, Zaphiropoulos PG (2006) PTCH mutations: distribution and analyses. Hum Mutat 27:215–219

Lo Muzio L (2008) Nevoid basal cell carcinoma syndrome (Gorlin syndrome). Orphanet J Rare Dis 3:32

Loncaster J, Swindell R, Slevin F, Sheridan L, Allan D, Allan E (2009) Efficacy of photodynamic therapy as a treatment for Gorlin syndrome-related basal cell carcinomas. Clin Oncol (R Coll Radiol) 21:502–508

Luande J, Henschke CI, Mohammed N (1985) The Tanzanian human albino skin. Natural history. Cancer 55:1823–1828

Manjima S, Naik Z, Keluskar V, Bagewadi A (2015) Multiple jaw cysts-unveiling the Gorlin-Goltz syndrome. Contemp Clin Dent 6:S102–S105

Mathias SD, Chren MM, Colwell HH, Yim YM, Reyes C, Chen DM, Fosko SW (2014) Assessing health-related quality of life for advanced basal cell carcinoma and basal cell carcinoma nevus syndrome: development of the first disease-specific patient-reported outcome questionnaires. JAMA Dermatol 150:169–176

Micali G, de Pasquale R, Caltabiano R, Impallomeni R, Lacarrubba F (2002) Topical imiquimod treatment of superficial and nodular basal cell carcinomas in patients affected by basal cell nevus syndrome: a preliminary report. J Dermatolog Treat 13:123–127

Michaelsson G, Olsson E, Westermark P (1981) The Rombo syndrome: a familial disorder with vermiculate atrophoderma, milia, hypotrichosis, trichoepitheliomas, basal cell carcinomas and peripheral vasodilation with cyanosis. Acta Derm Venereol 61:497–503

Muller EA, Aradhya S, Atkin JF, Carmany EP, Elliott AM, Chudley AE, Clark RD, Everman DB, Garner S, Hall BD, Herman GE, Kivuva E, Ramanathan S, Stevenson DA, Stockton DW, Hudgins L (2012) Microdeletion 9q22.3 syndrome includes metopic craniosynostosis, hydrocephalus, macrosomia, and developmental delay. Am J Med Genet A 158A:391–399

Pan S, Dong Q, Sun LS, Li TJ (2010) Mechanisms of inactivation of PTCH1 gene in nevoid basal cell carcinoma syndrome: modification of the two-hit hypothesis. Clin Cancer Res 16:442–450

Parren LJ, Frank J (2011) Hereditary tumour syndromes featuring basal cell carcinomas. Br J Dermatol 165:30–34

Pastorino L, Pollio A, Pellacani G, Guarneri C, Ghiorzo P, Longo C, Bruno W, Giusti F, Bassoli S, Bianchi-Scarra G, Ruini C, Seidenari S, Tomasi A, Ponti G (2012) Novel PTCH1 mutations in patients with keratocystic odontogenic tumors screened for nevoid basal cell carcinoma (NBCC) syndrome. PLoS ONE 7:e43827

Poblete Gutierrez P, Eggermann T, Holler D, Jugert FK, Beermann T, Grussendorf-Conen EI, Zerres K, Merk HF, Frank J (2002) Phenotype diversity in familial cylindromatosis: a frameshift mutation in the tumor suppressor gene CYLD underlies different tumors of skin appendages. J Invest Dermatol 119:527–531

Pricl S, Cortelazzi B, Dal Col V, Marson D, Laurini E, Fermeglia M, Licitra L, Pilotti S, Bossi P, Perrone F (2015) Smoothened (SMO) receptor mutations dictate resistance to vismodegib in basal cell carcinoma. Mol Oncol 9:389–397

Ragge NK, Salt A, Collin JR, Michalski A, Farndon PA (2005) Gorlin syndrome: the PTCH gene links ocular developmental defects and tumour formation. Br J Ophthalmol 89:988–991

Ramsay HM, Fryer AA, Hawley CM, Smith AG, Nicol DL, Harden PN (2003) Factors associated with nonmelanoma skin cancer following renal transplantation in Queensland, Australia. J Am Acad Dermatol 49:397–406

Ratcliffe JF, Shanley S, Ferguson J, Chenevix-Trench G (1995) The diagnostic implication of falcine calcification on plain skull radiographs of patients with basal cell naevus syndrome and the incidence of falcine calcification in their relatives and two control groups. Br J Radiol 68:361–368

Reifenberger J, Wolter M, Knobbe CB, Kohler B, Schonicke A, Scharwachter C, Kumar K, Blaschke B, Ruzicka T, Reifenberger G (2005) Somatic mutations in the PTCH, SMOH, SUFUH and TP53 genes in sporadic basal cell carcinomas. Br J Dermatol 152:43–51

Richmond-Sinclair NM, Pandeya N, Ware RS, Neale RE, Williams GM, van der Pols JC, Green AC (2009) Incidence of basal cell carcinoma multiplicity and detailed anatomic distribution: longitudinal study of an Australian population. J Invest Dermatol 129:323–328

Rubin AI, Chen EH, Ratner D (2005) Basal-cell carcinoma. N Engl J Med 353:2262–2269

Rudin CM, Hann CL, Laterra J, Yauch RL, Callahan CA, Fu L, Holcomb T, Stinson J, Gould SE, Coleman B, Lorusso PM, von Hoff DD, de Sauvage FJ, Low JA (2009) Treatment of medulloblastoma with hedgehog pathway inhibitor GDC-0449. N Engl J Med 361:1173–1178

Shanley S, Ratcliffe J, Hockey A, Haan E, Oley C, Ravine D, Martin N, Wicking C, Chenevix-Trench G (1994) Nevoid basal cell carcinoma syndrome: review of 118 affected individuals. Am J Med Genet 50:282–290

Shear M (2002) The aggressive nature of the odontogenic keratocyst: is it a benign cystic neoplasm? Part 1. Clinical and early experimental evidence of aggressive behaviour. Oral Oncol 38:219–226

Smith MJ, Beetz C, Williams SG, Bhaskar SS, O'Sullivan J, Anderson B, Daly SB, Urquhart JE, Bholah Z, Oudit D, Cheesman E, Kelsey A, McCabe MG, Newman WG, Evans DG (2014) Germline mutations in SUFU cause Gorlin syndrome-associated childhood medulloblastoma and redefine the risk associated with PTCH1 mutations. J Clin Oncol 32:4155–4161

Smyth I, Narang MA, Evans T, Heimann C, Nakamura Y, Chenevix-Trench G, Pietsch T, Wicking C, Wainwright BJ (1999) Isolation and characterization of human patched 2 (PTCH2), a putative tumour suppressor gene inbasal cell carcinoma and medulloblastoma on chromosome 1p32. Hum Mol Genet 8:291–297

Soto-Pena GA, Vega L (2008) Arsenic interferes with the signaling transduction pathway of T cell receptor activation by increasing basal and induced phosphorylation of Lck and Fyn in spleen cells. Toxicol Appl Pharmacol 230:216–226

Stacey SN, Sulem P, Gudbjartsson DF, Jonasdottir A, Thorleifsson G, Gudjonsson SA, Masson G, Gudmundsson J, Sigurgeirsson B, Benediktsdottir KR, Thorisdottir K, Ragnarsson R, Fuentelsaz V, Corredera C, Grasa M, Planelles D, Sanmartin O, Rudnai P, Gurzau E, Koppova K, Hemminki K, Nexo BA, Tjonneland A, Overvad K, Johannsdottir H, Helgadottir HT, Thorsteinsdottir U, Kong A, Vogel U, Kumar R, Nagore E, Mayordomo JI, Rafnar T, Olafsson JH, Stefansson K (2014) Germline sequence variants in TGM3 and RGS22 confer risk of basal cell carcinoma. Hum Mol Genet 23:3045–3053

Staples MP, Elwood M, Burton RC, Williams JL, Marks R, Giles GG (2006) Non-melanoma skin cancer in Australia: the 2002 national survey and trends since 1985. Med J Aust 184:6–10

Stockfleth E, Ulrich C, Hauschild A, Lischner S, Meyer T, Christophers E (2002) Successful treatment of basal cell carcinomas in a nevoid basal cell carcinoma syndrome with topical 5 % imiquimod. Eur J Dermatol 12:569–572

Surdu S, Fitzgerald EF, Bloom MS, Boscoe FP, Carpenter DO, Haase RF, Gurzau E, Rudnai P, Koppova K, Vahter M, Leonardi G, Goessler W, Kumar R, Fletcher T (2014) Polymorphisms in DNA repair genes XRCC1 and XRCC3, occupational exposure to arsenic and sunlight, and the risk of non-melanoma skin cancer in a European case-control study. Environ Res 134:382–389

Tang JY, Chiou AS, Mackay-Wiggan JM, Aszterbaum M, Chanana AM, Lee W, Lindgren JA, Raphael MA, Thompson BJ, Bickers DR, Epstein EH Jr (2014) Tazarotene: randomized, double-blind, vehicle-controlled, and open-label concurrent trials for basal cell carcinoma prevention and therapy in patients with basal cell nevus syndrome. Cancer Prev Res (Phila) 7:292–299

Wade TR, Ackerman AB (1978) The many faces of basal-cell carcinoma. J Dermatol Surg Oncol 4:23–28

Wadt KA, Aoude LG, Johansson P, Solinas A, Pritchard A, Crainic O, Andersen MT, Kiilgaard JF, Heegaard S, Sunde L, Federspiel B, Madore J, Thompson JF, Mccarthy SW, Goodwin A, Tsao H, Jonsson G, Busam K, Gupta R, Trent JM, Gerdes AM, Brown KM, Scolyer RA, Hayward NK (2014) A recurrent germline BAP1 mutation and extension of the BAP1 tumor predisposition spectrum to include basal cell carcinoma. Clin Genet

Wicking C, Gillies S, Smyth I, Shanley S, Fowles L, Ratcliffe J, Wainwright B, Chenevix-Trench G (1997) De novo mutations of the Patched gene in nevoid basal cell carcinoma syndrome help to define the clinical phenotype. Am J Med Genet 73:304–307

Youssef KK, Lapouge G, Bouvree K, Rorive S, Brohee S, Appelstein O, Larsimont JC, Sukumaran V, van de Sande B, Pucci D, Dekoninck S, Berthe JV, Aerts S, Salmon I, del Marmol V, Blanpain C (2012) Adult interfollicular tumour-initiating cells are reprogrammed into an embryonic hair follicle progenitor-like fate during basal cell carcinoma initiation. Nat Cell Biol 14:1282–1294

Zibat A, Uhmann A, Nitzki F, Wijgerde M, Frommhold A, Heller T, Armstrong V, Wojnowski L, Quintanilla-Martinez L, Reifenberger J, Schulz-Schaeffer W, Hahn H (2009) Time-point and dosage of gene inactivation determine the tumor spectrum in conditional Ptch knockouts. Carcinogenesis 30:918–926

Websites

www.scfa.edu.au. Accessed 21.12.15
www.americanskin.org. Accessed 21.12.15
www.pcds.org.uk. Accessed 21.12.15
www.cansa.org.za. Accessed 21.12.15
www.clinicaltrials.gov. Accessed 21.12.15

Genetic Testing for Rare Cancer: The Wider Issues

Chris Jacobs and Gabriella Pichert

Abstract

Identification of a potential genetic susceptibility to cancer and confirmation of a pathogenic gene mutation raises a number of challenging issues for the patient with cancer, their relatives and the health professionals caring for them. The specific risks and management issues associated with rare cancer types have been addressed in the earlier chapters. This chapter considers the wider issues involved in genetic counselling and genetic testing for a genetic susceptibility to cancer for patients, families and health professionals. The first part of the chapter will present the issues raised by the current practice in genetic counselling and genetic testing for cancer susceptibility. The second part of the chapter will address some of the issues raised by the advances in genetic testing technology and the future opportunities provided by personalised medicine and targeted cancer therapy. Facilitating these developments requires closer integration of genomics into mainstream cancer care, challenging the existing paradigm of genetic medicine, adding additional layers of complexity to the risk assessment and management of cancer and presenting wider issues for patients, families, health professionals and clinical services.

C. Jacobs (✉)
Department of Clinical Genetics, Guy's and St Thomas' NHS Foundation Trust, London, UK
e-mail: cjacobs@btinternet.com

C. Jacobs
University College London, London, UK

G. Pichert
London Bridge Hospital, London, UK

G. Pichert and C. Jacobs (eds.), *Rare Hereditary Cancers*,
Recent Results in Cancer Research 205, DOI 10.1007/978-3-319-29998-3_12

Keywords
Genetic counselling · Diagnostic genetic testing · Predictive genetic testing · Clinical genome sequencing · Cancer predisposition genes · Variant of unknown significance · Incidental findings · Informed consent · Direct to consumer testing

Contents

1 Introduction

The current model of genetic medicine involves identifying patients with a possible hereditary cancer from the phenotype (observable characteristics resulting from the interaction between genes and environment) and/or family history. For most types of cancer, referral to a genetics specialist is made following cancer treatment and often at the instigation of family members. In some cancers, there is growing evidence of a benefit to early identification of a pathogenic mutation (e.g. in *BRCA1* or *BRCA2* in patients with breast or ovarian cancer), resulting in increasing demand for rapid turnaround of genetic counselling and genetic testing.

Within current practice, testing of one of more individual genes will be offered following genetic counselling if the patient meets specified criteria and makes an informed decision to have the test. If a pathogenic mutation is identified in the patient with cancer (index patient), family members who may have inherited this mutation (at-risk relatives) can then be offered a predictive test following genetic counselling. This model of genetic medicine raises numerous practical, ethical and psychological issues for patients and families but relatively few challenges for referring health professionals, provided referral criteria are available and pathways of communication between specialist areas are clear and well developed.

Since mapping of the human genome in 2003, there have been rapid advances in scientific knowledge and technology around the importance of genomics in health care. Recognition of the potential benefit to patient outcomes through targeting of specific therapies has resulted in recommendations that the use of genetic technology shifts from the confined area of medical genetics into all aspects of health care (House of Lords Science and Technology Committee 2009).

Clinical genome sequencing (CGS) enables rapid characterisation of massive volumes of DNA and the potential to undertake testing of the whole genome. Alongside this, direct to consumer (DTC) genetic testing is becoming increasingly available through internet-based companies. These developments challenge the existing paradigm of genetic medicine, add additional layers of complexity to the risk assessment and management of cancer and present wider issues for patients, families, health professionals and clinical services in relation to rare cancers.

2 Identifying Patients with and at Risk of Hereditary Cancer

Whether or not patients with a potential hereditary cancer are referred to a genetics specialist is largely dependent on the knowledge, expertise and attitude of the referring health professional. This is particularly the case for patients with rare types of cancer.

Knowledge of genetics amongst physicians and nurses is low (Scheuner et al. 2008; Godino and Skirton 2012). Health professionals are not always confident to make a risk assessment (Metcalfe et al. 2010), are not always clear whose responsibility it is to make the referral (Lanceley et al. 2012) and do not consistently refer patients even if they have been identified (Grover et al. 2004; Daniels et al. 2009; Meyer et al. 2010).

Understanding the polygenic and multifactorial nature of cancer risk and the characteristics of hereditary cancer are essential skills for oncology practice. In the UK, National Occupational Standards have been developed in genetics and genomics education for non-genetics health professionals by the National Health Service (NHS) National Genetics and Genomics Education Centre[1], and training is available through NHS Health Education England.[2] In the USA, core competencies in genetic medicine have been integrated into oncology training requirements and ongoing educational programmes are provided by the American Society of Clinical Oncologists (ASCO) (Robson et al. 2015).

[1]http://www.geneticseducation.nhs.uk/for-practitioners-62/national-occupational-standards (last accessed 20.10.15).

[2]https://www.genomicseducation.hee.nhs.uk (last accessed 20.10.15).

3 Genetic Counselling About Hereditary Cancer

In North America, the UK and parts of Europe and Australasia genetic counselling is offered prior to genetic testing. Genetic counselling about hereditary cancer is usually provided by geneticists (medical specialists) and genetic counsellors (non-medical specialists), often with specialist education and expertise in cancer genetics.

Genetic counselling involves information-giving and education together with facilitating psychological adaptation and informed decision-making and promoting informed choice (ASHG 1975). The central ethos of genetic counselling is non-directiveness, and the focus tends to be on care of the individual within the wider family so that the implications for close and distant relatives are also addressed. Genetic counselling may or may not also involve genetic testing, depending on the wishes of the individual, their ability to give informed consent and the likelihood of identifying a genetic susceptibility to the cancer.

A number of practical and ethical issues are raised for patients investigating their family history, whether or not a genetic test is offered. For example, gathering the family history information required in order to generate a three-generation family pedigree can be difficult because family information may be sketchy, families have lost touch or the subject is too sensitive to broach. Testing in order to make information available for loved ones is a powerful motivator for genetic testing (Julian-Reynier et al. 1998). It can be extremely challenging for the index patient if relatives decide not to go ahead with testing once a pathogenic mutation has been identified. There may be different views within families about investigating the cause of the cancer, and once the outcome of genetic testing is known, there can be a tension between the duty to inform and the right not to know. It can be difficult for the patient with cancer to share the information with at-risk relatives, and there are well-documented barriers to family communication including lack of close relationship, reluctance to cause upset and lack of understanding risks and benefits and personal beliefs about the causes of family illness (Hughes et al. 2002; Forrest et al. 2003; Michie et al. 2003; Chivers Seymour et al. 2010).

One of the goals of genetic counselling is to facilitate informed consent. Confidentiality regarding genetics issues is extremely important, and patients may be deeply concerned about the protection of privacy for themselves and their relatives regarding the release of genetic information. Clear guidance regarding issues of consent and confidentiality in relation to sharing genetic information and genetic testing is available (Royal College of Physicians Royal College of Pathologists and British Society for Human Genetics 2011). Similarly, fear of discrimination regarding life insurance or employment may be a barrier for genetic testing. Currently in the UK, there is a concordant between the British government and the Association of British Insurers (ABI). This provides a moratorium on the use of predictive genetic test results by all insurers until 2017. The moratorium has been in place since 2001 and has been periodically extended in the past, although there is no guarantee that it will continue to be extended beyond 2017. The moratorium allows those who have had predictive testing for a genetic susceptibility to cancer to obtain significant levels of cover without disclosing the test results.[3] The guidance on this will vary from country to country, and it is important that health professionals are aware of how to access relevant information in order to inform patients.

There is a large body of research investigating the psychological impact of genetic testing for cancer susceptibility. Much of this work has focused on women with and at risk of hereditary breast cancer. These studies have shown that whilst there is a short-term increase in anxiety related to the genetic test result, there is no evidence of long-term adverse effects for the majority of patients (Meiser 2005). Two systematic reviews have concluded that whilst there is no change in psychological distress amongst individuals with cancer following genetic counselling, the psychological response is mediated by personal cancer experience (Hallowell et al. 2004; Vansenne et al. 2009).

Another area that may be addressed in genetic counselling relates to genetic testing for reproductive decision-making and testing of minors. Prenatal genetic testing and preimplantation genetic diagnosis may be available once a pathogenic mutation has been identified in a family and, if relevant, will be discussed during genetic counselling. Any discussion about genetic testing of children aims to ensure that action is taken in the best interests of the child, balancing the need to test a child to avert an adverse outcome (i.e. the occurrence of a cancer), against the anxiety and wishes of the parent and the loss of the child's future autonomy and privacy (Clarke 2010). Specific guidance regarding genetic testing of children is available within the UK (British Society for Human Genetics 2010) and the USA (Botkin et al. 2015).

Criteria for genetic testing tend to be locally determined, although there are some cancers where there are published and widely accepted genetic testing criteria (such as *TP53* testing). The decision to undertake genetic testing for rare cancers is often based on multidisciplinary team discussion. As outlined above, genetic testing raises many challenging issues for patients and families. Within current practice, these issues will be discussed during genetic counselling and referral for further support will be made where necessary.

4 Current Practice in Genetic Testing

4.1 Outcomes of Genetic Testing Available in Current Practice

The genetic test offered in current clinical practice will depend on whether or not there is a known pathogenic mutation in the family.

[3]https://www.abi.org.uk/News/News-releases/2011/04/Insurance-Genetics-Moratorium-extended-to-2017 (last accessed 16.11.15).

(a) **Diagnostic genetic testing** is generally offered to the index patient in order to try and identify a genetic mutation that could predispose to the cancers in the family. However as outlined below (under the heading 'types of diagnostic tests available in current practice'), there are some circumstances in which a diagnostic test will be offered to an individual who has not had cancer. There are three possible outcomes of diagnostic testing:

- **A pathogenic mutation is detected**: usually this resolves the question about the cause of cancer in the family. However, if there are unexplained cancers in the family, testing of other genes may be offered. If a pathogenic mutation is detected a predictive genetic test can usually be offered to at-risk relatives. Detection of a pathogenic mutation may also enable targeted cancer treatment, surveillance or risk-reducing options for the index patient.
- **No pathogenic mutation is detected**: predictive testing will not be offered to at-risk relatives. Depending on the cancer type and gene tested, a diagnostic test which reveals no pathogenic mutation in the index patient may enable more accurate risk assessment for other relatives based on the family history. However for some patients and families, the absence of a pathogenic mutation can be disappointing as it does not resolve questions about the cause of the cancer. This result can leave individuals and families feeling as uninformed as they were in the first place about the cancer risk.
- **A variant of unknown significance (VUS) is detected**: a VUS is a variation in the coding sequence of a gene where the effect of that change in the sequence is unknown. In many cases, the variation may be a single nucleotide substitution or missense variant resulting in a single amino acid change. Although some missense variants alter the function of the gene, the functional and therefore clinical significance for most variants is not known. Classification systems are in place for some genes, and there are some databases available to monitor variants that have previously been reported, but the data are sketchy. Risk assessment following identification of a VUS will usually be based on what is known about the variant and the family history. However, predictive testing for family members is not usually available following identification of a VUS (although there are some circumstances where predictive testing can be offered; see heading below 'Interpretation of genetic variants of unknown significance'). It is important that patients and relatives are not left with the misconception that a pathogenic mutation has been identified if in fact a VUS has been detected. The result inevitably presents a challenge to the diagnostic laboratory and the clinician in terms of interpretation, reporting and communication to the patient and family. Consequently, counselling patients once a VUS has been detected can be extremely challenging, and this is generally best managed by a specialist genetics health professional.

(b) **Predictive testing** becomes available for at-risk relatives if a pathogenic mutation is identified at diagnostic testing. There are two definitive outcomes of a predictive test:

- **The predictive test is positive,** i.e. the individual has inherited the pathogenic mutation.
- **The predictive test is negative,** i.e. the individual has *not* inherited the pathogenic mutation.

4.2 Types of Diagnostic Test Available in Current Practice

Several types of diagnostic genetic test may be available in current practice: (a) single gene testing, (b) multipanel testing, (c) founder mutation testing of particular ethnic groups and (d) diagnostic testing in an unaffected individual in specific rare circumstances.

(a) **Single gene testing**: until recently diagnostic testing involved the consecutive sequencing of the entire sequence of a single gene using Sanger technology. If no pathogenic mutation is found, the decision may be made to proceed with testing a further gene and so on. Single gene testing involves a process of clinical decision-making to determine the order of testing, and whether or not the cost of further testing is justified. Not only is this approach time-consuming for the laboratory and clinical service, but it is also expensive for the service provider and frustrating and anxiety-provoking for the patient and family who may have to wait for several years for testing to be completed, only to be left with an inconclusive result.

(b) **Multiple gene testing panels**: next-generation sequencing (NGS) is now being used in many laboratories to test for cancer susceptibility. This technology enables multiple genes to be examined simultaneously allowing for phenotypic targeting of specific groups of genes. This speeds up the process of genetic testing for patients and increases the likelihood of identifying a pathogenic mutation. However, there are disadvantages, such as increasing the possibility of discovering unexpected cancer risks, increasing the risk of identifying pathogenic mutations for which surveillance or risk-reducing measures are not available or the risk management is unclear and a greater risk of discovering a VUS.

(c) **Founder mutation testing—testing for pathogenic mutations that are common in particular ethnic groups**: There is a higher incidence of specific pathogenic (Founder) mutations within certain ethnic populations; for example, there are pathogenic *BRCA1/2 BRCA2* mutations that are known to be more prevalent in the Ashkenazi Jewish population, although the penetrance is lower than for other such mutations. In circumstances where a patient has not been affected with cancer but has a particular ethnic background, a genetic test may be available without first testing a relative with cancer.

(d) **Diagnostic testing of an unaffected individual**: very occasionally genetic testing may be offered to an unaffected individual without a pathogenic mutation having first been identified in an affected relative, for example where there is an unaffected relative who must be a carrier based on the analysis of the family history (an obligate carrier). Occasionally there may be other circumstances where this testing is offered. The current guidelines for Familial Breast Cancer in the UK (National Institute for Health and Care Excellence 2013) recommend testing an unaffected individual who has greater than 10 % chance of having inherited a *BRCA1* or *BRCA2* pathogenic mutation in a confirmed family history where there are no affected relatives available to test. Diagnostic testing of an unaffected individual raises additional complex and challenging issues, such as the difficulty of interpreting the risk for the individual tested if no mutation is detected.

4.3 Direct to Consumer Testing

There is a growing interest in and availability of direct to consumer testing (DTC). This is the purchase of genetic testing without any input from healthcare specialists, usually via the Internet. For example, 23andMe offers a personal genome service in the UK for £125.[4] Based on the examination of saliva, reports are offered on over 100 health conditions and traits.

Advocates of DTC are of the opinion that people have a right to know their genetic make-up and that this knowledge will empower them to better manage their health. Opponents point out that many companies, such as 23andMe, do not provide genetic counselling with their tests (Burton 2015) and that the clinical validity (the disease causing potential) and the clinical utility (the ability of the test result to enable the patient to make decisions that are beneficial to him or her) of many genetic changes have yet to be determined.

This type of testing raises huge challenges for health professionals and clinical services. The Association of Genetic Nurses and Counsellors (AGNC) in the UK has recently published helpful guidance for the general public and genetics services regarding DTC[5].

5 The Future of Genetic Testing

5.1 Clinical Genome Sequencing (CGS)

Advances in genetic testing have led to the growing availability of clinical genome sequencing (CGS). CGS includes whole exome and whole-genome sequencing of the tumour and/or the patient's genome (outlined in Chapter 1). CGS will result in a paradigm shift away from a small number of high-risk cancer patients being

[4]https://www.23andme.com/en-int/ (last accessed 01.05.15).

[5]http://www.agnc.org.uk/information-education/documents,-websites-downloads/ (last accessed 16.11.15).

referred to genetics services after treatment to large numbers of the population accessing genetic testing within mainstream clinical services. This will be particularly important for the management of patients with rare cancer syndromes and will lead to profound changes in the way a patient's cancer risk is assessed and how cancer is diagnosed and treated.

5.2 Targeted Treatment and Risk Management as a Result of CGS of the Tumour and/or the Patient's Genome

For individuals with cancer, these advances will enable targeted treatment and risk management. Pharmacogenomics will address efficacy as well as toxicity of cancer treatment in individual patients. For example, dihydropyrimidine dehydrogenase (DPD) deficiency may result in severe toxicity if patients with such a deficiency receive fluoropyrimidine as part of their cancer treatment (Thomas et al. 2015). Therefore, screening for DPD deficiency in patients who are about to receive fluoropyrimidine as part of their treatment may prove useful in the future. Cancer treatment will be tailored to pathways disrupted through pathogenic mutations specific for an individual cancer. A recent publication (Alexandrov et al. 2013) has shown that cancer genomes bear the signature of their mutational processes (with some of them present in many cancer types) which can be harnessed to develop specific cancer treatments. Furthermore, some mutational signatures correlate to ultraviolet light exposure or tobacco smoking, demonstrating the potential value of such signatures for cancer prevention.

There are already a number of pathway tailored cancer treatments available, such as the protein kinase inhibitor imatinib for chronic myeloid leukaemia (Roskoski 2015), poly(ADP-ribose) polymerase or PARP inhibitors for *BRCA1* and *BRCA2* deficient ovarian cancers and other solid tumours (Scott et al. 2015) and therapies that target the human epidermal growth factor receptor 2 (HER2) in breast cancers that overexpress HER2 (Hurvitz et al. 2013).

5.3 Challenges Around the Interpretation and Management of CGS Findings

CGS, in contrast to single gene testing, will generate huge amounts of data, giving rise to a number of challenges such as interpretation and decision-making regarding communication of the findings to patients and their families.

Classification of newly identified cancer predisposition genes (CPGs)
Cancer predisposition genes (CPG) identified by CGS have to be classified with regard to their cancer risks and the spectrum of cancers they cause in order to be clinically useful. Classifying CPGs is a complex and demanding procedure, given the rarity of most CPGs. Classification of CPGs requires correct interpretation of genetic data as well as validated functional assays (Rahman 2014a) of which there are only a few at the present time.

Interpretation of genetic variants of unknown significance
Discussing variants of unknown significance with a patient is challenging. The health professional needs to have a clear understanding of the likelihood that a particular variant is either harmless or disease causing. In addition, the health professional needs to be able to counsel the patient about appropriate cancer risk management options if the variant is detected. For instance, it is appropriate to discuss a bilateral risk-reducing mastectomy for a Class IV *BRCA* variant (for classification of variants see Chap. 1), whereas it would be inappropriate to discuss the same procedure with a patient who has a Class II variant or to offer predictive testing to relatives.

Management of incidental findings (IF)
The American College Medical Genetics and Genomics (ACMG) (Green et al. 2013) defines incidental findings (IF) as 'the result of a deliberate search for pathogenic or likely pathogenic alterations in genes that are not apparently relevant to the diagnostic indication for which the sequencing test was ordered'. Whether the cancer risks of such findings are the same as in pathogenic mutations identified in families with a substantial family history of cancer or suspicion of an inheritable form of cancer (i.e. multiple tumours in a young person) remains to be seen. The ACMG has recently issued guidelines for reporting IFs in clinical exome and genome sequencing (Green et al. 2013). They recommend a 'minimum list' of 25 CPGs where IFs should be reported to the ordering physician. In contrast, the European Society of Human Genetics (ESHG) advocates a targeted approach, i.e. examining only the parts of the genome relevant to the clinical question (Wright et al. 2013), and suggests developing guidelines for informed consent and testing minors with regard to disclosing IFs.

Informed consent
It is questionable whether it is ever possible to give fully informed consent for a test that could raise any number of possibilities. Hypothetical studies of patients' views about release of genetic information suggest disclosure of *any* result is preferred on the basis of the perceived medical advantages of disclosure over non-disclosure (Christenhusz et al. 2014). There is no consensus about how the issue of consent or disclosure of IFs should be approached, which is unsurprising given the differences in healthcare systems and societal attitudes around the world. Within the clinical setting, however, there is general agreement on i) the use and content of an informed consent form for whole-genome sequencing (Ayuso et al. 2013), ii) that discussion should take place about findings that will or will not be disclosed and iii) that clear, clinically important findings should be disclosed (Shked-Rafid et al. 2014). The ASCO guidelines (Robson et al. 2015) acknowledge the difficulty of providing informed consent for clinical genome sequencing but emphasise that the principle remains the same, i.e. individuals who undergo genetic susceptibility testing should provide educated pre test consent for such testing. The guidelines acknowledge that it is not feasible to discuss each gene individually as well as the potential implications of a pathogenic mutation or VUS, and suggest batching the

genes. The guidelines also point out that the pre test discussion will highlight the purpose of the test, the potential outcomes and the implications for the patient and family and the associated cancer risks, and explains the differences between well-understood high penetrance genes and less well-understood moderate penetrance genes, the possibility of unexpectedly identifying a deleterious gene mutation and the possible impact of this on the patient and family.

5.4 Examples of Development Projects that Are Implementing CGS

In the UK, the 100,000 Genome Project[6] was launched in 2012 to translate the knowledge gained from the Human Genome Project into benefits for patients with regard to prevention, diagnosis and treatment of diseases. A company was set up which is owned and funded by the UK Department of Health with the aim of sequencing 100,000 genomes from National Health Service patients until 2017 and linking their genomic data with their medical records. With regard to cancer, the programme focuses on breast, colon, lung ovarian and prostate cancer as well as chronic lymphatic leukaemia. This project will allow the set up a Genomics Service for the NHS and start the development of a UK Genomics Industry. The ultimate goal is to personalise medicine for individual patients.

Another such example is the Melbourne Genomics Health Alliance Demonstration Project in Australia. The project considers whether there are advantages to genome sequencing tests compared to the tests offered as part of usual care. The website[7] reports that to date there has been an increase in the rate of diagnosis of rare genetic conditions in childhood (including some cancers), agreement on common approaches to genetic testing and data management across all organisations involved and the establishment of multidisciplinary teams for interpreting the clinical significance of the genetic data.

There are other research studies underway across the world, and the findings from these studies will be hugely important in developing pathways and care models in clinical practice.

5.5 The Challenges of Integrating CGS Testing into Clinical Practice for Cancer Patients

There are a number of challenges that will need to be addressed prior to the integration of CGS into mainstream medicine. As yet there is limited evidence or experience of this and research is urgently required in order to design, develop and evaluate models of delivery, to develop clear pathways and to develop nationally

[6]http://www.genomicsengland.co.uk/ (last accessed 21.09.15).

[7]http://www.melbournegenomics.org.au/our-work/demonstration-project (last accessed 17.11.15).

agreed and evidence-based guidelines for the management of patients with mutations in cancer predisposition genes.

As of 2014, 114 germline CPGs have been identified (Rahman 2014a) and more CPGs are waiting to be detected. Emerging evidence demonstrates that mutated CPGs alter cellular pathways mostly through loss of function, as the overwhelming majority of known CPGs are tumour suppressor genes. There are, however, a few genes such as *RET* and *MET*, which increase cancer risks through a gain of function.

Identifying disrupted pathways opens up the possibility of targeted therapies. Some of these drugs have already completed clinical trials and are about to become routine treatment such as the PARP inhibitor olaparib for metastasized ovarian cancer (Alsop et al. 2014). Therefore, genetic testing will soon become part of cancer care.

So far, families with a history of cancer suggesting high-risk CPGs as their cause have been counselled, and quite often managed as well, within specialised genetic services (National Institute for Health and Care Excellence 2013). As the number of individuals eligible for CPG testing conferring high cancer risks is rapidly increasing and more treatments tailored to pathways disrupted by mutated CPGS are developed, oncologists, surgeons and other specialists treating these patients will become more involved in genetic testing and managing cancer risks in their patients. Furthermore, oncologists and other healthcare professionals order more and more multipanel gene tests through private companies.

One example of a research programme addressing this issue is 'Mainstreaming Cancer Genetics' which is currently in progress at the Institute of Cancer Research in partnership with the Royal Marsden NHS Foundation Trust (Rahman 2014b). The aim of this programme was to develop a single test targeting 94 CPGs and 248 single nucleotide polymorphisms to analyse all relevant genes faster and cheaper than before (now commercially available) and to develop the clinical infrastructure and education to safely deliver this new pathway of cancer care with an increased recognition of the benefits and implications of genetic testing in cancer.

What is still unclear is how genetic testing will be integrated into mainstream cancer medicine in practice; what impact this will have on clinical services; who will counsel patients about the implications of testing, facilitate informed consent and address the issues currently dealt with in pre- and posttest genetic counselling; what information will be communicated and how this will be framed; when this testing will take place (i.e. close to diagnosis or later in the treatment pathway); and what safety nets will be in place to ensure that relatives are aware of their risk and the risk management options available to them. Work is required to investigate the most effective models of delivering genetic testing in mainstream clinical practice and to educate and upskill the workforce to deliver these challenging developments.

6 Summary

This chapter has highlighted the wider issues involved for patients, families and health professionals in current and future practice of genetic testing. The benefits of the rapidly advancing technology in genetic testing for patients with rare cancer include an increased likelihood of identifying a cancer predisposition which may result in targeted therapy and the increased possibility of being able to offer predictive genetic testing to relatives in order to identify those at the highest risk. Challenges include the high possibility of identifying VUSs or IFs, the difficulty of obtaining informed consent, interpreting results and the limited availability of targeted treatment and surveillance options. Other challenges in implementing these technologies include educating health professionals, integrating the new technology into mainstream medicine in order to provide patients with sufficient information and support to be able to give informed consent, ensuring relatives continue to be aware of the risks to themselves (whatever the diagnostic test result) and managing the increased workload this will bring. Developing clear pathways enabling good communication between oncology and genetics, and the provision of education for health professionals and the general public will be essential for successful implementation.

References

Alexandrov BL, Nik-Zainai S, Wedge DC et al (2013) Signatures of mutational processes in human cancer. Nature 500(7463):415–421

Alsop K, Fereday S, Meldrum C et al (2014) BRCA mutation frequency and patterns of treatment response in BRCA mutation-positive women with ovarian cancer: A report from the Australian ovarian cancer study group. J Clin Oncol 21:2654–2663

ASHG (1975) Genetic counseling. Am J Hum Genet 27:240–242

Ayuso C, Millan J, Mancheno M, Dal-Re R (2013) Informed consent for whole-genome sequencing studies in the clinical setting. Proposed recommendations on essential content and process. Eur J Hum Genet 21(10):1054–1059

Botkin JR, Belmont JW, Berg JS et al (2015) Points to consider: ethical, legal, and psychosocial implications of genetic testing in children and adolescents. Am J Hum Genet 97(1):6–21

British Society for Human Genetics (2010) Report on the genetic testing of children 2010. British Society for Human Genetics

Burton A (2015) Are we ready for direct-to-consumer genetic testing? Lancet Neurol 14:138–139

Chivers Seymour K, Addlington-Hall J, Lucassen AM, Foster CL (2010) What facilitates or impedes family communication following genetic testing for cancer risk? A systematic review and meta-synthesis of primary qualitative research. J Genet Couns 19(4):330–342

Chrisitenhusz GM, Devriendt K, Peeters H et al (2014) The communication of secondary variants: interviews with parents whose children have undergone array-CHG testing Clin Genet 86 (3):207–216

Clarke A (2010) What is at stake in the predictive genetic testing of children? (2010). Fam Cancer 9(1):19–22

Daniels MS, Urbauer DL, Stanley JL et al (2009) Timing of BRCA1/BRCA2 genetic testing in women with ovarian cancer. Genet Med 11(9):624–628

Forrest K, Simpson SA, Wilson BJ et al (2003) To tell or not to tell: barriers and facilitators in family communication about genetic risk. Clin Genet 64(4):317–326

Godino L, Skirton H (2012) A systematic review of nurses' knowledge of genetics. J Nurs Educ Pract 2(3):173–184

Green RC, Berg JS, Grody WW et al (2013) ACMG recommendations for reporting of incidental findings in clinical exome and genome sequencing. Genet Med 15(7):565–574

Grover S, Stoffel EM, Bussone L et al (2004) Physician assessment of family cancer history and referral for genetic evaluation in colorectal cancer patients. Clin Gastroenterol Hepatol 2 (9):813–819

Hallowell N, Foster C, Eeles R et al (2004) Accommodating risk: responses to BRCA1/2 genetic testing of women who have had cancer. Soc Sci Med 59(3):553–565

House of Lords Science and Technology Committee (2009) Genomic medicine, 7 July

Hughes C, Lerman C, Schwartz M et al (2002) All in the family: evaluation of the process and content of sisters' communication about BRCA1 and BRCA2 genetic test results. Am J Med Genet 107(2):143–150

Hurvitz SA, Hu Y, O'Brien N, Finn RS (2013) Current approaches and future directions in the treatment of HER2-positive breast cancer. Cancer Treat Rev 39(3):219–229

Julian-Reynier C, Eisinger F, Chabal F et al (1998) Cancer genetic clinics: why do women who already have cancer attend? Eur J Cancer 34(10):1549–1553

Lanceley A, Eagle Z, Ogden G et al (2012) Family history and women with ovarian cancer: is it asked and does it matter?: an observational study. Int J Gynecol Cancer 22(2):254–259

Meiser B (2005) Psychological impact of genetic testing for cancer susceptibility: an update of the literature. Psychooncology 14(12):1060–1074

Metcalfe A, Pumphrey R, Clifford C (2010) Hospice nurses and genetics: implications for end-of-life care. J Clin Nurs 19(1–2):192–207

Meyer LA, Anderson ME, Lacour RA et al (2010) Evaluating women with ovarian cancer for BRCA1 and BRCA2 mutations: missed opportunities. Obstet Gynecol 115(5):945–952

Michie S, Smith JA, Senior V, Marteau TM et al (2003) Understanding why negative genetic test results sometimes fail to reassure. Am J Med Genet A 119A(3):340–347

National Institute for Health and Care Excellence (2013) Familial Breast Cancer: classification and care of people at risk of familial breast cancer and management of breast cancer and related risks in people with a family history of breast cancer CG164, London

Rahman N (2014a) Realizing the promise of cancer predisposition genes. Nature 505:302–308

Rahman N (2014b) Mainstreaming genetic testing of cancer predisposition genes. Clin Med 14 (4):436–439

Robson ME, Bradbury AR, Arun B et al (2015) American Society of Clinical Oncology Policy Statement Update: genetic and genomic testing for cancer susceptibility. J Clin Oncol (Aug 31)

Roskoski RJR (2015) A historical overview of protein kinases and their targeted small molecule inhibitors. Pharmacol Res 100:1–23

Royal College of Physicians Royal College of Pathologists and British Society for Human Genetics (2011) Consent and confidentiality in clinical genetic practice: guidance on genetic testing and sharing genetic information, 2nd edn. Report of the Joint Committee on Medical Genetics, London

Scheuner M, Sieverding P, Shekelle P (2008) Delivery of genomic medicine for common chronic adult diseases: a systematic review. J Am Med Assoc 299:1320–1334

Scott CL, Swisher EM, Kaufmann SH (2015) Poly (ADP-ribose) polymerase inhibitors: recent advances and future development. J Clin Oncol 33(12):1397–1406

Shked-Rafid S, Dheensa S, Crawford G et al (2014) Defining and managing incidental findings in genetic and genomic practice. J Med Genet 51(715):723 (Published online 16.09.14)

Thomas F, Hennebelle I, Delmas C et al (2015) Genotyping of a family with a novel deleterious DPYD mutation supports the pretherapeutic screening of DPD deficiency with dihydrouracil/uracil ratio. Clin Pharmacol Ther. doi:10.1002/cpt.210 [Epub ahead of print]

Vansenne F, Bossuyt PM, de Borgie CA (2009) Evaluating the psychological effects of genetic testing in symptomatic patients: a systematic review. Genet Test Mol Biomarkers 13:555–563

Wright CF, Middleton A, Burton H (2013) Policy challenges of clinical genome sequencing. BMJ 2013:347–353

Index

G. Pichert and C. Jacobs (eds.), *Rare Hereditary Cancers*,
Recent Results in Cancer Research 205, DOI 10.1007/978-3-319-29998-3

MIX
Papier aus verantwortungsvollen Quellen
Paper from responsible sources
FSC® C105338

If you have any concerns about our products,
you can contact us on
ProductSafety@springernature.com

In case Publisher is established outside the EU,
the EU authorized representative is:
Springer Nature Customer Service Center GmbH
Europaplatz 3, 69115 Heidelberg, Germany

Printed by Libri Plureos GmbH
in Hamburg, Germany